ANTIPLATELET THERAPY IN CLINICAL PRACTICE

CONTENTS

ANTIPLATELET THERAPY IN CLINICAL PRACTICE

Edited by

James J Ferguson III MD FACC
Associate Director, Cardiology Research
St Luke's Episcopal Hospital and
Texas Heart Institute
Houston, TX
USA

Nicolas AF Chronos MBBS MRCP FESC FACC
Director, Atlanta Cardiovascular Research Institute
Atlanta, GA
USA

Robert A Harrington MD FACC
Associate Professor
Director, Cardiovascular Clinical Trials
Duke Clinical Research Institute
Duke University Medical Center
Durham, NC
USA

MARTIN DUNITZ

© Martin Dunitz Ltd 2000

First published in the United Kingdom in 2000 by
Martin Dunitz Ltd
The Livery House
7–9 Pratt Street
London NW1 0AE

Reprinted 2000

A CIP record for this book is available from the British Library.

ISBN 1-85317-624-9

Distributed in the United States by:
Blackwell Science Inc.
Commerce Place, 350 Main Street
Malden MA 02148, USA
Tel: 1-800-215-1000

Distributed in Canada by:
Login Brothers Book Company
324 Salteaux Crescent
Winnipeg, Manitoba R3J 3T2
Canada
Tel: 1-204-224-4068

Distributed in Brazil by:
Ernesto Reichmann Distribuidora de Livros, Ltda
Rua Coronel Marques, 335
03440-000 São Paulo – SP
Brazil

Composition by Wearset, Boldon, Tyne and Wear.
Printed and bound in Great Britain by Biddles Ltd, Guildford and King's Lynn.

Contributors

K Martijn Akkerhuis MD
Thoraxcenter
Erasmus University and
University Hospital Rotterdam
Rotterdam
The Netherlands

Sonia Alamowitch MD
Department of Neurology
Tenon Hospital
75970 Paris Cedex 20
France

John Alexander MD
Cardiology Fellow
Duke Clinical Research Institute
Duke University Medical Center
Durham, NC 27710
USA

Richard C Becker MD
Professor of Medicine
Director, Coronary Care Unit
Director, Cardiovascular Thrombosis
Research Center
Division of Cardiovascular Medicine
University of Massachusetts Medical Center
Worcester, MA 01655-0214
USA

Scott D Berkowitz MD
Assistant Professor of Medicine and Pathology
Divisions of Hematology and Cardiology
Duke Clinical Research Institute
Duke University Medical Center
Durham, NC 27710
USA

Christopher P Cannon MD
Division of Cardiology
Brigham & Women's Hospital
Boston, MA 02115
USA

Zhi-Qang Chen MD
Department of Internal Medicine
University of Texas-Houston Medical School
Houston, TX 77030
USA

Nicolas AF Chronos MBBS MRCP FESC FACC
Director
Atlanta Cardiovascular Research Institute
Atlanta, GA 30342
USA

Jaap W Deckers MD PhD
Thoraxcenter
Erasmus University and
University Hospital Rotterdam
Rotterdam
The Netherlands

James J Ferguson III MD
Associate Director
Cardiology Research
St Luke's Episcopal Hospital and
Texas Heart Institute
Texas Medical Center
Houston, TX 77225-0345
USA

Desmond Fitzgerald MD FRCPI
Professor of Clinical Pharmacology
Royal College of Surgeons in Ireland
Dublin 2
Republic of Ireland

Richard Gallo MD
Institut de Cardiologie De Montréal
Montreal, PQ H1T 1C8
Canada

Eric Garbarz MD
Department of Cardiology
Tenon Hospital
75970 Paris Cedex 20
France

Robert A Harrington MD
Associate Professor of Medicine
Director, Cardiovascular Clinical Trials
Duke Clinical Research Institute
Duke University Medical Center
Durham, NC 27710
USA

Dean J Kereiakes MD FACC
Medical Director
The Carl and Edyth Lindner Center for
Clinical Cardiovascular Research,
Professor of Clinical Medicine
The University of Cincinnati College of
Medicine and Interventional Cardiologist
Ohio Heart Health Center
Cincinnati, OH 45219-2966
USA

Paul Kim MD
Fellow, Department of Cardiology
St Luke's Episcopal Hospital and
Texas Heart Institute
Texas Medical Center
Houston, TX 77225-0345
USA

Spencer B King III MD
The Andreas Gruentzig Cardiovascular
Center
Emory University Hospital
Atlanta, GA 30322
USA

Stephen L Kopecky MD
Associate Professor of Medicine
Mayo Medical School
Mayo Clinic
Rochester, MN 55905
USA

Weei-Chin Lin MD PhD
Instructor of Medicine
Division of Hematology and Medical
Oncology
Duke University Medical Center
Durham, NC 27710
USA

Alan B Lumsden MB ChB
Associate Professor
Head, General Vascular Surgery
Joseph B Whitehead Department of Surgery
Emory University School of Medicine
Atlanta, GA 30322
USA

Joel L Moake MD
Professor of Medicine
Baylor College of Medicine and
Associate Director
Biomedical Engineering Laboratory
Rice University
Houston, TX 77030
USA

Thomas L Ortel MD PhD
Associate Professor of Medicine
Division of Hematology
Assistant Professor of Pathology
Medical Director, Clinical Coagulation
Laboratory
Duke University Medical Center
Durham, NC 27710
USA

Vincenzo Pasceri MD
Department of Internal Medicine
University of Texas-Houston Medical School
Houston, TX 77030
USA

Martin Quinn MB BCh BAO MRCPI
Clinical Research Fellow
Department of Clinical Pharmacology
Royal College of Surgeons in Ireland
Dublin 2
Republic of Ireland

Etienne Roullet MD
Head, Department of Neurology
Tenon Hospital
75970 Paris Cedex 20
France

Mahomed Salame MD
The Andreas Gruentzig Cardiovascular Center
Emory University Hospital
Atlanta, GA 30322
USA

Andrew I Schafer MD
The Bob and Vivian Smith Professor and
Chairman
Department of Medicine
Baylor College of Medicine
Methodist Hospital
Houston, TX 77030
USA

Karsten Schrör MD
Direktor des Institutes für Pharmakologie
Heinrich Heine-Universität Düsseldorf
D-40225 Düsseldorf
Germany

Scott M Surowiec MD
Research Fellow
Division of Vascular Surgery
Joseph B Whitehead Department of Surgery
Emory University School of Medicine
Atlanta, GA 30322
USA

Pierre Theroux MD
Institut de Cardiologie De Montréal
Montreal, PQ H1T 1C8
Canada

Alec Vahanian MD
Professor of Cardiology
Head, Department of Cardiology
Tenon Hospital
75970 Paris Cedex 20
France

Michel Vayssairat MD
Head, Department of Vascular Medicine
Tenon Hospital
75970 Paris Cedex 20
France

Freek Verheugt MD
Professor of Cardiology
Academisch Ziekenhuis Nijmegen
Cardiologie
6500 HB Nijmegen
The Netherlands

Victor J Weiss MD
Endovascular Fellow
Division of Vascular Surgery
Joseph B Whitehead Department of Surgery
Emory University School of Medicine
Atlanta, GA 30322
USA

James T Willerson MD
Professor and Chairman
Department of Internal Medicine
University of Texas-Houston Medical School
Houston, TX 77030
USA

Pierre Zoldhelyi MD
Department of Internal Medicine
University of Texas-Houston Medical School
Houston, TX 77030
USA

Preface

On the verge of the new millennium, a number of major problems confront medicine today. The ever-increasing cost of healthcare is a major issue, fueled, in part, by our ever-expanding technical and pharmaceutical armamentarium. The *real* challenge we face is how to utilize new (and old) forms of therapy in the care of our patients appropriately.

There are few areas in Cardiology (or, for that matter, Medicine in general) that have witnessed the rapid advances we have seen in the field of antiplatelet therapy: the growing recognition of the benefits of aspirin therapy, and the substantive addition of IIb/IIIa antagonists and new thienopyridines. In one short decade, the 'standard of care' has expanded dramatically. And yet, with this abundance of new forms of therapy, come uncertainties as well. How good are they *really*? When and in whom are they most beneficial?

It is in hopes of addressing these questions that we have written this book. No, we do not have all the answers. What we have assembled in this book is a comprehensive approach to the data, both from the perspective of the individual compounds, and from the perspective of the clinical situations where they may prove useful. Yes, this is a somewhat daunting undertaking with clinical trials moving forward as rapidly as they have in recent years. But, this information is of crucial importance to the practicing physician at the bedside and to the clinical researcher of tomorrow. Antiplatelet therapy is a cornerstone of therapy in today's complex world of cardiovascular therapy; we hope you enjoy these initial steps on what will be an incredibly exciting journey in the decades to come.

James J Ferguson
Houston, TX, USA

Section I:

Coagulation and platelet function

1

A practical guide to blood coagulation
Andrew I Schafer

Introduction

The human coagulation system is an exquisitely regulated process that provides hemostasis at sites of vascular injury. It has evolved as a mechanism to prevent the loss of perfusion pressure and exsanguination wherever the integrity of the vascular system is disrupted. To achieve this, the hemostatic system is able to recognize injury to the vessel wall and to mobilize platelets and coagulation proteins to form a protective fibrin–platelet clot at the site of damage.

The process of hemostasis occurs with dazzling speed and precision, enabling the fibrin–platelet hemostatic plug to form in a highly localized manner, only where it is needed to staunch blood flow. The speed with which a hemostatic plug forms at the site of injury is a function of the interaction between coagulation proteins and platelets, wherein each of these two components of the hemostatic system is activated in an interdependent, synergistic and mutually self-amplifying manner. The localization of the hemostatic plug to the site of vascular intimal injury is a function of the ability of adjacent normal endothelium, which lines the intimal surface of the entire circulatory tree, to perform antithrombotic properties.

The major components of the hemostatic system are: coagulation proteins, platelets, and the vessel wall. These three components are completely interdependent and act in concert:

(1) To promote blood fluidity under normal circumstances; and
(2) To produce a clot at a site of vascular damage.

Breakdown in any one of several critical constituents of this system can lead to clinical hemostatic disorders that range from life-threatening bleeding diatheses to fatal thrombotic events.

Coagulation cascade

The coagulation proteins arose during evolution through gene duplication and mutation, and they represent a family of proteins with common, unified structural domains that possess diverse functional properties. The plasma coagulation proteins normally circulate in their inactive forms, referred to as 'zymogens' or 'proenzymes'. The classical concept of the mechanism of fibrin formation is the 'cascade' or 'waterfall' model of the coagulation process, which was described separately in 1964 by Macfarlane[1] and by Davie and Ratnof.[2] This model, which has generally held up to subsequent investigation, proposes that, in response to vascular injury, coagulation zymogens become sequentially activated to active enzymes, referred to as 'serine proteases', by a linked series of reactions in which each serine protease that is formed catalyses the subsequent zymogen–protease transition. Zymogens are converted to their active enzyme forms by the cleavage of one or two peptide bonds. Thus, the coagulation cascade is a biochemical amplifier, since it permits a small, initiating stimulus to generate large quantities of the end-product, namely fibrin.[3]

The traditional view of the coagulation cascade is that it comprises two independent and alternative pathways (the 'intrinsic pathway' and the 'extrinsic pathway'), which converge upon the 'common pathway' of coagulation that is initiated by the activation of factor X. Activated factor X (factor X_a) is the protease that catalyses the conversion of prothrombin to thrombin, with factor V serving as an essential cofactor in this reaction. Thrombin then acts at the end of the common pathway of coagulation to convert fibrinogen to fibrin. Fibrinogen, which is soluble in plasma, is composed of 2 Aα, 2 Bβ and to 2 γ chains.[4] The protein circulates as a disulfide-linked dimer. The aminotermini of the Aα and Bβ chains (termed 'fibrinopeptide A' and 'fibrinopeptide B', respectively) are cleaved simultaneously by thrombin. Thus, the thrombin-generated fibrin monomers that are formed expose a D-domain at the carboxyterminus and an E-domain at the aminoterminus. Fibrin polymerization then occurs to form protofibrils. Finally, the fibrin clot is stabilized by activated factor XIII (factor XIII_a), formed from plasma zymogen factor XIII by thrombin itself. Factor XIII_a catalyses the covalent cross-linking of fibrin polymers by a transamidation reaction.

The traditional view of the coagulation cascade was that the intrinsic and extrinsic pathways of coagulation, which converge upon factor X activation, are equally important and independent (alternative) events. This aspect of the coagulation cascade model has undergone significant revision in recent years.

The intrinsic pathway, also known as the 'contact activation' pathway, is initiated when factor XII is converted to its active enzyme form by limited proteolysis.[5,6] One mechanism whereby this action can be initiated is through autoactivation of factor XII on negatively charged surfaces. The process of contact activation requires the presence of two other proteins, prekallikrein and high-molecular-weight kininogen, to achieve maximal rates. Activated factor XII (factor XII_a) converts the plasma zymogen factor XI to its corresponding serine protease, factor XI_a. In the presence of calcium, factor XI_a then serves as the activator for factor IX. Factor IX_a thus generated becomes one of the activators of factor X to initiate the common pathway. The activation of factor X to factor X_a by factor IX_a requires factor VIII as an essential cofactor.

The extrinsic pathway of coagulation is initiated by the exposure of tissue factor to circulating blood, hence this pathway is also referred to as the 'tissue factor pathway' of coagulation.[7–9] Tissue factor is an integral membrane protein of many types of cells and is not normally exposed to circulating blood.[10] However, since it is a normal constituent of subendothelial components of the vessel wall, appearing on the surfaces of vascular smooth muscle cells and fibroblasts, it is exposed at sites of vascular intimal damage where endothelium is lost. Furthermore, while it is not normally expressed on the surfaces of endothelial cells and leukocytes, perturbation of these cell types by various mediators of injury can lead to the surface expression of tissue factor on these cells.[11] Tissue factor serves as the essential cofactor for activated factor VII (factor VII_a) and the factor VII_a–tissue factor complex can then activate factor X to initiate the common pathway of coagulation. The exact mechanism of factor VII activation remains unclear, although it is likely that trace amounts of factor VII$_a$ actually circulate in blood, unlike the other coagulation factors that are entirely proteolytically inert in their zymogen forms in fluid phase plasma.[12,13] Under normal circumstances, however, where tissue factor is unavailable, plasma factor VII$_a$ is rendered hemostatically incompetent. It is only upon vascular injury, whereupon tissue factor is exposed, that plasma factor VII$_a$ can bind to tissue factor, leading to rapid autocatalytic conversion of factor VII to factor VII$_a$. This amplifies the hemostatic response by generating even more factor VII$_a$–tissue factor complexes.[14]

In recent years, it has become apparent that the intrinsic and extrinsic pathways of coagulation are not entirely separate alternative systems to activate factor X. Nevertheless, in clinical coagulation laboratory testing, the two major screening tests still measure effectively the integrity of each of these pathways separately. Thus, the activated partial thromboplastin time (aPTT) measures the integrity of the intrinsic and common pathways of coagulation, while the prothrombin time (PT) measures the integrity of the extrinsic and common pathways of coagulation. Physiologically, however, important interactions occur between the extrinsic and intrinsic pathways that make several facets of the classical model oversimplified and untenable.[15] The factor VII$_a$–tissue factor complex can activate not only factor X but also factor IX. Thus, the factor VII$_a$–tissue factor complex can activate factor X either directly or indirectly via activation of factor IX Kinetic studies have indicated that factor IX is actually the preferred substrate for the enzymatic action of the factor VII$_a$–tissue factor complex when both factors IX and X are presented simultaneously to it. There is also now growing evidence that coagulation is predominately initiated in vivo by the extrinsic (tissue factor) pathway. Thus, the intrinsic (contact activation) pathway likely serves as an amplifying arm to the coagulation cascade rather than an important initiator. This may explain long-standing clinical observations that patients with inherited deficiencies of the contact activation factors (e.g. factor XII, prekallikrein, and high-molecular-weight kininogen) never have bleeding problems, even when provoked by surgery or trauma.[16] These relationships, including the pivotal role of thrombin in sustaining the cascade by feedback activation of coagulation factors, are depicted Figure 1.1.

Platelet activation

In normal circulation, the only stationary cells that flowing blood constituents are exposed to are endothelial cells that line the intimal surface of the entire circulatory tree. In the presence of healthy endothelium, platelets circulate passively in their inactive forms. Platelets are cytoplasmic fragments of bone marrow megakaryocytes. These terminal cell fragments are anucleate, and therefore possess minimal, if any, capacity to synthesize new protein. Following release from the bone marrow, platelets circulate with an average life-span of about 7–10 days, and senescent platelets are finally cleared predominately by the spleen.[17,18] Although they are only cytoplasmic fragments, platelets possess the explosive ability to become activated at sites of injury; indeed they can become critical components of the hemostatic plug, as shown by the serious bleeding disorders that result from quantitative or qualitative platelet abnormalities. Furthermore, hyper-reactivity of platelets, which is usually induced by abnormalities of the intimal surface of the vessel wall, can lead to the development of predominately platelet thrombi,

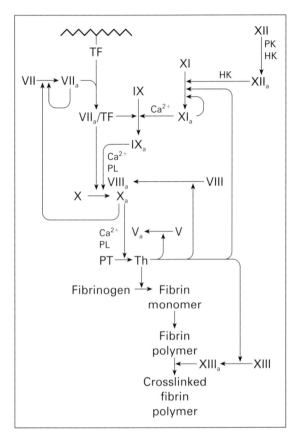

Figure 1.1
*The coagulation cascade. This scheme
emphasizes recent understanding of: (i) the
importance of the tissue factor pathway in
initiating clotting in vivo; (ii) the interactions
between pathways; and (iii) the pivotal role of
thrombin in sustaining the cascade by feedback
activation of coagulation factors. HK, high-
molecular-weight kininogen; PK, prekallikrein; PL,
phospholipid; PT, prothrombin; TF, tissue factor;
Th, thrombin. (From Schafer,[3] used with
permission.)*

tially bridges the intimal gap created by focal
endothelial denudation.[19,20] Platelets adhere to
subendothelial constituents of the vessel wall,
particularly collagen. The process of platelet
adhesion is mediated primarily by von Willebrand factor (vWF), which is present in both
plasma and in the extracellular matrix of the
subendothelial vessel wall. The large vWF
multimers that thus serve as the 'molecular
glue' for platelet adhesion bind to specific
receptors on the platelet surface, which are
located in the platelet membrane glycoprotein
(Gp) Ib-IX-V complex. High levels of shear
stress on the arterial side of the circulation
promote the interaction between vWF and
platelet membrane Gp Ib, presumably either
through subtle changes in the vWF molecule
and or its platelet Gp Ib receptor.[21] Adhesion
is also facilitated by platelet binding directly to
collagen via specific platelet membrane collagen receptors.

Following adhesion, the adherent platelets
undergo activation. Platelet activation is partly
mediated by the generation of thromboxane
A_2, which is rapidly synthesized de novo after
free arachidonic acid is liberated from platelet
membrane phospholipid pools by phospholipases. Thromboxane A_2 is oxygenated by the
enzyme cyclo-oxygenase to prostaglandin
endoperoxides and then converted by thromboxane synthase to thromboxane A_2. Thromboxane A_2 is not only a potent activator and
aggregator of platelets but also a vasoconstrictor, thus having dual hemostatic actions.
Adherent platelets also become activated by
degranulation, whereby they release (secrete)
preformed constituents of specific cytoplasmic
granules. Hemostatically active constituents of
the dense granules (dense bodies) of platelets
include adenosine diphosphate (ADP) and
fibrinogen.

The products of arachidonic acid metabolism and granule secretion then mediate the

especially in high-shear, arterial regions of the
circulation.

With loss of endothelium at a site of vascular damage, circulating platelets rapidly
undergo the process of adhesion, forming a
monolayer of adherent platelets that essen-

final phase of platelet activation, that of platelet aggregation. In this process, additional circulating platelets are recruited to the site of vascular injury, where platelet plugs are formed through platelet–platelet interactions that eventually lead to an occlusive thrombus. The occlusive platelet plug is anchored by the fibrin mesh that develops simultaneously, as discussed later in this chapter. Platelet aggregation is mediated by fibrinogen, which can be derived either from circulating plasma or from the platelet granule releasate. At higher shear levels, vWF itself, which is also the ligand that mediates adhesion, can serve as the 'molecular glue' of aggregation.[21] Fibrinogen or vWF bind to specific platelet membrane surface receptors that are located in the Gp IIb–IIIa complex. The heterodimeric platelet Gp IIb–IIIa complex is not exposed in its active form on the platelet surface unless platelets are activated. More detailed discussion of the mechanisms of platelet activation are provided in subsequent chapters.

Coagulation–platelet interactions

Following vascular injury, activation of the coagulation cascade and activation of platelets do not occur independently. The sequential cascade of reactions that convert plasma zymogens to their enzymes forms in the coagulation system is effective physiologically only when these factors are assembled in complexes on cell membrane surfaces.[15] The formation of coagulation enzyme complexes on cell membranes greatly enhances their rates of reaction by localizing and concentrating the complex components on the membranes. Furthermore, complex formation on the membranes sequesters the activated clotting factors from inhibition by physiological regulators of coag-

ulation (see later text). Several of the reactions of the coagulation cascade require calcium, and calcium ions facilitate the interaction of coagulation proteins with negatively charged surface membrane phospholipids.

The 'activated' cell membrane is the critical element in coagulation complex formation and function. The assembly of coagulation proteins on cell surfaces requires the availability of membranes containing phospholipids. Acidic phospholipid surfaces that promote coagulation reactions are not normally exposed on unactivated endothelial cell or blood cell membranes. Vascular injury, however, triggers the translocation of acidic phospholipid head groups to expose these procoagulant membrane components on the surfaces of activated cells. In vivo, the procoagulant membrane surface upon which these reactions proceed is considered to be contributed primarily by platelets, specifically in their activated forms. Other circulating blood cells, including monocytes and lymphocytes, as well as vascular cells, may also contribute to this membrane surface system. The final result of the propagation of coagulation through the activities of the membrane-dependent enzyme complexes is the activation of prothrombin to thrombin. Thrombin, in turn, activates additional circulating platelets to expose additional acidic phospholipid membrane surfaces to amplify and propagate these reactions (Figure 1.2).[16] Thus, the focal availability of critical membrane phospholipid components at sites of vascular damage and thrombin generation serves not only to accelerate the coagulation cascade but also to localize blood clotting to areas of injury.

The availability of activated platelet membrane surfaces is particularly important in the assembly of the so-called 'Xase' ('tenase') complex, which leads to the activation of factor X, and also to the so-called 'prothrombi-

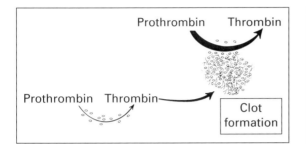

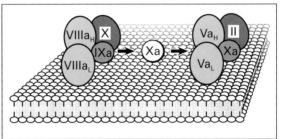

Figure 1.2
Reciprocal interaction between thrombin generation and platelet activation. Membranes of activated platelets facilitate thrombin generation by providing a surface for assembly of coagulation factors. Conversely, thrombin is a potent activator of platelets, thus acting to promote and amplify activation of the coagulation system. This reciprocal interaction results in the accelerated and tightly focused formation of a hemostatic plug composed of platelets and fibrin. (From Schafer,[16] used with permission.)

Figure 1.3
Possible mechanism of product flux between successive reaction centers of coagulation. Assembly of Xase and prothrombinase complexes on a cell membrane surface requires the transfer of factor Xa between reaction centers by diffusion along the same membrane surface. See text for details. (From Mann et al[23], modified with permission.)

nase' complex, which leads to the activation of prothrombin to thrombin.[22] Each of these complexes (Xase and prothrombinase) consists of a zymogen, serine protease and an activated cofactor protein – all of which are assembled on the platelet membrane surface in the presence of calcium ions. Thus, these aspects of the coagulation cascade described above proceed on the surfaces of activated platelets (and possibly other activated cell types) as shown in Figure 1.3. Here, the assembly of the two successive enzyme complexes (the Xase and prothrombinase complexes) is shown to occur on one cell membrane surface.[23,24] The Xase complex (consisting of the zymogen factor X, the serine protease factor IX_a, and the cofactor factor VIII_a) generates activated factor X (factor X_a). Factor Xa then joins the prothrombinase complex (now consisting of the serine protease factor X_a, the zymogen prothrombin

(factor II) and the cofactor factor V_a). The prothrombinase complex on activated platelet membrane surfaces then efficiently generates thrombin, which, as already noted, can perpetuate the reactions by activating additional neighboring platelets to provide expansion of cell surface area for further reactions.

Physiological antithrombotic mechanisms

In order to maintain blood fluidity within the circulation under normal circumstances, it is essential for the coagulation system and platelets to remain inactive. Furthermore, at a focal site of vascular injury, hemostasis must be localized precisely to prevent propagation of the clot to uninjured regions of the circulation. Therefore, multiple physiological antithrombotic mechanisms have evolved to control blood clotting. Inherited or acquired defects in any one of several of these physiological antithrombotic systems can lead to

	Antithrombotic activity	Mechanism(s) of action
Coagulation protein binding	Glycosaminoglycans	Bind AT and catalyse AT neutralization of thrombin and other activated coagulation factors
	Thrombomodulin	Binds thrombin (thereby removing it from circulation) and activates protein C
	TFPI	Binds and inhibits TF-factor VII$_a$ complex and factor X$_a$
Fibrinolytic activation	t-PA	Activates plasminogen to plasmin
	PA binding sites (annexin II, u-PAR)	Bind plasminogen activators, thereby localizing and amplifying fibrinolysis
	Plasminogen binding sites	Bind plasminogen, thereby localizing and amplifying fibrinolysis
Platelet inhibition (and vasodilation)	Prostacyclin (PGI$_2$)	Inhibits platelet aggregation by stimulating platelet adenylyl cyclase and raising platelet cAMP; causes vasorelaxation by raising vascular SMC cAMP
	Nitric oxide (NO)	Inhibits platelet adhesion and aggregation by stimulating platelet guanylyl cyclase and raising platelet cGMP; causes vasorelaxation by raising vascular SMC cGMP
	Carbon monoxide (CO)	Same as nitric oxide
	ADPase	Inhibits platelet activation by breakdown of ADP to AMP

AT, antithrombin (III); TFPI, tissue factor pathway inhibitor; t-PA, tissue plasminogen activator; PA, plasminogen activator; cAMP, cyclic AMP; cGMP, cyclic GMP; SMC, smooth muscle cell.

Table 1.1
Antithrombotic (thromboresistant) properties of vascular endothelium.

serious thrombotic problems clinically. The 'guardian' of blood fluidity is the vascular endothelium, which normally elaborates an armamentarium of antithrombotic mediators.[25] The activity of these diverse antithrombotic mechanisms depends upon the integrity of endothelium. The focal nature of thrombotic disease can be explained by organ-dependent variations in the levels of endothelial cell inhibitors that regulate the coagulation cascade, platelet activation, or fibrinolysis.[26]

Under normal circumstances, quiescent endothelial cells present a highly thromboresistant surface to flowing blood throughout the circulation. This property of endothelium is constitutively effected by the elaboration of the mediators listed in Table 1.1 that prevent fibrin accumulation and platelet activation.[11]

Physiological anticoagulant systems

At least three major physiological anticoagulant systems operate to reduce fibrin accumulation in the circulation: antithrombin III (now more commonly referred to as simply 'antithrombin'); protein C/protein S; and tissue factor pathway inhibitor. These anticoagulants act at different points in the coagulation cascade so that, as shown in Figure 1.4, essentially they blanket the entire coagulation system to quench fibrin formation. A 'hypercoagulable state' exists whenever coagulation enzyme production exceeds enzyme neutralization.[27]

Antithrombin is the major protease inhibitor of the coagulation cascade.[28-31] It inhibits not only thrombin but also other activated coagulation factors, including factors X_a, IX_a, XI_a and XII_a. Antithrombin inactivates thrombin and the other coagulation enzymes by forming a complex between the active site of the protease and the reactive center (Arg393 and Ser394) of antithrombin.[32] Although this reaction occurs relatively sluggishly, it is greatly accelerated in the presence of heparin. In fact, heparin works as a pharmacologic anticoagulant primarily by acting as a catalyst for the neutralization of thrombin by antithrombin. Heparin and heparin sulfate proteoglycans are normally present in the vessel wall and, therefore, antithrombin inactivation of thrombin and other coagulation

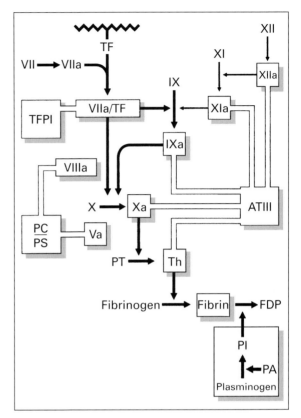

Figure 1.4
Sites of action of the major physiological antithrombotic pathways. Antithrombin (AT); protein C/protein S (PC/PS); tissue factor pathway inhibitor (TFPI); fibrinolytic system, consisting of plasminogen, plasminogen activator (PA); and plasmin (PI). (From Schafer,[26] modified with permission.)

proteases is most likely to occur physiologically on vascular surfaces rather than in fluid-phase plasma.

Protein C is a vitamin K-dependent anticoagulant protein that must be activated to 'activated protein C' (APC).[33] The physiological activator of protein C is thrombin itself, producing a negative feedback loop whereby thrombin generates its own inactivator. Rapid protein C activation requires the formation of a high-affinity complex between thrombin and thrombomodulin, a glycosaminoglycan on the surface of intact endothelial cells.[34] APC then acts as a physiological anticoagulant by inactivating the two key cofactors of the Xase and prothrombinase complexes, factors V_a and VIII_a, respectively. The essential cofactor of APC is protein S, another vitamin K-dependent glycoprotein.

Tissue factor pathway inhibitor (TFPI) is a Kunitz-type plasma protease inhibitor that blocks tissue factor-induced coagulation in the extrinsic pathway.[35] Circulating plasma TFPI is largely bound to lipoproteins. TFPI has inhibitory activity not only against the factor VII_a-tissue factor complex but also against factor X_a.

Fibrinolytic system

Any thrombin activity that escapes the inhibitory effects of the physiological anticoagulant systems noted above can convert fibrinogen to fibrin. An endogeneous fibrinolytic system is then activated to digest rapidly intravascular fibrin and thereby maintain the patency of the vasculature.[36] Endogenous fibrinolysis is dependent primarily upon endothelial cells. The inactive plasma zymogen protein, plasminogen, is acted upon by tissue-type plasminogen activator (t-PA) and urokinase-type plasminogen activators (u-PA) produced by endothelial cells. Both t-PA and u-PA are serine proteases. They convert plasminogen to the active serine protease enzyme, plasmin. Plasmin then digests fibrin (and fibrinogen) into fibrin(ogen) degradation products. The products of plasmin-induced cleavage of non-covalently cross-linked fibrin and fibrinogen are indistinguishable, while plasmin cleavage of cross-linked fibrin yields additional degradation products, including D dimers. The fibrinolytic system has its own control mechanisms: these include plasminogen activator inhibitors (including PAI-1, PAI-2, PAI-3 and protease nexin) and α_2-antiplasmin, a circulating inhibitor which directly inactivates plasmin itself.

Physiological antiplatelet systems

Several endothelium-derived mediators are potent platelet inhibitors that act to maintain circulating platelets in their quiescent states under normal circumstances.[25] These include prostacyclin (prostaglandin I_2 or PGI_2), nitric oxide (NO), possibly carbon monoxide (CO), and endothelial ecto-ADPase. In addition to the platelet inhibitory functions of these mediators, they also directly or indirectly act as vasodilators. Thus, each of these endogenous antiplatelet agents promotes blood fluidity by inhibiting platelets and causing vasodilation.

Prostacyclin[37,38] is the product of arachidonic acid metabolism by endothelial cells (in contrast to thromboxane A_2, a product of arachidonic acid metabolism by platelets). Prostacyclin inhibits platelets by activating platelet adenylyl cyclase and thereby raising the intracellular levels of cyclic AMP (cAMP). Elevated levels of cAMP within the platelet produce global inhibition of platelet activation pathways. Prostacyclin similarly causes vasodilation by raising cAMP levels in vascular smooth muscle cells, which leads to vasorelaxation.

Nitric oxide (NO), a major constituent of what was previously referred to as endothelium-derived relaxing factor, is a by-product of the conversion of L-arginine to L-citrulline by NO syntheses.[39,40] NO is a potent activator of soluble guanylyl cyclase, and thereby raises intracellular cyclic GMP (cGMP) levels in both platelets and vascular smooth muscle cells. Elevation of cGMP leads to platelet inhibition and vasorelaxation. Carbon monoxide (CO) has also been identified recently as an endogenous, simple, diatomic gaseous product of the vessel wall.[41] It acts as a platelet inhibitor and vasodilator through cGMP, as does NO. ADPase, is a membrane-associated ectonucleotidase, which has been recently identified in endothelial cells as CD39.[42] ADP, released by platelets and other cells, is an activator of platelets as already described. Endothelial ecto-ADPase metabolizes this platelet agonist and thereby maintains platelets in their resting states. While ADPase does not have intrinsic vasodilator properties, it can exert this action indirectly by generating vasodilator adenosine through sequential dephosphorylation of ATP to ADP to AMP to adenosine by an enzyme chain of ectonucleotidases at the luminal surface. Thus, prostacyclin, NO, CO, and ADPase all represent locally active, endothelium-derived platelet inhibitors that are also vasodilators, thereby promoting blood fluidity.

References

1. Macfarlane RG. An enzyme cascade in the blood clotting mechanism and its function as a biochemical amplifier. *Nature* 1964;**202**: 498–9.
2. Davie EW, Ratnoff OD. Waterfall sequence of intrinsic blood coagulation. *Science* 1964;**145**: 1310–12.
3. Schafer AI. Coagulation cascade: an overview. In: Loscalzo J, Schafer AI (eds) *Thrombosis and Hemorrhage* (Blackwell Scientific: Boston. 1994) 3–12.
4. Doolittle RF. The structure and evolution of vertebrate fibrinogen. *Ann NY Acad Sci* 1983;**408**:13–27.
5. Bouma BN, Griffin JH. Human blood coagulation factor XI. Purification, properties, and mechanism of activation by activated factor XII. *J Biol Chem* 1977;**252**:6432–7.
6. Fujikawa K, Heimark RL, Kurachi K, Davie EW. Activation of bovine factor XII (Hageman factor) by plasma kallikrein. *Biochemistry* 1980;**19**:1322–30.
7. Nemerson Y. Tissue factor and hemostasis. *Blood* 1988;**71**:1–8.
8. Edgington TS, Mackman N, Brand K, Ruf W. The structural biology of expression and function of tissue factor. *Thromb Haemost* 1991;**66**:67–79.
9. Nakagaki T, Foster DC, Berkner KL, Kisiel W. Initiation of the extrinsic pathway of blood coagulation: evidence for the tissue factor dependent autoactivation of human coagulation factor VII. *Biochemistry* 1991;**30**: 10819–24.
10. Drake TA, Morrissey JH, Edgington TS. Selective cellular expression of tissue factor in human tissues. Implications for disorders of hemostasis and thrombosis. *Am J Pathol* 1989;**134**:1087–97.
11. Cines DB, Pollak ES, Buck CA, et al. Endothelial cells in physiology and in the pathophysiology of vascular disorders. *Blood* 1998; **91**:3527–61.
12. Lecompte MF, Rosenberg I, Gitter C. Membrane insertion of prothrombin. *Biochem Biophys Res Commun* 1984;**125**:381–6.
13. Spicer EK, Horton R, Bloem L, et al. Isolation of cDNA clones coding for human tissue factor: primary structure of the protein and cDNA. *Proc Natl Acad Sci USA* 1987;**84**: 5148–52.
14. Mann KG, Krishnaswamy S, Lawson JH. Surface-dependent hemostasis. *Semin Hematol* 1992;**29**:213–26.
15. Jenny NS, Mann KG. Coagulation cascade: an overview. In: Loscalzo J, Schafer AI (eds) *Thrombosis and Hemorrhage*, 2nd edn (Williams & Wilkins: Baltimore, in press).
16. Schafer AI, The primary and secondary hypercoagulable states. In: Schafer AI (ed.) *Molecular Mechanisms of Hypercoagulable States* (Landes Bioscience: Austin, 1997) 1–48.
17. Kaushansky K. Regulation of megakaryopoiesis, In: Loscalzo J, Schafer AI. *Thrombosis and Hemorrhage*, 2nd edn (Williams & Wilkins: Baltimore, in press).
18. Dale GL. Platelet turnover. In: Loscalzo J, Schafter AI (eds) *Thrombosis and Hemorrhage*, 2nd edn (Williams & Wilkins: Baltimore, in press).
19. Schafer AI. Antiplatelet therapy. *Am J Med* 1996;**101**:199–209.
20. Schafer AI. Antiplatelet therapy with glycoprotein IIb/IIIa receptor inhibitors and other novel agents. *Tex Heart Inst J* 1997;**24**:90–6.
21. Kroll MH, Hellums JD, McIntire LV, Schafer AI, Moake JL. Platelets and shear stress. *Blood* 1996;**88**:1525–41.
22. Kung C, Hayes E, Mann KG. A membrane-mediated catalytic event in prothrombin activation. *J Biol Chem* 1994;**269**:25838–48.
23. Mann KG, Nesheim ME, Church WR, Haley P, Krishnaswamy S. Surface-dependent reactions of the vitamin K-dependent enzyme complexes. *Blood* 1990;**76**:1–16.
24. Kalafatis M, Swords NA, Rand MD, Mann KG. Membrane-dependent reactions in blood coagulation: role of the vitamin K-dependent

enzyme complexes. *Biochim Biophys Acta* 1994;**1227**:113–29.

25. Schafer AI. Vascular endothelium: in defense of blood fluidity [editorial]. *J Clin Invest* 1997;**99**:1143–4.

26. Weiler-Guettler H, Christie PD, Beeler DL, et al. A targeted point mutation in thrombomodulin generates viable mice with a prethrombotic state. *J Clin Invest* 1998;**101**:1983–91.

27. Schafer AI. Hypercoagulable states: molecular genetics to clinical practice. *Lancet* 1994;**344**:1739–42.

28. Howell WH, Holt E. Two new factors in blood coagulation – heparin and proantithrombin. *Am J Physiol* 1918;**47**:328–41.

29. Abildgaard U. Antithrombin and related inhibitors of coagulation. In: Poller L (ed.) *Recent Advances in Blood Coagulation* (Churchill Livingstone: Edinburgh, 1981) 151–73.

30. Petersen TE, Dudek-Wojciechowska G, Sottrup-Jensen L et al. Primary structure of antithrombin III (heparin cofactor). Partial homology between antitrypsin and antithrombin III. In: Collen D, Wiman B, Verstraeta M (eds) *The Physiological Inhibitors of Blood Coagulation and Fibrinolysis* (Elsevier Science Publishers: Amsterdam, 1979) 43–54.

31. Bock SC, Wion KL, Vehar GA, Lawn RM. Cloning and expression of the cDNA for human antithrombin III. *Nucleic Acids Res* 1982;**10**:8113–25.

32. Bjork I, Danielsson A, Fenton JW, Jornvall. The site in human antithrombin for functional proteolytic cleavage by human thrombin. *FEBS Lett* 1981;**126**:257–60.

33. Dahlbäck B. The protein C anticoagulant system: inherited defects as basis for venous thrombosis. *Thromb Res* 1995;**77**:1–42.

34. Esmon CT. Molecular events that control the protein C anticoagulant pathway. *Thromb Haemost* 1993;**70**:29–35.

35. Broze GJ Jr. Tissue factor pathway inhibitor and the revised theory of coagulation. *Annu Rev Med* 1995;**46**:103–12.

36. Collen D, Lijnen HR. Molecular basis of fibrinolysis, as relevant for thrombolytic therapy. *Thromb Haemost* 1995;**74**:167–71.

37. Meade EA, Jones DA, Zimmerman GA, McIntyre TM, Prescott SM. Prostaglandins and related compounds. Lipid messengers with many actions. *Handbook Lipid Res* 1996;**8**:285.

38. Weksler BB, Marcus AJ, Jaffe EA. Synthesis of prostaglandin I_2 (prostacyclin) by cultured human and bovine endothelial cells. *Proc Natl Acad Sci USA* 1977;**74**:3922–6.

39. Stamler JS, Singel DJ, Loscalzo J. Biochemistry of nitric oxide and its redox-activated forms. *Science* 1992;**258**:1898–902.

40. Loscalzo J, Welch G. Nitric oxide and its role in the cardiovascular system. *Prog Cardiovasc Dis* 1995;**38**:87–104.

41. Christodoulides N, Durante W, Kroll MH, Schafer AI. Vascular smooth muscle cell heme oxygenases generate guanylyl cyclase-stimulatory carbon monoxide. *Circulation* 1995;**91**:2306–9.

42. Marcus AJ, Broekman MJ, Drosopoulos JHF, et al. The endothelial cell ecto-ADPase responsible for inhibition of platelet function in CD39. *J Clin Invest* 1997;**99**:1351–60.

2

Platelet physiology

James J Ferguson, Martin Quinn and Joel L Moake

Introduction

Coagulation and the action of platelets is of major significance in many aspects of atherosclerotic disease.[1,2] Appreciating the full potential of antiplatelet therapy requires familiarity with the basic physiologic concepts of platelet function. This chapter will review the role of platelets in the process of coagulation. The purpose of this introduction is to serve as a framework for subsequent chapters describing specific forms of antiplatelet therapy.

Thrombosis

Historically, our understanding of coagulation has been based on the observed blood-clotting aberrations that occur in various deficiency states.[3] The physiology of coagulation has traditionally included the intrinsic pathway (with all required factors present in the blood) and also the extrinsic pathway (with at least some extravascular factors required), both of which culminate in the common pathway.

The traditional concept of separate extrinsic, intrinsic, and common coagulation pathways has, however, been revised in recent years, as described in Chapter 1. A newer, unified concept presents three major steps that are involved in coagulation: namely, initiation; amplification; and propagation (Figure 2.1).[1,2] In the initiation phase, the impetus for coagulation is the exposure of tissue factor (TF) at an initial site of injury that combines with factor VIIa to activate a small amount of factor IX. Factor IXa then activates a small amount of factor X, which goes on to generate a small amount of thrombin. The end result of the initiation phase is the generation of a small amount of thrombin after tissue injury. This small amount of thrombin is the 'spark' that initiates coagulation. The thrombin produced serves to activate platelets and promote the assembly of coagulation factors and cofactors on the platelet surface as part of the subsequent amplification and propagation stages of coagulation.

During the amplification phase, the small amounts of thrombin that were generated initially activate factor XI, which then activates factor IX (through the classic intrinsic system). In conjunction with an activated platelet membrane and factor VIIIa, small quantities of thrombin feed back to generate large amount of the complex of factors Va, VIIIa, and IXa on the platelet membrane. The end result of the amplification phase is that the small amount of thrombin generated in the preceding phase goes on to generate large amounts of the complexes necessary for coagulation to proceed. These complexes are the fuel for the fire of coagulation.

Finally, during the propagation phase, factor X associates with the already assembled complex of factor VIIIa on the surface of an activated platelet membrane, generating factor Xa. Factor Xa, in turn, associates with the already assembled complex of factor Va on the surface of an activated platelet membrane to form the prothrombinase complex, which converts prothrombin (factor II) to thrombin (factor IIa). Finally, thrombin acts to cleave fibrinogen and form fibrin. The end result of the propagation phase is that the preassembled complexes in the amplification phase go on to form fibrin. The process of coagulation is

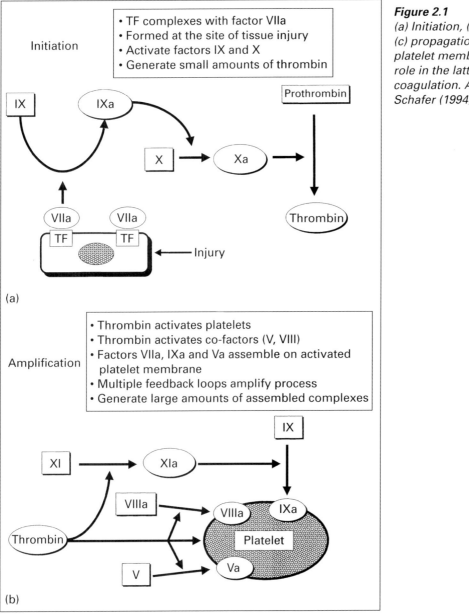

(a)

(b)

Figure 2.1
(a) Initiation, (b) amplification, (c) propagation: The activated platelet membrane plays a key role in the latter two stages of coagulation. Adapted from Schafer (1994).

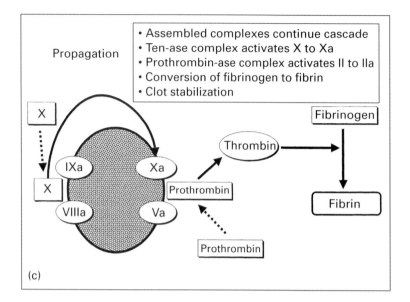

- Assembled complexes continue cascade
- Ten-ase complex activates X to Xa
- Prothrombin-ase complex activates II to IIa
- Conversion of fibrinogen to fibrin
- Clot stabilization

(c)

tremendously accelerative; the spark and the fuel combine on the 'fuse' of the platelet membrane in an explosive generation of thrombin and fibrin formation.

Overview of platelet physiology

Platelets are small, disc-shaped elements found in large numbers in the blood that play a pivotal role in atherosclerotic and thrombotic processes (Figure 2.2). In human beings, platelets are anucleate cell fragments shed by megakaryocytes in the bone marrow. As a result of higher shear forces at the vessel wall, platelets tend to circulate toward the outer margin of the vessel in proximity to the wall.

At a site of arterial injury, the endothelial barrier separating the vessel wall contents from the circulating blood is broken. Platelets adhere to exposed collagen, von Willebrand factor (vWF), and fibrinogen by specific cell receptors: glycoprotein (GP)Ib and GPIa-IIa.

Adherent platelets are then activated by several independent mediators, including collagen, thromboxane, serotonin, epinephrine (adrenaline), adenosine diphosphate (ADP), and thrombin. Strong activators, such as collagen and thrombin, appear primarily responsible for initial platelet activation at sites of arterial injury in vivo. Activated platelets degranulate and secrete chemotaxins, clotting factors, and vasoconstrictors, thereby promoting thrombin generation, vasospasm, and additional platelet accumulation. The release of internally stored ADP and thromboxane 'amplifies' the process of platelet activation by secondary feedback loops. In addition, activated platelets change shape and extrude pseudopodia, thus increasing the surface area on which thrombin production can occur (Figure 2.3).

As mentioned previously, the platelet phospholipid membrane acts as a cofactor that greatly facilitates coagulation.[2] The regulatory role of the phospholipid membrane may seem

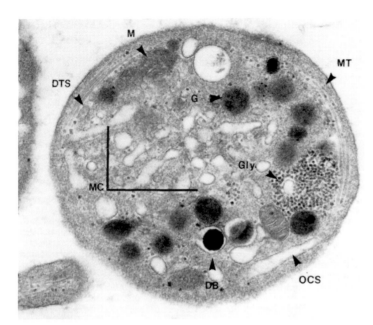

Figure 2.2
Normal resting platelet. M – mitochondria. G – granules, DB – dense bodies, OCS – open canalicular system, DTS – dense tubular system, MC – membrane complex, MT – microtubules, Gly – glycogen particles. From Mehta JL, Conti CR (eds) Thrombosis and platelets in Myocardial Ischemia. (Philadelphia: FA Davis, 1987)

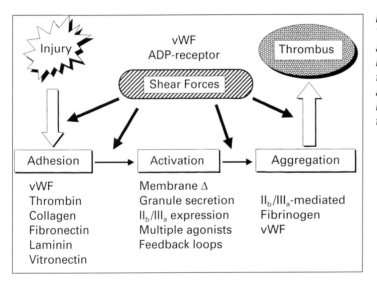

Figure 2.3
The processes of adhesion, activation, and aggregation, with key mediators highlighted. Shear forces may play a role in facilitating all three of these steps, mediated largely through von Willebrand factor and ADP receptors.

relatively insignificant given the ubiquitous nature of such membranes within the body. However, a specific type of phospholipid membrane is required for the coagulation process. Predominantly negatively charged membranes (rich in phosphatidylserine and phosphatidylinositol) provide the surface on which the enzymes of the coagulation cascade function with maximum efficiency; when activated, platelets alter their cell membranes to

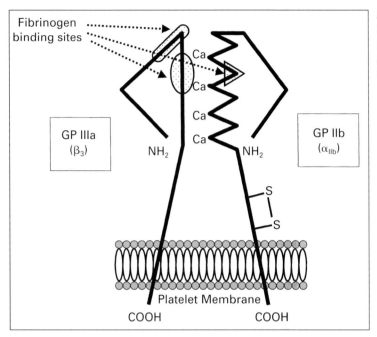

Fibrinogen binding sites

GP IIIa (β_3)

NH$_2$

Ca
Ca
Ca
Ca

NH$_2$

GP IIb (α_{IIb})

S
S

Platelet Membrane

COOH   COOH

Figure 2.4
Schematic structure of GP IIb/IIIa. COOH – carboxy terminal, NH$_2$ – amino terminal, Ca – calcium binding sites.

conform exactly to these requirements. Thus activated platelet membranes constitute the primary source of phospholipid surface on which the coagulation cascade proceeds. Even though it may extend into the fluid phase from the platelet membrane, the coagulation cascade operates at a considerable disadvantage if an activated platelet membrane is not present.

In the presence of platelet activation, previously inactive GPIIb-IIIa receptors on the platelet membrane surface undergo structural modification and become receptive to ligand binding. The GPIIb-IIIa receptor is the most numerous receptor found on the platelet surface, with approximately 40 000–80 000 receptors per platelet, and represents the final common pathway for platelet aggregation (Figure 2.4).[3,4] Once activated, the GPIIb-IIIa receptor becomes available to bind fibrinogen and vWF, which act to cross-link platelets and promote the generation of a platelet mass (and

a large surface of platelet membrane) at the site of vascular injury. Over the ensuing hours of continuing platelet activation, additional GPIIb-IIIa receptors stored within the platelets are extruded to the surface and became available for ligand binding. As the arborizing mass of platelets grows at the initial site of vascular injury, large amounts of activated platelet membrane accumulate, providing an ideal milieu for thrombus formation. Furthermore, as the activated platelets within the platelet mass degranulate, they release vasoactive substances and platelet factor 4, thus limiting the actions of endogenous (and exogenous) heparin.

Platelet adhesion

Hemostasis is initiated when endothelial cells are damaged, and platelets adhere to the collagen and von Willebrand factor (vWF)

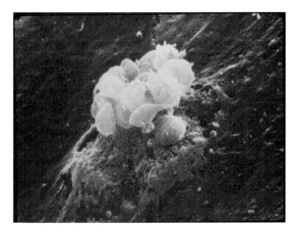

Figure 2.5
Adherent platelets at the site of endothelial injury.

multimers in the subendothelium. These events occur in flowing blood, with platelets exposed to different shear stresses in different areas of the circulation. vWF is a multivalent, multimeric protein that is essential for platelet adhesion to the subendothelium of damaged blood vessels. vWF has binding sites for the GPIb component of platelet GPIb-IX-V, for GPIIb-IIIa, and for several types of collagen (I, III, and VI). Platelets adhere initially to subendothelial vWF multimers via GPIb receptors, and interact with collagen via GPIa-IIa receptors, which are integral membrane proteins. GPIb is a disulfide-linked heterodimer that is complexed to other smaller platelet integral membrane proteins, GPIX and GPV. vWF multimers bind to the GPIb molecules extending from the exterior surface of the platelet membrane (Figure 2.5).

Platelet activation

Platelet activation and subsequent aggregation is complex and many of the underlying intracellular signals have yet to be defined. It is the process by which the normally smooth, discoid platelet is transformed into an irregular spherical particle with numerous pseudopodia projecting from its surface (Figure 2.6). Coincident with these morphological changes, the activated platelet acquires the ability to bind the plasma protein, fibrinogen. There are many different agonists that induce platelet activation. Thrombin, collagen and thromboxane A_2 (TXA$_2$) are all strong agonists and can produce aggregation independent of secretion. Adenosine diphosphate (ADP) and serotonin are intermediate agonists, while epinephrine, is effective only at supraphysiological concentrations. Also, physical stimuli such as high fluid shear stress induce platelet activation and subsequent aggregation. This may be an important means of platelet activation at the site of a severe coronary stenosis where fluid shearing forces are quite large. The latter response is mainly mediated through vWF binding to its membrane receptor GPIb-IX. High shear stresses induce a conformational change in the GPIb-IX receptor, or vWF, that allows vWF to bind. vWF binding provokes several intracellular signals including an increase in Ca^{2+} and TXA$_2$ formation, which result in GPIIb-IIIa activation[5] (Figure 2.7).

Several platelet agonists are generated or released at the site of platelet activation. TXA$_2$ is produced from arachidonic acid released by the action of phospholipase A_2 in activated platelets. Arachidonic acid is metabolized to the intermediate product prostaglandin (PG)H$_2$ by the enzyme cyclo-oxygenase. PGH$_2$ is further metabolized by a P_{450} enzyme, thromboxane synthase, to thromboxane A_2.[6,7] Thromboxane A_2 has a very short half-life (approx 30 s) as it is rapidly hydrolysed to thromboxane B_2, which is inactive. TXA$_2$ mediates its effects through specific G-protein-linked membrane receptors PGH$_2$, the TXA$_2$ precursor, also stimulates these receptors.[8]

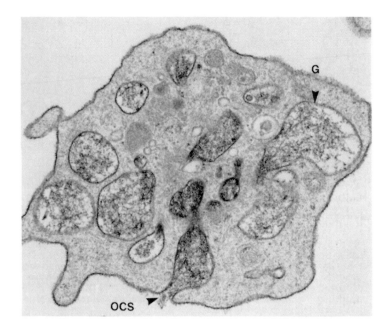

Figure 2.6
An activated, secretory platelet. The granules (G) have become dilated and swollen, and have fused, in places, with the open canicular system (OCS).

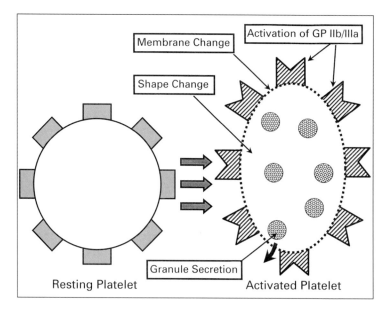

Figure 2.7
The process of platelet activation results in a shape change, a change in the structure of the platelet membrane, a change in the conformation of GP IIb/IIIa that allows it to bind ligands, and secretion of the platelet granule contents.

Two separate isoforms of the TXA$_2$ receptor, TXRα and TXRβ, have been identified. These have been cloned from platelet mRNA and expressed in a cell line.[9] In expression systems, both receptors are linked to phospholipase C, while TXRα activates, TXRβ inhibits adenylate cyclase. The two cloned receptors differ in several respects from the two receptor subtypes previously identified in intact platelets with the use of specific receptor antagonists, since only one of these was linked to the activation of phospholipase C, platelet aggregation and secretion, and the other to platelet shape change and calcium flux.[10] While this pharmacological evidence suggests that both isoforms are expressed in platelets, the presence of the two receptors has not been confirmed at the protein level.

Two other activators released on cell activation are ADP and serotonin, which are present in the platelet dense-granules. ADP acts through binding to low- and high-affinity membrane receptors. These receptors are members of the P2 family of nucleotide receptors, which are further classified into P2X (ion-channel receptors) and P2Y (G-protein-linked receptors). Recently, three separate platelet ADP receptors have been proposed, based on research with antagonists of the different nucleotide receptors. These include a $P2X_1$ ion-channel receptor that mediates the early transmembrane flux of calcium but does not appear to affect shape change or aggregation; aP2TAC G-protein linked receptor coupled to the ADP-induced inhibition of adenylate cyclase and aggregation; and a $P2Y_1$ receptor coupled to the activation of phospholipase C, which results in increased inositol triphosphate levels, the mobilization of intracellular calcium and platelet shape change.[11] These investigators have recently cloned the $P2Y_1$ receptor from platelet cDNA.[12]

Thrombin is generated by the coagulation cascade on the surface of the platelet as the platelet aggregate provides a focal point for the assembly of coagulation enzymes, including the prothrombinase complex of factor V, X, Ca^{2+} and phospholipid.[13] Thrombin interacts with at least two receptors on platelets, a protease activated receptor (PAR-1) and a high-affinity site on GPIb.[14] PAR-1 is one of a novel class of receptors that act as substrates for cell-activating enzymes. Thrombin binds to a sequence within the extracellular tail of PAR-1 that resembles the thrombin binding site on the anticoagulant, hirudin.[15] Thrombin cleaves the extracellular tail, generating a novel amino-terminal that acts as the ligand for the receptor and activates the cell. Indeed, small peptides comprising as few as six amino acids corresponding to the new amino-terminal can activate platelets.[16]

Platelets may also be activated by collagen present in the extracellular matrix, which is exposed at sites of endothelial damage. The tertiary and quaternary structure of collagen is important in this method of activation and aggregation. Nevertheless platelets can adhere to monomeric collagen, particularly types I and III without activation. The circulating platelets adhere directly to the exposed collagen via their $\alpha_2\beta_1$ receptors. This results in an increase in intracellular Ca^{2+} activation of phospholipase C and phosphorylation of several intracellular proteins, leading to secretion and full platelet activation.[17] GPVI also plays a role as GPVI-deficient platelets have a reduced response to fibrillar collagen and do not respond to a triple helical analog of collagen that induces full platelet activation and aggregation in an $\alpha_2\beta_1$-independent manner. The interaction of collagen with the GPVI receptor is required for several intracellular signaling events, including the phosphorylation of p72[syk] and p125[FAK], and activation of phospholipase C. Kehrel and colleagues propose a two-site, two-step model of activation with initial adhesion to collagen via $\alpha_2\beta_1$ and subsequent interaction with GPVI, which induces full platelet activation.[18] Finally, platelets also interact with collagen through their GPIb-IX receptors. Circulating vWF binds to exposed collagen and consequently expresses a binding site for the GPIb-IX receptor.[5]

Epinephrine, a weak agonist, acts through the G-protein-linked α_2-adrenergic receptor to

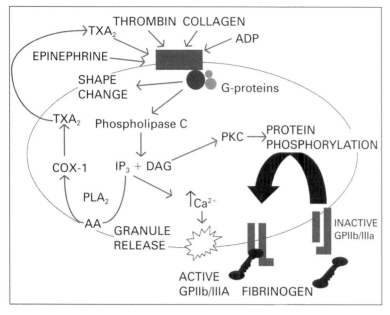

Figure 2.8

Agonist binding to specific membrane receptors results in the activation of phospholipase C, which releases inosital triphosphate (IP_3) and diacyl glycerol (DAG). IP_3 increases intracellular Ca^{2+}. The increased Ca^{2+} activates phospholipase A_2 (PLA_2) and causes granule release. PLA_2 releases arachidonic acid (AA) from the plasma membrane, which is converted to thromboxane A_2 (TXA_2) by cyclo-oxygenase (COX). DAG activates protein kinase C (PKC). This leads to phosphorylation of various intracellular proteins and results in activation of GPIIb/IIIa.

stimulate aggregation and inhibition of adenylate cyclase. The level of epinephrine required to induce platelet activation is supraphysiological, although it may act synergistically with other agonists, and, indeed, can overcome the inhibitory activity of aspirin in vivo. In a canine model of coronary stenosis, an infusion of epinephrine overcame the inhibitory effects of aspirin on clot formation.[19]

Many platelet agonists, such as thrombin, thromboxane, epinephrine and ADP, act through the superfamily of seven transmembrane G-protein linked receptors. Agonist binding causes signaling into the cell that results in shape change, secretion and aggregation. These signals are mediated through mobilization of calcium from intracellular stores via activation of phospholipase C and inosital triphosphate production. The increase in Ca^{2+} triggers phospholipase A_2 activation and release of arachidonic acid from the cell membrane, which is subsequently converted into TXA_2 (see Figure 2.8). Phospholipase C generates diacylglycerol, which activates protein kinase C, one of the pathways that result in GPIIb-IIIa activation.[20] The response is mimicked by phorbol esters, although the aggregation induced is delayed and is of a lesser extent than seen with potent agonists like thrombin, suggesting that other mechanisms are involved. Several different G-proteins differently transduce these signals.[21] Recently, a genetically modified mouse model in which a G-protein α-subunit, $G\alpha_q$, was disrupted has been described.[22] The animals had increased bleeding times and were protected from collagen and adrenaline (epinephrine)-induced thromboembolism. Their platelets failed to aggregate to any known agonists, although agonist-induced platelet shape change was unaffected. Agents such as the calcium ionophore A23187, which bypass the surface receptor G-protein pathways, also induced platelet aggregation. These findings indicate that $G\alpha_q$ is required for platelet aggregation and that other platelet G-proteins are required for shape change.

Platelet aggregation

Platelet aggregation is mediated through a platelet surface receptor, glycoprotein (GP)IIb-IIIa, which is one of a family of adhesion receptors called integrins (Figure 2.4).[23] These calcium-dependent heterodimers composed of two non-covalently linked subunits, an α and a β subunit, which in the case of GPIIb-IIIa, are α_{IIb} and β_{III}. Integrins play an important role in many diverse physiological processes including cell adhesion and migration, wound healing, bone remodeling, tumorogenesis and thrombosis. They act as receptors for adhesion proteins, which in the case of GPIIb-IIIa include fibrinogen, von Willebrand factor (vWF), fibronectin and vitronectin (Figure 2.9). The β_{III} subunit of GPIIb-IIIa is the smaller of the two is composed of a single polypeptide chain with a large extracellular amino terminus, a short transmembrane segment and a carboxyterminal intracellular tail. The α-chain is composed of two subunits, an extracellular heavy chain, αIIb_a, joined by a disulfide bond to the transmembrane and intracellular portion of the light chain, αIIb_b.[24] The importance of the receptor in thrombosis is demonstrated by the bleeding disorder, Glanzmann's thromboasthenia, in which patients lack a functional receptor and consequently their platelets fail to bind fibrinogen or to aggregate upon activation.[25] These patients usually have a mild hemostatic defect that is characterized by minor bleeding events and marked prolongation of their bleeding time; however, major bleeding events can also occur.

GPIIb-IIIa is the most abundant receptor on the platelet surface with 40 000–80 000 complexes per platelet.[26] Under resting conditions, the platelet GPIIb-IIIa does not recognize, or has a very low affinity for fibrinogen. Upon platelet activation, however, GPIIb-IIIa expresses a high affinity for its ligands. Binding of fibrinogen cross-links adjacent platelets, resulting in platelet aggregation. Platelet activation may also increase the surface density of receptors by releasing stores of GPIIb-IIIa, which is present within platelet α- and dense-granules, where some of the receptors are already complexed with fibrinogen.[27] Thus, secretion of these granules upon stimulation not only provides an increased receptor number but also a fibrinogen-occupied receptor.

Virtually all known platelet agonists induce a fibrinogen binding site in GPIIb-IIIa, thus activation of GPIIb-IIIa is often considered the final common pathway of platelet activation. The ligand affinity of GPIIb-IIIa is carefully regulated in order to prevent inadvertent platelet aggregation. The control of its affinity is exerted by signals transmitted through the intracellular tails of the receptor and deletion of parts of the intracellular tails of either subunit produces a constitutively active or inactive receptor.[28–32] Similarly short peptide sequences based on a highly conserved region in the αIIb tail (KVGFFKR) can induce receptor activation, TXA_2 production and platelet aggregation suggesting that this sequence is important in receptor activation.[33] The means by which these signals enable fibrinogen binding are not known, however there are clues. Certain monoclonal antibodies, such as PAC-1, bind only to the active receptor, indicating that activation or the increased affinity for fibrinogen occurs as a result of a conformational change in the receptor.[34] This has been confirmed using fluorescence energy transfer experiments where relative movement of labeled antibodies bound to the two subunits have been detected, which is again consistent with a conformational change with

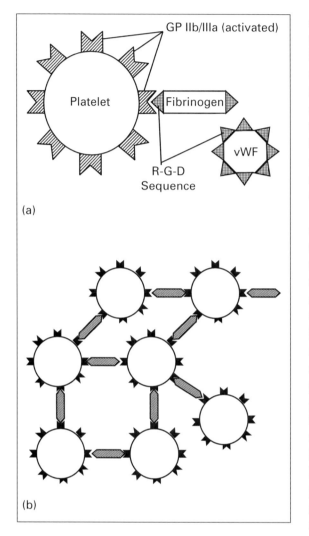

(a)

(b)

Figure 2.9
*(a) The primary ligands for activated GP IIb/IIIa
are fibrinogen (a dimeric molecule) and von
Willebrand factor (vWF, a multimeric molecule).
Both contain multiple copies of the arginine-
glycine-aspartic acid (R-G-D) amino acid
sequence.*
*(b) Platelet aggregation proceeds as adjacent
platelets are cross-linked by fibrinogen (shown)
or vWF. The end result is a large mass of
activated platelet membrane concentrated at the
site of injury, greatly facilitating thrombus
formation, but keeping it largely confined to the
original area of injury.*

activation.[35] This conformational change is
thought to result in exposure of the fibrinogen
binding site, which is cryptic in the inactive
receptor, thus allowing circulating fibrinogen
to bind. Interestingly, such activation does not
appear necessary for platelets to recognize
solid-phase fibrinogen. It is possible that the
fibrinogen, when it adheres to a surface,
undergoes a conformational change that
allows it to be recognized by the inactive
receptor.

Additional conformational changes in the
receptor are induced upon ligand binding, and
these are referred to as ligand-induced binding
sites or LIBS.[36] LIBS have been identified as
the appearance of neoepitopes detected by
monoclonal antibodies upon ligand binding.
Conversely, a monoclonal antibody, Mab2,
has been identified that will bind only to the
unoccupied receptor.[37] Ligand-induced conformational changes may be important for
platelet responses subsequent to ligand occupancy of GPIIb-IIIa. The monoclonal antibody, D3, which recognizes a LIBS on the β of
the receptor, inhibits clot retraction, although
it simultaneously promotes fibrinogen
binding.[38,39] In a similar way, Mab2 prevents
platelet aggregation but fails to inhibit fibrinogen binding, suggesting that the site recognized by the antibody is involved in events
subsequent to ligand binding that are necessary for full aggregation.[37]

These studies with monoclonal antibodies
suggest that conformational changes in GPIIb-
IIIa are involved in both ligand recognition
and so called 'outside-in' signaling. Indeed, far
from being a passive adhesion receptor for fibrinogen, GPIIb-IIIa provokes an array of intracellular signals.[40] These include the very visible
cytoskeletal rearrangement, pseudopodia formation and spreading on solid-phase fibrinogen. Within the platelet this 'outside-in'
signaling through GPIIb-IIIa results in the for-

mation of focal adhesion complexes of signaling proteins that amplify existing activation events, such as TXA_2 production and inositol phosphate metabolism.[41,42] Phosphorylation of focal adhesion kinase and several additional late tyrosine phosphorylations also occurs and may, likewise, be dependent on GPIIb-IIIa clustering and/or ligand binding.[43] The degree of activation triggered through the platelet GPIIb-IIIa receptor is most evident when platelets bind to solid-phase fibrinogen coated on a plate, an interaction that does not require preceding activation of the platelet or the GPIIb-IIIa, yet results in platelet spreading, TXA_2 formation and tyrosine phosphorylation of multiple proteins.

Fibrinogen is a hexapeptide made up of three different pairs of identical subunits (α, β and γ) and has six different sites that potentially interact with the receptor, two arginine-glycine-aspartate (RGD) domains at residues 95–97 and 572–574, respectively in each of two α-chains and a dodecapeptide in the carboxy terminus (residues 400–411) of each γ-chain. Chemical cross-linking studies demonstrate that the RGD sequence and the dodecapeptide bind to separate sites on the integrin.[44-46] However, the binding of RGD and the dodecapeptide is mutually exclusive and both prevent fibrinogen binding, suggesting that they each recognize the ligand recognition site. Fibrinogen from transgenic mice, deficient in the dodecapeptide sequence, was unable to support platelet aggregation, although the mutated fibrinogen can support clot retraction.[47] Similarly, studies with other fibrinogen mutants demonstrate that the dodecapeptide sequence is the primary receptor binding domain.[48] When fibrinogen is coated on a surface, platelets adhere to it. This adhesion is mediated initially by unactivated GPIIb-IIIa receptors and results in signaling into the platelet, as indicated by spreading of

the adherent platelet over the surface. The γ-chain dodecapeptide sequence supports this adhesion but requires platelet activation for firm irreversible adhesion to the surface. RGD-containing fibrinogen fragments do not support adhesion but intact fibrinogen supports full adhesion independent of aggregation. Under conditions of flow, only the intact fibrinogen molecule supports adhesion. Thus although the γ-chain peptide is important in platelet–platelet and platelet–surface interactions, other sites within the intact fibrinogen molecule are necessary for normal platelet function.[49]

GPIIb-IIIa ligand binding is not restricted to fibrinogen; indeed, other adhesive ligands including vWF, fibronectin, vitronectin and thrombospondin, which also contain RGD domains, bind to the receptor. Nevertheless, fibrinogen is the principle ligand in vivo owing to its high concentration in plasma. These adhesion proteins interact differently with the receptor, although they all bind through the RGD sequence. For example, the anti-LIBS antibody D3 induces fibrinogen and vWF binding but fails to induce vitronectin binding.[50] This finding suggests that the receptor may express different conformations that differentiate between ligands, adding further to the complexity of ligand receptor interactions. It is important to note that ligands other than fibrinogen and receptors other than GPIIb-IIIa are important for platelet function. For example, vWF binding to GPIIb-IIIa and GPIb-IX mediates shear stress-mediated platelet activation and the vWF-GPIb-IX interaction initiates the adhesion of platelets to areas that are denuded of endothelium. So, even when there is complete inhibition GPIIb-IIIa, platelets still form an adherent monolayer over damaged endothelium. This may explain the low incidence of serious bleeding problems in the majority of patients receiving GPIIb-IIIa antagonists and in patients with Glanzmann's thrombasthenia.

Platelet thrombus formation

It is hypothesized that platelet thrombosis in the regions of the arterial circulation narrowed by atherosclerosis or vasoconstriction, and consequently subjected to abnormally elevated levels of fluid shear stress, may be produced by two different mechanisms.[51] These are:

1. Direct platelet aggregation produced by high shear stress in constricted small arteries and arterioles that have intact endothelial lining cells; and
2. A pathological amplification of normal hemostatic platelet adhesion and subsequent aggregation reactions at sites of vascular injury, endothelial desquamation and subendothelial exposure.

Direct shear stress-induced platelet aggregation

Direct platelet aggregation in response to pathologically elevated shear stress depends on the presence of plasma vWF multimers, the platelet vWF receptor complexes GPIb-IX-V and GPIIb-IIIa, Ca^{2+}, and adenosine diphosphate (ADP).[52–54] Fibrinogen may be the bridging ligand effecting platelet aggregation at shear stresses below ~12 dynes/cm^2;[55] however, at shear stresses greater than 10–12 dynes/cm^2, platelet aggregation depends only upon vWF as the bridging ligand, and is independent of plasma or platelet fibrinogen.[53–55] The linking of GPIb-IX-V complexes on adjacent platelets by vWF multimers leads to the cohesive interplatelet interactions induced by ristocetin in stirred platelet-rich plasma (PRP) in vitro. In PRP under static or stirred conditions, vWF binding to GPIIb-IIIa in the presence of chemical agonists other than ristocetin

(or botrocetin) is minimal.[56] If high shear stresses are applied to platelets in blood or plasma, however, vWF binds to platelets GPIb-IX-V complexes, and then to GPIIb-IIIa molecules, resulting in direct shear-induced platelet aggregate formation.[57,58] Moreover, larger vWF multimers support shear-induced platelet aggregation more effectively than smaller multimers.[52,54] ADP released from platelets and red blood cells is also required for shear stress-induced platelet aggregation, probably by potentiating the activation of platelet GPIIb-IIIa. When platelets are pretreated with epinephrine before shearing, the aggregation response is enhanced.[59,60]

The predominant effect of elevated fluid shear stress is likely to be on platelet vWF receptors, rather than on plasma vWF, causing a transient state of platelet glycoprotein receptivity for vWF.[52,58] These shear-sensitive platelet membrane components may be a part of the GPIb-IX-V complex.[61–63]

Elevations of platelet cyclic AMP, as induced by endothelial cell-derived prostacyclin (PGI$_2$), or elevations of platelet cyclic GMP, as induced by endothelial cell-derived nitric oxide (NO), inhibit shear stress-induced platelet aggregation.[64,65] In contrast, inhibition of cyclo-oxygenase and therefore, of platelet thromboxane A$_2$, production, by acetylsalicylic acid (aspirin) has little effect on direct platelet aggregation in response to shear stress.[64] This latter observation may account for the relative lack of potency of aspirin as antithrombotic therapy in some arterial thrombotic disorders.

Except for the profound inhibitory effects of EDTA, which causes the de-assembly of GPIIb-IIIa, most anticoagulants have little effect on shear stress-induced platelet aggregation. One study shows that the extent of shear-induced platelet aggregation in a cone-and-plate viscometer is similar using PRP anticoagulated with sodium citrate, recombinant hirudin, unfractionated heparin, or low-molecular-weight heparin (LMWH).[66] Other studies have suggested a modest inhibitory effect of unfractionated heparin on shear-induced platelet aggregation,[67] and of combined hirudin and LMWH on shear-dependent platelet thrombus formation using ex vivo perfused vessels.[68] Shear stress-induced platelet aggregation is unequivocally inhibited by fibrinolytic agents, because of plasmin-mediated proteolysis of vWF multimers.[69]

Pathological adhesion/aggregation

Physiologic time-averaged mean shear stress levels in the human arterial circulation are about 20–30 dynes cm^2, and pathologic levels (i.e. as in a stenosed coronary or cerebral artery) may reach over 350 dynes/cm^2.[51,70-72] The latter clinical situation is often associated with platelet thrombus formation.

As described already, pathologic stenosis can lead to direct shear-induced aggregation of platelets from the blood in constricted arteries. In addition, the adhesion of blood platelets onto exposed atherosclerotic subendothelium in a region of endothelial cell desquamation (e.g. after atherosclerotic plaque rupture) can lead to extensive subsequent platelet aggregation and thrombus formation. These responses require fluid shear stresses. With pathologically elevated shear stresses (over 30 dynes/cm^2), platelet thrombus formation depends on the initial binding of vWF multimers to platelet GPIb-IX-V complexes in order to attract and localize platelets onto the exposed subendothelium. Subendothelium vWF binding to activated platelet GPIIb-IIIa complexes then completes the platelet immobilization onto the injured site.[51,55,57,73-80] Most

endothelial vWF has been secreted from the previously overlying endothelial cells, and is associated with collagen and other components.[81] Upon exposure of subendothelium, vWF from the plasma also becomes rapidly insolubilized onto the subendothelial matrix components,[73,74] as does vWF secreted from platelet α granules.[66,82,83] Larger vWF multimers are more effective than smaller vWF multimers at promoting platelet adhesion and subsequent aggregation and thrombus formation,[76] as is the case with direct shear stress-induced platelet aggregation. In association with platelet adherence via GPIb-IX-V complexes to subendothelial vWF multimers, collagen fibrils may interact with platelet GPIa-IIa receptors to accentuate platelet intracellular signaling and GPIIb-IIIa activation. Both fibrinogen and vWF multimers can serve as bridging molecules between activated GPIIb-IIIa complexes on adjacent platelets to support the platelet cohesion, or aggregation, process.[66,83] Platelet thrombus formation promotes factor VII activation, the assembly of activated coagulation factors, and fibrin polymer formation.[84] The activation of coagulation is a secondary event that occurs in vivo a short time after platelet adhesion and aggregation.[85,86]

Acetylsalicylic acid (aspirin) treatment of blood does not inhibit platelet thrombus formation in a parallel-plate flow chamber,[66,87] although it has been reported to have a modest inhibitory effect in other flow systems.[88] PGI$_2$ derived from endothelial cells, however, inhibits platelet thrombus formation on subendothelium under flowing conditions.[89]

Summary

This chapter has provided an overview of platelet physiology with specific emphasis on platelet activation and aggregation. Significant recent major advances have taken place in the world of antiplatelet therapy; an adequate understanding of normal platelet function is necessary to understand what exactly these new forms of therapy are doing and how they may best be utilized.

References

1. Roberts HR, Lozier JN: New perspectives on the coagulation cascade. *Hosp Pract* 1992;**27**:97–112.

2. Schafer AI: Coagulation cascade: an overview, in Loscalzo J, Schafer AI (eds). *Thrombosis and Hemorrhage* (Boston, Blackwell Scientific, 1994) 3–12.

3. Lefkovits J, Topol EJ: Platelet glycoprotein IIb/IIIa receptor antagonists in coronary artery disease. *Eur Heart J* 1996;**17**:9–18.

4. Lefkovits J, Plow EF, Topol EJ: Platelet glycoprotein IIb/IIIa receptors in cardiovascular medicine. *N Engl J Med* 1995;**332**:1553–59.

5. Kroll M, Hellums J, McIntire L, Schafer A, Moake J: Platelets and shear stress. *Blood* 1996;**88**:1525–41.

6. Reilly M, Fitzgerald GA: Cellular activation by thromboxane A_2 and other eicosanoids. *Eur Heart J* 1993;**14**:88–93.

7. FitzGerald GA: Mechanisms of platelet activation thromboxane A_2 as an amplifying signal for other agonists. *Am J Cardiol* 1991; **68**:11B–15B.

8. Halushka PV, Allan CJ, Davis-Bruno KL: Thromboxane A_2 receptors. *J Lipid Med Cell Signal* 1995;**12**:361–78.

9. Hirata T, Ushikubi F, Kakizuka A, Okuma M, Narumiya S: Two thromboxane A_2 receptor isoforms in human platelets: opposite coupling to adenylyl cyclase with different sensitivity to Arg^{60} to Leu mutation. *J Clin Invest* 1996; **97**:949–56.

10. Takahara K, Murray R, FitzGerald GA, Fitzgerald DJ: The response to thromboxane A_2 analogues in human platelets: discrimination of two binding sites linked to distinct effector systems. *J Biol Chem* 1990;**265**: 6836–44.

11. Jin J, Daniel J, Kunapuli S: Molecular basis for ADP-induced platelet aggregation: the P2Y1 receptor mediates ADP-induced intracellular calcium mobilization and shape change in platelets. *J Biol Chem* 1998;**273**:2030–34.

12. Daniel J, Dangelmaier C, Jin J, Ashby B, Smith J, Kunapuli S: Molecular basis for ADP-induced platelet activation: evidence for three distinct ADP receptors on human platelets. *J Biol Chem* 1998;**273**:2024–29.

13. Swords N, Mann K: The assembly of the pro-thrombinase complex on adherent platelets. *Arterioscler Thromb* 1993;**13**:1602–12.

14. Jamieson GA: Pathophysiology of platelet thrombin receptors. *Thromb Haemost* 1997; **78**:242–46.

15. Ray A, Hegde LG, Gupta JB: Thrombin receptor: a novel target for antiplatelet drug development. *Thromb Res* 1997;**87**:37–50.

16. Chiu PJ, Tetzloff GG, Foster C, Chintala M, Sybertz EJ: Characterization of in vitro and in vivo platelet responses to thrombin and thrombin receptor-activating peptides in guinea pigs. *Eur J Pharm* 1997;**321**:129–35.

17. Keely PJ, Parise LV: The $\alpha_2\beta_1$ integrin is a necessary co-receptor for collagen-induced activation of Syk and the subsequent phosphorylation of phospholipase Cγ2 in platelets. *J Biol Chem* 1996;**271**:26 668–76.

18. Kehrel B, Wierwille S, Clemetson K, Anders O, Steiner M, Knight CG, et al: Glycoprotein VI is a major collagen receptor for platelet activation it recognizes the platelet-activating quaternary structure of collagen, whereas CD36, glycoprotein IIb/IIIa, and von Willebrand factor do not. *Blood* 1998;**91**:491–99.

19. Folts JD, Rowe GG: Epinephrine potentiation of in vivo stimuli reverses aspirin inhibition of platelet thrombus formation in stenosed canine coronary arteries. *Thromb Res* 1988;**50**: 507–16.

20. Blockmans D, Deckmyn H, Vermylen J: Platelet activation. *Blood Reviews* 1995; **9**:143–56.

21. Brass LF, Manning DR, Cichowski K, Abrams CS: Signaling through G proteins in platelets to the integrins and beyond. *Thromb Haemost* 1997;**78**:581–89.

22. Offermanns S, Toombs C, Hu Y, Simon M: Defective platelet activation in Gα_q-deficient

mice. *Nature* 1997;**389**:183–86.

23. Cox D, Aoki T, Seki J, Motoyama Y, Yoshida K: The pharmacology of the integrins. *Medic Res Rev* 1994;**14**:195–228.

24. Calvete JJ: On the structure and function of platelet integrin $\alpha_{IIb}\beta_3$, the fibrinogen receptor. *Proc Soc Exper Biol Med* 1995;**208**:346–60.

25. George JN, Caen JP, Nurden AT: Glanzmann's thrombasthenia: the spectrum of clinical disease. *Blood* 1990;**75**:1383–95.

26. Wagner CL, Mascelli MA, Neblock DS, Weisman HF, Coller BS, Jordan RE: Analysis of GPIIb-IIIa receptor number by quantification of 7E3 binding to human platelets. *Blood* 1996;**88**:907–14.

27. Nurden P, Humbert M, Piotrowicz RS, Bihar C, Poujol C, Nurden AT, et al: Distribution of ligand-occupied $\alpha_{IIb}\beta_3$ in resting and activated human platelets determined by expression of a novel class of ligand-induced binding site recognized by monoclonal antibody AP6. *Blood* 1996;**88**:887–99.

28. O'Toole T, Mandelman D, Forsyth J, Shattil SJ, Plow EF, Ginsberg MH: Modulation of the affinity of integrin $\alpha_{IIb}\beta_3$ (GPIIb-IIIa) by the cytoplasmic domain of alpha IIb. *Science* 1991;**254**:845–47.

29. O'Toole T, Katagiri Y, Faull RJ, et al: Integrin cytoplasmic domains mediate inside-out signal transduction. *J Cell Biol* 1994;**124**:1047–59.

30. Wang R, Shattil SJ, Ambruso DR, Newman PJ: Truncation of the cytoplasmic domain of β_3 in a variant form of Glanzmann thrombasthenia abrogates signaling through the integrin alpha(IIb)beta3 complex. *J Clin Invest* 1997;**100**:2393–403.

31. Peter K, Bode C: A deletion in the alpha subunit locks platelet integrin alpha IIb beta 3 into a high-affinity state. *Blood Coag Fibrinolysis* 1996;**7**:233–36.

32. Shattil SJ, Gao J, Kashiwagi H: Not just another pretty face: regulation of platelet function at the cytoplasmic face of integrin $\alpha_{IIb}\beta_3$. *Thromb Haemost* 1997;**78**:220–25.

33. Stephens G, O'Luanaigh N, Reilly D, Harriott P, Walker B, Fitzgerald D, et al: A sequence within the cytoplasmic tail of GPIIb independently activates platelet aggregation and thromboxane synthesis. *J Biol Chem* 1998;**273**:20317–22.

34. Shattil SJ, Hoxie JA, Cunningham M, Brass LF: Changes in the platelet membrane glycoprotein IIb-IIIa complex during platelet activation. *J Biol Chem* 1985;**260**:11107–14.

35. Sims PJ, Ginsberg MH, Plow EF, Shattil SJ: Effect of platelet activation on the conformation of the plasma membrane glycoprotein IIb-IIIa complex. *J Biol Chem* 1991;**266**:7345–52.

36. Kouns WC, Kirchhofer D, Hadvary P, Edenhofer A, Weller T, Pfenninger G, et al: Reversible conformational changes induced in glycoprotein IIb-IIIa by a potent and selective peptidomimetic inhibitor. *Blood* 1992;**80**:2539–47.

37. Quinn MJ, Cox D, Theroux P, Fitzgerald D: Interaction of antagonists with the platelet GP IIb-IIIa: characterization of two monoclonal antibodies that detect drug binding. *J Am Coll Cardiol* 1998;**331**:353A [Abstract].

38. Frelinger A, Du XP, Plow E, Ginsberg M: Monoclonal antibodies to ligand-occupied conformers of integrin $\alpha_{IIb}\beta_3$ (glycoprotein IIb-IIIa) alter receptor affinity, specificity, and function. *J Biol Chem* 1991;**266**:17106–11.

39. Frelinger A, Cohen I, Plow EF, Smith MA, Roberts J, Lan SC, et al: Selective inhibition of integrin function by antibodies specific for ligand-occupied receptor conformers. *J Biol Chem* 1990;**265**:6346–52.

40. Yamada KM, Miyamoto S: Integrin transmembrane signaling and cytoskeletal control. *Curr Opin Cell Biol* 1995;**7**:681–89.

41. Fox JE, Lipfert L, Clark EA, Reynolds CC, Austin CD, Brugge JS: On the role of the platelet membrane skeleton in mediating signal transduction. Association of GP IIb-IIIa, pp60c-src, pp62c-yes, and the p21ras GTPase-activating protein with the membrane skeleton. *J Biol Chem* 1993;**268**:25973–84.

42. Shattil S, Haimovich B, Cunningham M, Lipfert L, Parsons JT, Ginsberg MH, et al: Tyrosine phosphorylation of pp125FAK in platelets requires coordinated signaling through integrin and agonist receptors. *J Biol Chem* 1994;**269**:14738–45.

43. Miyamoto S, Akiyama SK, Yamada KM: Synergistic roles for receptor occupany and aggregation in integrin transmembrane function. *Science* 1995;**267**:883–85.

44. D'Souza S, Ginsberg MH, Burke TA, Lam SC,

Plow EF: Localization of an Arg-Gly-Asp recognition site within an integrin adhesion receptor. *Science* 1988;242:91–93.

45. D'Souza S, Ginsberg MH, Lam SC, Plow EF: Chemical cross-linking of arginyl-glycyl-aspartic acid peptides to an adhesion receptor on platelets. *J Biol Chem* 1988;263:3943–51.

46. Plow EF, D'Souza SE, Ginsberg MH: Ligand binding to GPIIb-IIIa: a status report. *Semin Thromb Hemost* 1992;18:324–32.

47. Holmback K, Danton MJ, Suh TT, Daugherty CC, Degen JL: Impaired platelet aggregation and sustained bleeding in mice lacking the fibrinogen motif bound by integrin $\alpha_{IIb}\beta_3$. *EMBO J* 1996;15:5760–71.

48. Farrell DH, Thiagarajan P, Chung DW, Davie EW: Role of fibrinogen alpha and gamma chain sites in platelet aggregation. *Proc Natl Acad Sci USA* 1992;89:10729–32.

49. Savage B, Bottini E, Ruggeri M: Interaction of integrin $\alpha_{IIb}\beta_3$ with multiple fibrinogen domains during platelet adhesion. *J Biol Chem* 1995;270:28812–17.

50. Mondoro TH, Wall CD, White MM, Jennings LK: Selective induction of a glycoprotein IIIa ligand-induced binding site by fibrinogen and von Willebrand factor. *Blood* 1996;88:3824–30.

51. Kroll MH, Hellums JD, McIntyre LV, Schafer AI, Moake JL: Platelets and shear stress. *Blood* 1996;88:1525–41.

52. Moake JL, Turner NA, Stathopoulos NA, Nolasco LH, Hellums JD: Involvement of large plasma von Willebrand factor (vWF) multimers and unusually large vWF forms derived from endothelial cells in shear stress-induced platelet aggregation. *J Clin Invest* 1986;78:1456–1460.

53. Peterson DM, Stathopoulos NA, Giorgio TD, Hellums JD, Moake JL: Shear-induced platelet aggregation requires von Willebrand factor and platelet membrane glycoproteins Ib and IIb-IIIa. *Blood* 1987;69:625–28.

54. Moake JL, Turner NA, Stathopoulos NA, Nolasco LH, Hellums JD: Shear-induced platelet aggregation can be mediated by vWF released from platelets, as well as by exogenous large or unusually large vWF multimers, requires adenosine diphosphate, is resistant to aspirin. *Blood* 1988;71:1366–74.

55. Ikeda Y, Handa M, Kawano K, Kamata T, Murata M, Araki Y, et al: The role of von Willebrand factor and fibrinogen in platelet aggregation under varying shear stress. *J Clin Invest* 1991;87:1234.

56. Schullek J, Jordan J, Montgomery RR: Interaction of von Willebrand factor with human platelets in the plasma milieu. *J Clin Invest* 1984;73:421.

57. McCrary JK, Nolasco LH, Hellums JD, Kroll MH, Turner NA, Moake JL: Direct demonstration of radiolabeled von Willebrand factor binding to platelet glycoprotein Ib and IIb-IIIa in the presence of shear stress. *Ann Biomed Eng* 1995;23:787–93.

58. Konstantopoulos K, Chow TW, Turner NA, Hellums JD, Moake JL: Shear stress-induced binding of von Willebrand factor to platelets. *Biorheology* 1997;34:57–61.

59. Goto S, Ikeda Y, Murata M, Handa M, Takahashi E, Yoshioka A, et al: Epinephrine augments von Willebrand factor-dependent shear-induced platelet aggregation. *Circulation* 1992;86:1859.

60. Wagner CT, Kroll MH, Chow TW, Hellums JD, Schafer AI: Epinephrine and shear stress synergistically induce platelet aggregation via a mechanism that bypasses vWF-GPIb interaction. *Biorheology* 1996;33:209–29.

61. Roth GJ: Developing relationships: arterial platelet adhesion, glycoprotein Ib, and leucine-rich glycoproteins. *Blood* 1991;77:5.

62. Modderman PW, Admiraal LG, Sonnenberg A, von demBrone AEGK: Glycoprotein V and Ib-IX form a noncovalent complex in the platelet membrane. *J Bio Chem* 1992;267:364.

63. Lopez JA: The platelet glycoprotein Ib-IX complex. *Blood Coagul Fibrin* 1994;5:97.

64. Hardwick RA, Hellums JD, Peterson DM, Moake LJ, Olson JD: The effect of PGI$_2$ and theophyline on the response of platelets subjected to shear stress. *Blood* 1981;58:678.

65. Durante W, Schafer AI, Hrobolich JK, Claure RA, Mendelsohn ME, Kroll MH: Endothelium-derived relaxing factor inhibits shear stress-induced platelet aggregation. *Platelets* 1993;4:135.

66. Alevriadou BR, Moake JL, Ruggeri ZM, Turner NA, Folie BJ, Phillips MD, et al: Real-time analysis of shear dependent thrombus for-

mation and its blockade by inhibitors on von Willebrand factor binding to platelets. *Blood* 1993;**81**:1263–76.

67. Wurzinger LJ, Opitz R, Schmid-Schobein H: Effect of anticoagulants on shear-induced platelet alterations. *Thromb Res* 1987;**49**:133.

68. van Zanten GH, de Graaf S, Slootweg PJ, Heijnen HFG, Connolly TM, de Groot PG, et al: Increased platelet deposition on atherosclerotic coronary arteries. *J Clin Invest* 1994;**93**:615.

69. Kamat SG, Michelson AD, Benoit SE, Moake JL, Rajasekhar D, Hellums JD, et al: Fibrinolysis inhibits shear stress-induced platelet aggregation. *Circulation* 1995;**92**:1399–407.

70. Tangelder GJ, Slaff DW, Arts T, Reneman RS: Wall shear rate in arterioles in vivo: least estimates from platelet velocity profiles. *Am J Physiol* 1988;**254**:H1059.

71. Strony J, Beaudoin A, Brands D, Adelman B: Analysis of shear stress and hemodynamic factors in a model of coronary artery stenosis and thrombosis. *Am J Physiol Heart Circ Physiol* 1993;**265**:H1787.

72. Strony J, Phillips M, Brands D, Moake J, Adelman B: Aurin-tricarboxylic acid in a canine model of coronary artery thrombosis. *Circulation* 1990;**81**:1106–1114.

73. Weiss HJ, Baumgartner HR, Tschopp TB, Turitto VT, Cohen D: Correction by factor VIII of the impaired platelet adhesion to subendothelium in von Willebrand's disease. *Blood* 1978;**51**:267.

74. Weiss HJ, Turitto VT and Baumgartner HR: Effect of shear rate on platelet interaction with subendothelium in citrated and native blood: shear rate-dependent decrease of adhesion in von Willebrand disease and the Bernard Soulier syndrome. *J Lab Clin Med* 1978;**92**:750.

75. Baumgartner HR, Tschopp TB, Meyer D: Shear rate dependent inhibition of platelet adhesion and aggregation on collagenous surfaces by antibodies to human factor VIII/von Willebrand factor. *Br J Haematol* 1980; **44**:127.

76. Sixma JJ, Sakariassen KS, Beeser-Visser NH, Ottenhof-Rovers M, Bolhuis PA: Adhesion of platelet to human artery subendothelium: effect of factor VIII-von Willebrand factor of various multimeric composition. *Blood* 1984; **63**:128.

77. Turitto VT, Weiss HJ, Baumgartner HR: Decreased platelet adhesion on vessel segments in von Willebrand's disease: a defect in initial attachment. *J Lab Clin Med* 1983;**102**:551.

78. Turitto VT, Weiss HJ, Baumgartner HR: Platelet interaction with rabbit subendothelium in von Willebrand's disease: altered thrombus formation distinct from defective platelet adhesion. *J Clin Invest* 1984;**74**:1730.

79. Savage B, Salivar E, Ruggeri ZM: Initiation of platelet adhesion by arrest onto fibrinogen or translocation on von Willebrand factor. *Cell* 1996;**84**:289–97.

80. Tschopp TB, Weiss HJ, Baumgartner HR: Decreased adhesion of platelets to subendothelium in von Willebrand's disease. *J Lab Clin Med* 1974;**83**:296.

81. Stel HV, Sakariassen KS, De Groot PG, Van Mourik JA, Sixma JJ: von Willebrand factor in the vessel wall mediates platelet adherence. *Blood* 1985;**65**:85.

82. Weiss JH, Turitto VT, Baumgartner HR: Platelet adhesion and thrombus formation on subendothelium in platelets deficient in glycoproteins IIb-IIIa, Ib, and storage granules. *Blood* 1986;**67**:322.

83. Sakariassen K, Nievelstein P, Colleer B, Sixma J: The role of platelet membrane glycoproteins Ib and IIb-IIIa in platelet adherence to human artery subendothelium. *Br J Haematol* 1986; **63**:681.

84. Weiss HJ, Turitto VT, Baumgartner HR: Role of shear rate and platelets in promoting fibrin formation on rabbit subendothelium. *J Clin Invest* 1986;**78**:1072.

85. Kirchhofer D, Tschopp TB, Steiner BT, Baumgartner HR: Role of collagen-adherent platelet in mediating fibrin formation in flowing whole blood. *Blood* 1995;**86**:3815.

86. Turitto VT, Baumgartner HR: Initial deposition of platelets and fibrin on vascular surfaces in flowing blood, in Coleman RW, Hirsch J, Marder VJ, Salzman ED (eds), *Hemostasis and Thrombosis* (3rd edn.), (Philadelphia, PA: Lippincott, 1994) 805.

87. Grabowski EF: Platelet aggregation in flowing blood at a site of injury to an endothelial cell monolayer: quantification and real-time imaging with TAB monoclonal antibody. *Blood* 1990;**75**:390.

88. Baumgartner HR, Muggli R, Tschoop TB, Turitto VT: Platelet adhesion, release and aggregation in flowing blood: effects of surface properties, and platelet function. *Thromb Haemost* 1976;35:124.

89. Tschoop TB, Baumgartner HR: Platelet adhesion and mural platelet thrombus formation on aortic subendothelium of rats, rabbits and guinea pigs correlate negatively with the vascular PGI$_2$-production. *J Lab Clin Med* 1981;98:402.

3

Laboratory assessment of platelet function

Joel L Moake

Introduction

Excessive bleeding can result from either decreased platelet numbers or defective platelet function, especially in association with trauma or surgery. Laboratory determination of whole blood platelet counts has long been automated and reliable. In contrast, effective evaluation of platelet function has been elusive and controversial. This chapter will describe briefly the techniques that have been used most commonly by clinicians during the past generation, and then will review in more detail the newer methods . . . including more advanced systems designed to study platelet function under flowing conditions analogous to those encountered in vivo. The discussion will include descriptions of several assays that will soon become widely available in hospital clinical pathology laboratories.

Summary of normal platelet function in hemostasis

Hemostasis is initiated when endothelial cells are damaged, and platelets adhere to the collagen and von Willebrand factor (vWf) multimers in the subendothelium. These events occur in flowing blood, with platelets exposed to different shear stresses in different areas of the circulation. vWf is a multivalent, multimeric protein that is essential for platelet adhesion to the subendothelium of damaged blood vessels. vWf has binding sites for the glycoprotein (GP) GPIb component of platelet GPIb-IX-V, for GPIIb-IIIa, and for several types of collagen (I, III, and VI).

Platelets initially adhere to subendothelial vWf multimers via GPIb receptors, and interact with collagen via GPIa-IIa receptors. These are integral membrane proteins. GPIb is a disulfide-linked heterodimer that is complexed to other smaller platelet integral membrane proteins, GPIX and GPV. vWf multimers bind to the GPIb molecules extending from the exterior surface of the platelet membrane.

Following platelet–subendothelial adherence, platelets are activated to generate and transmit internal chemical signals. These transducing signals include: G proteins; the effector enzymes phospholipase C, phospholipase A_2, adenylyl cyclase, protein kinase C, and tyrosine kinases; and the second messengers inositol triphosphate, Ca^{2+}, diacylglycerol, thromboxane A_2, cyclic AMP and cyclic GMP. An important result of platelet activation is the increased exposure of binding sites for fibrinogen and vWf on platelet surface GPIIb-IIIa complexes.

One example of platelet signaling is the following: membrane lipases hydrolyse arachidonic acid from ester bonds in platelet membrane phospholipids. Platelet fatty acid cyclo-oxygenase, the enzyme that is irreversibly inhibited when it is acetylated by aspirin, rapidly converts arachidonic acid to cyclic endoperoxides (PGG_2 and PGH_2), and then via thromboxane synthetase to thromboxane A_2 (TXA_2). TXA_2 is a short-lived compound that potentiates the release of adenosine diphosphate (ADP), serotonin and Ca^{2+} from platelet-dense granules, as well as several proteins from α-granules. These latter include: platelet-derived growth factor that is mitogenic for smooth muscle cells and fibroblasts; platelet factor 4 that is cationic and capable of binding negatively charged heparin molecules; and fibrinogen and vWf multimers that attach, along with their plasma forms, to activated GPIIb-IIIa complexes on platelet surfaces. The result is platelet–platelet cohesion, or aggregation, of platelets onto those already adherent to subendothelial vWf and collagen.

Thrombin generated by activated coagulation pathways, together with epinephrine (adrenaline), amplify platelet release and aggregation. Any TXA_2 that leaks from activated platelets may potentiate platelet aggregation and stimulate vasoconstriction locally before it is hydrolysed non-enzymically into an inactive end-product, thromboxane B_2.

Most common tests of platelet function during the past 25 years

Bleeding time

This test aspires to be an in vivo measurement of the vWf-dependent adhesion and subsequent aggregation of platelets on locally injured vascular subendothelium, with minimal involvement of coagulation factor activation and fibrin polymer formation. A blood pressure cuff is inflated on the upper arm to a pressure of 40 mmHg, and a disposable, automated device inflicts a cut of standardized length on the volar surface of the forearm.[1–3] The wound is blotted gently with filter paper and the time elapsed until bleeding ceases is noted (normally about 3–9 minutes).

In a patient with a platelet count below 100,000/μl, the bleeding time is variable and difficult to interpret. A prolonged bleeding time in a patient with a platelet count above 100,000/μl supposedly indicates either impaired platelet function or deficient or defective subendothelial vWf factor multimers (as in the von Willebrand's disease subtypes). It is a common experience, however, that even in individuals with platelet counts above 100,000/μl the bleeding time can vary according to the depth of the cut produced by the technician or physician performing the test.[42] For example, the bleeding time can range from normal to prolonged in patients: ingesting aspirin;[2,4–6] treated with heparin or warfarin;[3] with different subtypes of von Willebrand's disease;[7] with hemophilia A[8–10] or other coagulation factor defects;[11–15] and with varying local skin thickness or vascular patterns. The test can also vary serially over time in the same individual, even in patients with known von Willebrand's disease subtypes who have clinical abnormalities of vWf-mediated platelet-subendothelial adhesion.[7] Furthermore, the bleeding time lengthens with decreasing hematocrit,[16–18] probably because red blood cells in oozing blood are involved in displacing platelets laterally toward exposed subendothelial surfaces to function in adhesion and aggregation reactions. The observations summarized thus far account for the reluctance of many physicians to base clinical decisions on 'bleeding times' that are of dubious reproducibility and dependent upon vascular, rheological, and coagulation events in addition to in vivo platelet adhesion and aggregation.

Platelet aggregometry

Another familiar test of platelet function is platelet aggregometry,[19] an in vitro spectrophotometric measurement of platelet cohesion usually performed using citrated PRP stirred at a very low shear rate in a small cuvette. Substances that induce the binding of vWf multimers to platelet GPIb-IX-V complexes (e.g. ristocetin or botrocetin), activate platelet GPIIb-IIIa complexes to bind fibrinogen (e.g. ADP or thrombin), or induce the release of platelet ADP (collagen or arachidonic acid) cause platelets to cohere or aggregate from the PRP. This results in increased light transmission through the plasma. The rate and extent of the increase in light transmission in response to added agonists are recorded on moving chart paper.

Platelet aggregometry usually requires several hours for a technician to perform using patient and control PRP samples that must be freshly prepared by gentle centrifugation of citrated whole blood. Any inadvertent ex vivo injury or activation of platelets may result in aggregation profiles that are confusing or misleading.

Platelet aggregometry provides information on platelet clumping under conditions different from those in normal flowing blood. Nevertheless, aggregometry is capable of detecting a deficiency or defect of vWf in patients with von Willebrand's disease subtypes, as well as rare abnormalities of GPIb-IX-V (Bernard-Soulier syndrome) or GPIIb-IIIa (Glanzmann's thromboasthenia). The relationship between aggregometry abnormalities and clinical bleeding in these disorders is well established. Aggregometry can also detect suppressed arachidonic acid-induced aggregation, which is characteristic of aspirin inhibition of platelet fatty acid cyclo-oxygenase. In contrast to test results with von Willebrand's disease,

Bernard-Soulier syndrome and Glanzmann's thromboasthenia patients, however, the relationship between the acquired aspirin-induced platelet aggregation abnormality and clinical bleeding is not firmly established.

A small percentage of patients anticoagulated with heparin in therapeutic, prophylactic or even 'keep open' dosages will develop thrombocytopenia (heparin-induced thrombocytopenia or HIT). Low-molecular weight heparin, however, may be less likely to produce thrombocytopenia than unfractionated heparin.[20] Heparin attaches to positively charged platelet factor-4 molecules that are secreted from the α-granules of activated platelets onto, or near, their outer membrane surfaces. In susceptible patients, IgG antibodies are produced and bind, via their Fab regions, to the heparin/platelet factor 4 complexes. The Fc portions of these IgG antibodies interact with Fc receptors on the platelet surfaces and activate platelets via internal signaling molecules, including arachidonic acid released from platelet membrane phospholipids. Arachidonic acid is converted to cyclic endoperoxides and TXA_2, ADP and other platelet granule contents are secreted, ADP induces the binding of fibrinogen to activated platelet GPIIb-IIIa complexes, and intravascular platelet aggregation occurs.[21-28] The consequences are thrombocytopenia that becomes progressively more severe over the course of several days, often accompanied by arterial or recurrent venous thrombosis (*heparin-induced thrombocytopenia/thrombosis* or *HITT*). Discontinuation of heparin leads to a reversal of intravascular aggregation as the heparin is catabolized and excreted, and the platelet count returns to normal within days.

As yet there is no generally accepted laboratory test that detects HIT. An aggregometry-type test, with several different concentrations of heparin added to heat-inactivated patient serum that is mixed with normal platelets or PRP, has been used widely.[28-31] The test has limited sensitivity, however. A variant of this test, with ^{14}C-serotonin release from radio-labeled platelets as the endpoint of the assay, has been claimed to be superior.[29-31] This modified assay has not, however, gained wide acceptance.

Newer tests
Modified whole blood platelet aggregation

A rapid and simple variation of aggregometry, using whole blood, has recently been developed by Coller et al.[32] This test is designed to monitor platelet function in patients receiving anti-arterial thrombotic therapy with intravenous and oral agents that block platelet GPIIb-IIIa complexes. In this new assay, a sample of patient or control citrated whole blood is mixed with fibrinogen-coated polystyrene beads. Platelets are stimulated with a thrombin receptor-activating peptide, and activated platelet GPIIb-IIIb molecules bind to and agglutinate the fibrinogen-coated beads. The agglutination is monitored as an increase in transmission of infrared light through the sample. The extent of blockade of platelet GPIIb-IIIa complexes by intravenous chimeric monoclonal 7E3 Fab antibodies (abciximab, ReoPro), or the cyclic peptide, integrilin, or by any of the several oral agents now in clinical trials may be determined quickly using this new method.

An equally rapid and even more generally useful method for assessing platelet function in whole blood is provided by **combining aggregometry and flow cytometry.** Citrated or

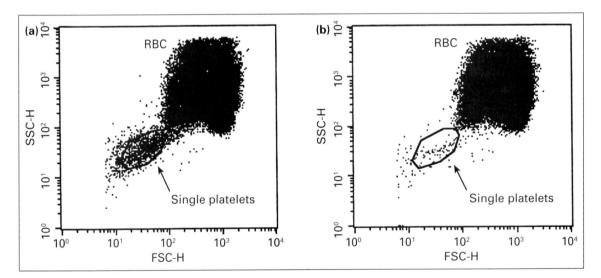

Figure 3.1
Whole blood aggregometry. The disappearance of single platelets into platelet aggregates can be seen by comparing flow cytometry patterns before (a) and after (b) the addition of 5 µm ADP to a sample of normal citrated whole blood.

heparinized patient whole-blood samples are stirred at 37°C in an aggregometer cuvette in the presence of the agonist to be evaluated (e.g. ADP, ristocetin, collagen, arachidonic acid, etc.). A 10 μl aliquot is removed before and after addition of the agonist, fixed immediately in formaldehyde, and analysed using flow cytometry. The disappearance of single platelets into aggregates can be detected easily in the flow cytometer, even in the presence of RBC[33] (Figure 3.1). This test system utilizes equipment already available in most clinical pathology laboratories, and the methodology allows ready detection of:

(1) Congenital platelet disorders (e.g. Bernard Soulier syndrome or Glanzmann's thrombasthenia);
(2) Blockade of GPIIb-IIIa by therapeutic agents;
(3) Possible blockade of platelet purine receptors (which bind ADP) by a new class of compounds under development;[34] and
(4) Suppression of large vWf multimer binding to platelet GPIb-IX-V complexes in the presence of ristocetin or botrocetin by recombinant vWf fragments capable of attaching directly to GPIb.[35]

Evaluation of direct shear stress-induced platelet aggregation: viscometers

Direct shear-induced platelet aggregation in a viscometer is inhibited by any agent that blocks the binding of vWf multimers to the GPIb component of platelet GPIb-IX-V complexes or to platelet GPIIb-IIIa molecules. These agents include:

(1) Monoclonal antibodies to GPIb;
(2) Aurin tricarboxylic acid polymers (which bind to vWf and prevent vWf multimer attachment to platelet GPIb);
(3) Recombinant fragments of vWf that include the GPIb binding site, bind directly to GPIb in the absence of any stimulus, and block the attachment of large vWf multimers to platelet GPIb;[35]
(4) Monoclonal antibodies (c7E3, ReoPro), cyclic peptides, or other compounds that block vWf binding to platelet GPIIb-IIIa complexes;
(5) Substances that metabolize ADP or prevent ADP interaction with platelet purine receptors; or
(6) Compounds that prevent ADP-induced vWf binding to GPIIb-IIIa (ticlopidine or clopodigrel).

There are several rotational viscometer prototypes;[36–40] some have been modified to apply pulsatile shear stress,[41] while others have been adapted to allow real-time optical measurements of platelet aggregation and calcium flux.[42] The two designs in most common use are:

(1) A stationary bob within a rotating concentric cylinder (the Couette viscometer); and
(2) A rotating cone whose center is in proximity (approx. 25 μm) to the center of a flat plate (the cone-and-plate viscometer).

Both designs generate a constant and uniform shear stress within the citrated or heparinized PRP or whole blood being tested. Platelet–surface interactions are minimized by coating the shear stress-generating surfaces with silicone or another non-thrombogenic material. The cone-and-plate viscometer (Figure 3.2a) offers the advantage of an open suspension, allowing rapid removal of samples for analyses. The shear rate in this system is nearly constant throughout the liquid between the cone and the plate; it is directly proportional to the rotations per minute of the cone, and inversely proportional to the gap angle between the cone and the plate. The gap angle used to generate

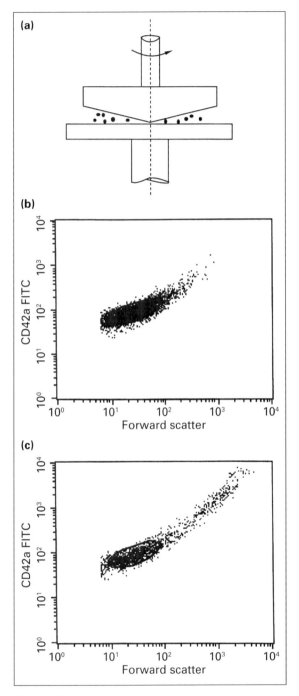

Figure 3.2
Direct shear stress-induced aggregation. (a) cone-and-plate viscometer; (b) pre-shear sample; (c) post-shear sample.

arterial-level shear forces is typically in the range of 0.30–1.00°, and the viscosity (in poise) of a suspension of cells is constant through the range of shear stresses applied experimentally. A constant shear stress can, therefore, be applied to anticoagulated PRP or whole blood placed into the rotational viscometer by imposing and maintaining a constant number of revolutions per minute of the cone on the plate. This type of rotational viscometer is capable of generating shear stresses ranging from less than 2 dynes/cm^2 (as in the venous system) to 20–30 dynes/cm^2 (arterial) to greater than 200 dynes/cm^2 (as occurs in stenosed arteries).

Shear stress promotes platelet aggregation by increasing both the number and efficiency of platelet–platelet collisions. Increased collision efficiency at higher shear stresses may result from the direct effects of shear stress on platelets (perhaps specifically on GPIb-IX-V and GPIIb-IIIa molecules) to induce the vWf multimer binding that results in platelet aggregation.[40,43] Shear-induced aggregation is evaluated by quantifying the disappearance of single platelets into platelet clumps following application of shear stress by the viscometer. The instrument used with the viscometer to quantify shear-induced platelet aggregation can either be an electronic particle counter (e.g. a Coulter counter)[36,37,42] or, more recently, a flow cytometer[33] (Figure 3.2b, c).

The viscometers presently in use are expensive; however, it is anticipated that, before long, a small and relatively inexpensive viscometer will be commercially available for widespread use in clinical pathology laboratories.

Evaluation of platelet adhesion and aggregation under flowing conditions: perfusion chambers

Most studies of shear-induced platelet-collagen interactions in perfusion chambers have used

Epifluorescence microscopy   3D representation

(a)

(b)

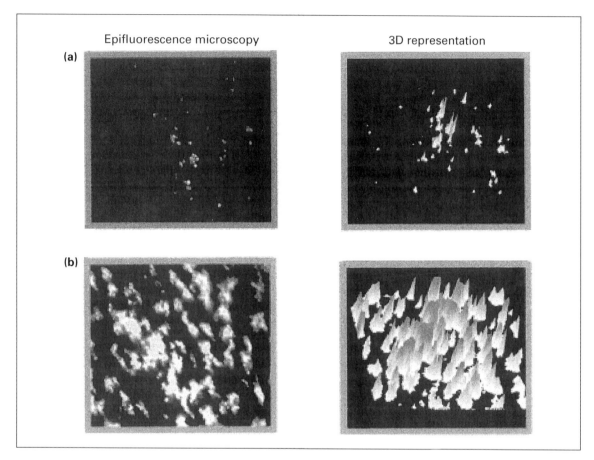

Figure 3.3
Adhesion followed by aggregation in real time. Perfusion of citrated whole blood over collagen/vWf.
(a) Adhesion at 15 sec; (b) adhesion at 60 sec.

morphometric or radioactive techniques to evaluate platelet accumulation at the end of an experiment. Recently, parallel plate perfusion of anticoagulated whole blood at 37°C over bovine collagen type I combined with computerized epifluorescence videomicroscopy has allowed the observation, videotaping, and three-dimensional representation of platelet adhesion followed by aggregation in **real time** (Figures 3.3 and 3.4). This methodology is consistent with studies of transverse sections of human coronary atheromatous plaques demonstrating that the 'thrombogenicity' of excised plaques subjected to 64 dynes/cm^2 shear stress in a parallel plate perfusion chamber results from the interaction of platelets with vWf, as well as plaque collagens type I and III.

vWf in plasma becomes rapidly insolubilized from flowing whole blood onto the exposed subendothelium of human arteries, as

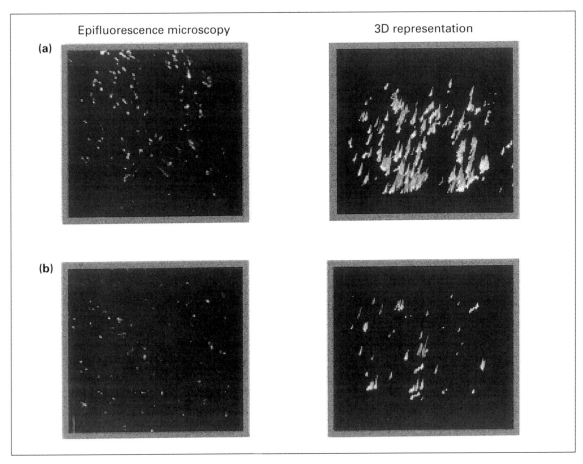

Figure 3.4
Adhesion followed by aggregation in real time. Citrated whole blood perfused over collagen type I/vWf in the presence of (a) c7E3 or (b) integrilin, both at 60 sec.

well as onto collagenous and non-collagenous components of the vessel wall. In vitro experiments indicate that vWf multimers are instantaneously immobilized onto slides coated with bovine collagen type I. Only a small quantity of vWf immobilized onto collagen is sufficient to initiate platelet adhesion via the GPIb component of GPIb-IX-V.[44–47]

In the parallel plate flow chamber, the number of individual platelets per unit area, a measure of platelet adhesion, increases during an initial 15-second exposure to 1500–3000 s^{-1} wall shear rate (60–120 dynes/cm^2 wall shear stress). Platelet aggregates develop at these sites of initial platelet adhesion after 30–60 seconds of flow. In this system, the total number of platelets deposited from normal blood onto collagen-coated slides using various anti-coagulants (0.38% citrate, 10 U/ml unfractionated porcine heparin, 1 U/ml low molecular weight heparin, or 200 U/ml recombinant hirudin) is not significantly different.

Platelet adhesion onto vWf/collagen-coated surfaces can be inhibited by monoclonal antibodies to GPIb, aurin tricarboxylic acid polymers, or recombinant fragments of vWf that bind to GPIb and block the binding of large vWf multimers to the GPIb component of platelet GPIb-IX-V. In the presence of GPIIb-IIIa blockade (e.g. c7E3, or ReoPro; integrilin), which inhibit the binding of fibrinogen and vWf multimers to GPIIb-IIIa, platelet adhesion is minimally inhibited. In contrast, subsequent platelet aggregation is almost eliminated (Figure 3.4). ADP promotes platelet aggregation subsequent to initial adhesion, but blockade of platelet cyclo-oxygenase by aspirin has no significant effect on either platelet adhesion or aggregation under the conditions of most perfusion experiments.

Collagen fibrils activate platelets already adherent to vWf multimers that have been insolubilized onto the collagen. This activation, which is likely to occur via platelet receptors GPIa-IIa and GPVI,[48] potentiates the activation of platelet GPIIb-IIIa complexes necessary for platelet binding of fibrinogen and vWf, and for associated platelet aggregation.

Evaluation of platelet thrombus formation under flowing conditions: the 'In Vitro Platelet Function Analyzer (PF-100)'

A recently developed commercial system[49,50] enables rapid laboratory analysis of platelet thrombus formation on equine collagen type I under high shear conditions. This system requires the presence of vWf multimers, and platelet GPIb-IX-V and GPIIb-IIIa receptors. Citrated whole blood is placed in a small bench-top instrument and aspirated at 37°C and 5000–6000 s^{-1} (~200–240 dynes/cm^2) through the aperture of a nitrocellulose membrane impregnated with collagen type I plus either ADP or epinephrine. Within 2–3 minutes, the membrane aperture normally becomes completely occluded, stopping blood flow as the end point of the test. Occlusion of the aperture under these test conditions requires:

(1) The immobilization of vWf multimers onto membrane-bound collagen;
(2) Platelet adhesion to the immobilized vWf mediated via the GPIb component of platelet GPIb-IX-V complexes;
(3) Platelet activation, at least partially dependent on the generation of cyclo-oxygenase-generated arachidonic acid metabolites; and
(4) Platelet aggregation mediated via the bridging of GPIIb-IIIα complexes on adjacent platelets by vWf multimers from the blood.

Fibrinogen is not required in this process. Development of the occlusive platelet thrombus is impeded in an aspirinized individual if the more 'gentle' agonist, epinephrine, instead of ADP, is on the nitrocellulose membrane along with equine collagen type I.

Although the 'In Vitro Platelet Function Analyzer' cannot provide direct observation and evaluation of platelet adhesion, followed by aggregation in real time, it provides a rapid practical assessment of overall platelet hemostatic function. This test can be modified for use in thrombocytopenic and anemic patients. Furthermore, using the collagen plus epinephrine membrane, it may be capable of detecting inhibition of platelet cyclo-oxygenase by aspirin.

Summary

The bleeding time, although widely used as a rapid, inexpensive test of in vivo platelet adhesion and aggregation, is difficult to perform with consistency and to interpret with confidence. In vitro testing of platelet aggregation using PRP is laborious and subject to ex vivo artifacts. A rapid evaluation of aggregation in whole blood in response to a variety of added agonists can be performed using the combination of an aggregometer and flow cytometer. This latter system is a considerable improvement on the PRP aggregation method long in use.

Viscometry allows the analysis of direct shear-induced platelet aggregation. Parallel-plate perfusion systems provide evaluation (some in real time) of platelet adhesion followed by aggregation. These techniques analyse platelet function under flowing conditions; however, they require sophisticated instruments and laboratory skills. A new commercial instrument designed for clinical pathology laboratories (the 'PFA-100 In Vitro Platelet Function Analyzer')[50] provides a promising technique for the evaluation of overall platelet function under flowing conditions (although not in real time).

Acknowledgments

The development of some of the concepts presented in this chapter was supported by NIH grants HL-32200, NS-23327, HL-18584 and HL-54169, and grants from the Advanced Technology Program of the State of Texas. The figures were prepared by Ms Nancy A. Turner, and the manuscript by Ms Andrea Bethel.

References

1. Buchanan GR and Holtkamp CA. A comparative study of variables affecting bleeding time using two disposable devices. *Am J Clin Path* 1989;**91**:45–51.
2. Mielke CH, Kaneshiro MM, Maher JA, Weiner JM, Rapaport SI. The standardized normal Ivy bleeding time and it prolongation by aspirin. *Blood* 1969;**34**:204–15.
3. Rodgers RPC, Levin J. A critical reappraisal of the bleeding time. *Semin Thromb Hemost* 1990;**16**:1–20.
4. Mielke CH. Aspirin prolongation of the bleeding time: influence of venostasis and direction of incision. *Blood* 1982;**60**:1139–42.
5. Stuart MJ, Miller ML, Davey FR. The post aspirin bleeding time: a screening test for evaluation of haemostatic disorders. *Br J Haematol* 1979;**43**:649–59.
6. Deykin D, Janson P, McMahon L. Ethanol potentiation of aspirin-induced prolongation of the bleeding time. *N Engl J Med* 1982;**306**:852–4.
7. Abildgaard CF, Suzuki Z, Harrison J, Jefcoat K, Zimmerman TS. Serial studies in von Willebrand's disease: variability versus 'variants'. *Blood* 1980;**56**:712–16.
8. Buchanan GR, Holtkamp CA. Prolonged bleeding time in children and young adults with hemophilia. *Pediatrics* 1980;**66**:951–5.
9. Eyster ME, Gordon RA, Ballard JO. The bleeding time is longer than normal in hemophilia. *Blood* 1981;**58**:719–23.
10. Smith PS, Baglini R, Meissner GF. The prolonged bleeding time in hemophilia A: comparison of two measuring techniques and clinical association. *Am J Clin Pathol* 1985;**83**: 211–15.
11. Breederveld K, van Royen EA, ten Cate JE. Severe factor V deficiency with prolonged bleeding time. *Thromb Diath Haemorrh* 1974;**32**:538–48.
12. Ly B, Solum NO, Venerod AM, Dahl O, Hagen I, Orstavik KH. A syndrome of factor VII deficiency and abnormal platelet release reaction. *Scand J Haematol* 1978;**21**:206–14.
13. Brody JI. Prolonged bleeding times with factor IX and XI deficiency and von Willebrand syndromes. *Am J Med Sci* 1975;**269**:19–24.
14. Winter M, Needham J, Barkham P. Factor XI deficiency and platelet defect. *Haemostasis* 1983;**13**:83–8.
15. Edgin RA, Metz EN, Fromkes JJ, Beman FM. Acquired factor X deficiency with associated defects in platelet aggregation. A response to corticosteroid therapy. *Am J Med* 1980; **69**:137–9.
16. Hellem AJ, Borchgrevink CF, Ames DB. The role of red cells in haemostasis: the relation between haematocrit, bleeding time and platelet adhesiveness. *Br J Haematol* 1961; **7**:42–50.
17. Small M, Lowe GDO, Cameron E, Forbes CD. Contribution of the haematocrit to the bleeding time. *Haemostasis* 1983;**13**:379–84.
18. Fernandez F, Goudrable C, Sie P, Ton-That D, Durant JM. Low haematocrit and prolonged bleeding time in ureamic patients. Effect of red cell transfusions. *Br J Haemtol* 1985;**59**: 139–48.
19. Born GVR. Aggregation of blood platelets by adenosine diphosphate and its reversal. *Nature* 1962;**194**:927.
20. Vitoux J-F, Mathieu J-F, Roncato M, Fiessinger J-N, Aich M. Heparin-associated thrombocytopenia. Treatment with low molecular weight heparin. *Thromb Haemost* 1986; **55**:37–9.
21. Amiral J, Bridey F, Dreyfus M, et al. Platelet factor 4 complexed to heparin is the target for antibodies generated in heparin-induced thrombocytopenia. *Thromb Haemost* 1992;**68**: 95–96.
22. Horne KM III. The effect of secreted heparin-binding proteins on heparin binding to platelets. *Thromb Res* 1993;**70**:91–98.
23. Chong BH, Pitney WR, Castaldi PA. Heparin-induced thrombocytopenia: association of thrombotic complications with heparin-dependent IgG antibody that induces thromboxane syn-

thesis and platelet aggregation. *Lancet* 1982;**2**: 1246–9.

24. Chong BH, Fawaz I, Chesterman CN, Berndt MC. Heparin-induced thrombocytopenia: mechanisms of interaction of the heparin-dependent antibody with platelets. *Br J Haematol* 1989;**73**:325–40.

25. Chong BH, Pilgrim RL, Cooley MA, Chesterman CN. Increased expression of platelet IgG Fc receptors in immune heparin-induced thrombocytopenia. *Blood* 1993;**81**:988–93.

26. Horsewood P, Hayward CPM, Warkentin TE, Kelton JG. Investigation of the mechanisms of monoclonal antibody-induced platelet activation. *Blood* 1991;**78**:1019–26.

27. Anderson GP, Anderson CL. Signal transduction by the platelet Fc receptor. *Blood* 1990;**76**:1165–72.

28. Kelton JG, Sheridan D, Brain H, Powers PJ, Turpie AG, Carter CJ. Clinical usefulness of testing for a heparin-dependent platelet aggregating factor in patients with suspected heparin-associated thrombocytopenia. *J Lab Clin Med* 1984;**103**:606–12.

29. Kelton JG, Sheridan D, Santos A, Smith K, Steeves K, Smith C. Heparin-induced thrombocytopenia: laboratory studies. *Blood* 1988;**72**:925–30.

30. Sheridan D, Carter C, Kelton JG. A diagnostic test for heparin-induced thrombocytopenia. *Blood* 1986;**67**:27–30.

31. Chong BH, Burgess J, Ismail F. The clinical usefulness of the platelet aggregating test for the diagnosis of heparin-induced thrombocytopenia. *Thromb Haemost* 1993;**69**:344–353.

32. Coller BS, Lang D, Scudder LE. A rapid and simple platelet function assay to assess GPIIb-IIIa receptor blockade. *Circulation* 1997;**95**:860–7.

33. Chow TW, Turner NA, Chintagumpala M, McPherson PD, Nolasco LH, Rice L, et al. Increased von Willebrand factor binding to platelets in single episode and recurrent types of thrombotic thrombocytopenic purpura. *Am J Hematol* 1998;**57**:293–302.

34. Hechler B, Leon C, Vial C, Vigne P, Frelin C, Cazenave J-P, Gachet C. The P2Y$_1$ receptor necessary for adenosine 5'-diphosphate-induced platelet aggregation. *Blood* 1998;**92**:152–9.

35. Sugimoto M, Ricca G, Hrinda ME, Schreiber AB, Searfoss GH, Bottini E, Ruggeri ZM. Functional modulation of the isolated glycoprotein Ib-binding domain of von Willebrand factor expressed in *Escherichia coli*. *Biochem* 1991;**30**:5202–9.

36. MacCallum RN, O'Bannon W, Hellums JD, Alfrey CP, Lynch EC. Viscometric instruments for studies on red blood cell damage. In: Gabelnick HL, Litt M (eds) *Rheology of Biological Systems* (Springfield, Charles C. Thomas, 1973) 70.

37. Belval T, Hellums JD, Solis RT. The kinetics of platelet aggregation induced by fluid-shearing stress. *Microvas Res* 1984;**28**:279–88.

38. Giorgio TD, Hellums JD. A cone-and-plate viscometer for the continuous measurement of blood platelet activation. *Biorheology* 1988;**25**:605–24.

39. Fukuyama M, Sakai K, Itagaki I, Kawano K, Murata M, Kawai Y, et al. Continuous measurement of shear-induced platelet aggregation. *Thromb Res* 1989;**54**:253–60.

40. Hellums JD. 1993 Whitaker lecture: Biorheology in thrombosis research. *Ann Biomed Eng* 1994;**22**:445–55.

41. Sutera SP, Nowak MD, Joist JH, Zeffren DI, Bauman JE. A programmable, computer controlled cone-plate viscometer for the application of pulsatile shear stress to platelet suspensions. *Biorheology* 1988;**25**:449–59.

42. Chow TW, Hellums JD, Moake JL, Kroll MH. Shear stress-induced von Willebrand factor binding to platelet glycoprotein Ib initiates calcium influx associated with aggregation. *Blood* 1992;**80**:113–20.

43. Goto S, Salomon DR, Ikeda Y, Ruggeri ZM. Characterization of the unique mechanisms mediating the shear-dependent binding of soluble von Willebrand factor to platelets. *J Biol Chem* 1995;**270**:23352–61.

44. Baruch D, Denis C, Marteaux C, Schoevaert D, Coulombel L, Meyer D. Role of von Willebrand factor associated with extracellular matrices in platelet adhesion. *Blood* 1991;**77**:519–27.

45. Olson JD, Zaleski A, Hermann D, Flood PA. Adhesion of platelets to purified solid-phase von Willebrand factor: Effects of wall shear rate, ADP, thrombin, and ristocetin. *J Lab Clin Med* 1989;**114**:6–18.

46. Badimon L, Badimon JJ, Rand J, Turitto VT, Fuster V. Platelet deposition on von Willebrand factor-deficient vessels. Extra-corporeal perfusion studies in swine with von Willebrand's disease using native and heparinized blood. *J Lab Clin Med* 1987;**11**:634–47.

47. Bolhuis PA, Sakariassen KS, Sander HJ, Bouma BN, Sixma JJ. Binding of factor VIII-von Willebrand factor to human arterial subendothelium precedes increased platelet spreading. *J Lab Clin Med* 1981;**97**:568–76.

48. Verbley MW, Morton LF, Knight CG, de Groot PG, Barnes MJ, Sixma JJ. Simple collagen-like peptides support platelet adhesion under static but not under flow condition: interaction via α2β1 and von Willebrand factor with specific sequences in native collagen is a requirement to resist shear forces. *Blood* 1998;**91**:3808–16.

49. Kundu SK, Heilmann EJ, Sio R, Garcia C, Ostgaard RA. Characterization of an in vitro platelet function analyzer, PFA-100. *Clin Appl Thromb Hemost* 1996;**2**:241–9.

50. Dietrich GV, Schueck R, Menges T, Kiesenbauer NP, Fruehauf A-C, Marquardt I. Comparison of four methods for the determination of platelet function in whole blood in cardiac surgery. *Thromb Res* 1998;**89**:295–301.

4

Inherited and acquired disorders of platelet function
Weei-Chin Lin, Thomas L Ortel and Scott D Berkowitz

Introduction

Platelets are essential for normal hemostasis. Their function depends not only on mechanical plugging but also on activation and signal amplification. In order to carry out their function in hemostasis, platelets must perform a sequence of actions namely, adhesion, activation, secretion, and aggregation. (The readers are referred to Chapter 2 for the detailed description of these actions.) These processes will be reviewed only briefly here. The emphasis of this chapter is platelet disorders according to their qualitative and quantitative aspects, which are then subclassified to congenital and acquired disorders.

Adhesion

Wherever a subendothelial matrix is exposed owing to endothelial damage, platelets respond by adhering to these surfaces. Adhesion is dependent on the physical interaction between platelets, von Willebrand factor (vWF), and collagen. The receptor for vWF on platelets is the glycoprotein Ib-IX-V (GPIb-IX-V) complex.[1] The collagen receptor function is carried out by several different glycoproteins on platelets, including GP Ia-IIa complex, GPIV, GPIIb, and GPVI.

Activation and secretion

After platelets adhere to exposed subendothelial surface, they are activated and able to secrete mediators such as adenosine phosphate (ADP), serotonin and thromboxane A_2 (TXA$_2$), which further attract and activate more platelets. This secretion enables platelets to amplify the response and form an effective thrombus. To prevent activation in the unstimulated situation, pre-formed agonists or mediators are secluded within granules in platelets. Dense granules contain serotonin and ADP, and α-granules contain fibrinogen and thrombospondin.

Platelet activation is a very complex process and involves fundamental cellular signal transduction.[2] Many extracellular stimuli can activate platelets including thrombin, plasmin, platelet-activating factor, collagen, catecholamines, ADP, vWF, prostaglandin endoperoxidases and TXA$_2$. These activators bind to specific receptors on the surface of platelets and activate platelets. Most of these receptors are G protein-coupled, that is, they transduce the signal into the cells through a family of guanosine triphosphate-(GTP)-binding regulatory proteins (G proteins). The G proteins can activate two enzymes, phospholipase C (PLC) and adenylyl cyclase, which in turn generate second messengers including inositol 1,4,5-triphosphate (IP$_3$), *sn*-1,2-diacylglycerol (DAG) and cyclic adenosine monophosphate (cAMP). These secondary messengers then induce other cellular responses and activate the cells. IP$_3$ releases calcium and activates calcium-dependent enzymes including phospholipase A_2 (PLA$_2$). DAG activates protein kinase C, and cAMP can activate cAMP-dependent protein kinases. PLA$_2$ can further release arachidonic acid (AA) from membrane phospholipids. AA is metabolized by cyclo-oxygenase and lipoxygenase to form a group of eicosanoids, including prostaglandin G_2 (PGG$_2$), prostaglandin H_2 (PGH$_2$) and TXA$_2$, which are potent platelet agonists, and in turn amplify the cycle of activation. With the action of cyclo-oxygenase, AA forms PGG$_2$ which is metabolized by peroxidase to form PGH$_2$. PGH$_2$ is then converted to TXA$_2$ by TXA$_2$ synthetase. Any defect that occurs in the process of activation can, potentially, lead to a clinical platelet disorder, especially if involving AA and prostaglandin metabolism.

Aggregation

When platelets are activated, their membrane protein complex glycoprotein (GP) IIb-IIIa (GPIIb-IIIa) undergoes confirmational change and becomes able to bind its ligand, fibrinogen. Platelets also spread on subendothelium and attain closer proximity to each other.[3] Then platelets are bridged by fibrinogen through this ligand–receptor interaction and become aggregated. The activated platelets can secrete substances such as ADP and TXA$_2$, which can recruit more platelets to form a plug and establish primary hemostasis. The primary plug is then strengthened and modified by secondary and tertiary hemostasis processes, including fibrin deposition and cross-linking through the coagulation system. A defect in GPIIb-IIIa complex causes Glanzmann's thrombasthenia and leads to abnormality in platelet aggregation.

Laboratory diagnosis

Patients with different underlying platelet disorders usually present with similar bleeding signs and symptoms. Laboratory studies play a very important role in defining the actual abnormality in the differential diagnosis. The basic screening tests for platelet disorders include platelet count, blood smear, and bleeding time. A prolonged bleeding time despite a normal platelet count suggests a qualitative platelet disorder if von Willebrand disease has been excluded. A decreased platelet count indicates a quantitative defect, although mild to moderate thrombocytopenia is common in some qualitative disorders such as Bernard-Soulier syndrome and gray platelet syndrome. Since the mid 1960s, platelet aggregation study has been the mainstay of the tests for classifying the qualitative platelet disorders. This test measures, either in platelet-rich plasma or whole blood, the degree of platelet aggregation in response to various agonists. Each disorder has a characteristic pattern of platelet aggregation curves (Figure 4.1). Most disorders of platelet function are qualitative but a few affect the numbers of platelets, that is they are quantitative.

Qualitative platelet disorders

Congenital disorders of platelet function are listed in Table 4.1.

Congenital disorders of platelet adhesion

Bernard-Soulier syndrome

The molecular defect of Bernard-Soulier syndrome lies in GP Ib-IX-V complex. GPIb-IX-V complex comprises four transmembrane subunits: GPIbα, GPIbβ, GPIX, and GPV. These four polypeptides arise from four distinct genes residing in different regions of the genome. Together, they form a complex on the surface

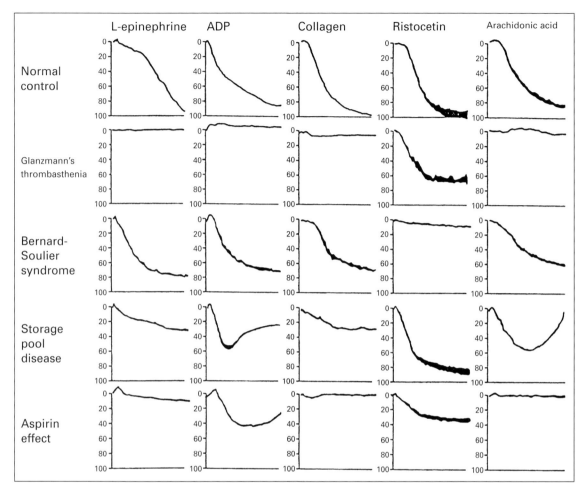

Figure 4.1
Platelet aggregation studies for various diseases.
Source: adapted from Hathaway WE, Goodnight SH Jr, p. 99.

of platelets, bind vWF and mediate adhesion to the blood vessel wall. Beside mechanical adhesion, the binding of vWF to the GPIb-IX-V complex also transduces signals inside the cells and facilitates the ability of thrombin to activate platelets. The GPIb-IX-V complex also constitutes the major attachment site between plasma membrane and cytoskeleton through actin-binding protein.[5]

The Bernard-Soulier syndrome, first described in 1948,[6] is a very rare congenital platelet disorder. There are only about 100 cases reported in literature so far. The condition is characterized by a prolonged bleeding time, thrombocytopenia and very large but fragile platelets. These patients present with frequent mucosal or cutaneous bleeding, usually since childhood. The degree of throm-

Disorders		Defect(s)	Inheritance
Disorders of platelet adhesion	Bernard-Soulier syndrome	GPIb-IX	AR
	Pseudo-von Willebrand disease	Intrinsic GPIb defect; increased binding of vWF	AD
	Deficiencies of platelet collagen receptor	GPIa-IIa	
Disorders of platelet aggregation	Glanzmann's thromboasthenia	GPIIb-IIIa	AR
Defects in platelet activation/ secretion	Cyclo-oxygenase deficiency	Cyclo-oxygenase	AR
	Thromboxane synthetase deficiency	Thromboxane synthetase	
	Impaired release of AA		
	Impaired response to thromboxane A_2		
	Defects in phosphotidylinositol metabolism		
	Defects in calcium mobilization		
Storage pool defects	α-Granule deficiency (α-storage pool deficiency, gray platelet syndrome)	α-Granule	AR
	Dense-granule deficiency (δ-storage pool deficiency)	Dense-granule	AD
	Combined α, δ storage pool deficiency	α- and dense-granules	AD
Disorders of platelet procoagulant activity	Scott syndrome	? Phosphatidylserine translocase	AR

AR: autosomal recessive, AD: autosomal dominant; AA: arachidonic acid

Table 4.1
Congenital platelet disorders.

bocytopenia is quite variable, and may fluctuate over time even on the same patient. In a Baumgartner chamber in which blood is perfused through subendothelium at various rates, Bernard-Soulier platelets fail to adhere at high shear rates, but adhesion is normal at low shear rates.[7] The platelet adhesion at high shear rates has been shown to depend on vWF interaction. Platelet aggregation response to ristocetin is absent, but the response to other agonists, such as ADP and collagen is normal (see Figure 4.1). The GPIb-IX-V complex binds to intracellular cytoskeleton and presumably stabilized plasma membrane. The interaction between GPIb and the cytoskeleton is not only important for membrane stability but also plays a role in platelet reshaping upon activation. This is because the phosphorylation of cytoplasmic region of GP Ibβ can regulate actin polymerization. The GPIb-IX-V complex also binds to thrombin, and the Bernard-Soulier platelets have a decreased response to thrombin.

The genetic defects in Bernard-Soulier syndrome are heterogeneous. Lopez and co-workers have shown that surface expression of GPIbα, GPIbβ and GPIX requires the presence of all three components.[8] Mutations of any of these three genes can, theoretically, lead to Bernard-Soulier syndrome. In most of the cases reported, Bernard-Soulier syndrome is transmitted in autosomal recessive pattern, and among these families consanguinity is common. Autosomal dominant inheritance has been reported in only one family.[9]

Bernard-Soulier syndrome was often misdiagnosed as idiopathic thrombocytopenic purpura (ITP) owing to a prolonged bleeding time and thrombocytopenia. Definitive diagnosis requires a platelet aggregation study: the Bernard-Soulier syndrome is characterized by an isolated defect in ristocetin-induced agglutination (see Figure 4.1). Patients with Bernard-Soulier syndrome can be treated with platelet transfusion in case of major bleeding, however alloimmunization can occur, so transfusion should be minimized. Desmopressin (1-desamino-8-D-arginine vasopressin, DDAVP) is able to induce the release of vWF from vascular endothelial storage sites, and is used for patients with von Willebrand disease. DDAVP may shorten the bleeding time of some, but not all, patients with Bernard-Soulier syndrome.[1]

Pseudo-von Willebrand disease

When mutation occurs in the GPIb gene and the mutation is located near the vWF binding domain, it may cause the platelets to have an abnormally high affinity to vWF and deplete the functional high-molecular-weight vWF multimers from plasma. This condition is termed pseudo-von Willebrand disease, or a platelet-type von Willebrand disease. These patients have clinical symptoms similar to patients with von Willebrand disease including mucocutaneous hemorrhage, decreased vWF multimers and intermittent thrombocytopenia. Nevertheless, platelet morphology is normal. The genetic defect is a single base mutation (G to T) within the vWF binding domain of GPIbα gene,[10] this causes a codon change from glycine to valine at position 233. It is inherited as an autosomal dominant condition. The thrombocytopenia is probably caused by an increased sensitivity of platelet aggregation, as demonstrated by a ristocetin-induced platelet aggregation assay. Thus DDAVP, which induces the release of vWF, or the transfusion of cryoprecipitate, that is rich in vWF, can aggravate the thrombocytopenia.

Deficiencies of platelet collagen receptor

The interaction between vWF and GPIb-IX-V is important for platelet adhesion at a high shear rate. Under low-shear conditions, other factors such as collagen, fibronectin and laminin are more important for initial platelet adhesion. Mutations in these receptors also lead to bleeding diathesis. Glycoprotein Ia-IIa (GPIa-IIa, VLA-2 receptor) is an integrin receptor and has been shown to bind collagen.[11] A monoclonal antibody against GPIa-IIa can inhibit collagen-induced platelet aggregation.[12] Moreover, a congenital GPIa-IIa deficiency has been reported.[13] The patients had a prolonged bleeding time and easy bruisability and, although their platelets were normal in number, they contained only 20% of GPIa and adhered poorly to collagen. The other two glycoproteins that can bind collagen are GPIV and GPVI. Deficiency in these two glycoproteins leads to very mild bleeding disorder.[14,15]

Congenital disorders of platelet aggregation

Glanzmann's thrombasthenia

Glanzmann's thrombasthenia is a congenital disorder with autosomal recessive inheritance.[16] It is rare and usually associated with consanguity. The molecular defect can be in either GPIIb or GPIIIa and results in absence of a functional GPIIb-IIIa receptor. GPIIb-IIIa is activated by agonists (e.g. collagen, thrombin, ADP, epinephrine (adrenaline) and serotonin), and activated GPIIb-IIIa is the receptor for RGD-containing molecules such as fibrinogen and fibronectin, and mediates platelet aggregation.

Patients with Glanzmann's thrombasthenia have normal platelet morphology and count. The ristocetin-induced platelet agglutination is normal, but platelets fail to aggregate in response to all other agonists (see Figure 4.1). Glanzmann's thrombasthenic platelets are able to adhere to the subendothelial matrix, but unable to spread on the matrix and form microthrombi. These patients have a bleeding diathesis present since early childhood.

The molecular genetics of Glanzmann's thrombasthenia have been well worked out. Mutations in either GPIIb or GPIIIa gene will affect the surface expression of the whole complex. Caen has classified Glanzmann's thrombasthenia into three types.[17] Type I Glanzmann's thrombasthenia has undetectable level of surface GPIIb-IIIa, whereas type II patients have some but markedly diminished levels (10–20%) of surface GPIIb-IIIa and have less severe clinical manifestations than type I. The third class, called Glanzmann's thrombasthenia variants, have qualitative rather than quantitative defects of the GPIIb-IIIa complex. The mutations in Glanzmann's thrombasthenia variants do not significantly affect the expression of protein but affect the function, such as binding RGD peptides or fibrinogen. Several different Glanzmann's thrombasthenia variants have been reported. Their platelets fail to aggregate to either ADP, collagen, epinephrine or thrombin, but have 50–100% of GPIIb-IIIa level. Ginsberg described a variant called the Cam variant,[18] which has a point mutation in RGD binding site of GPIIIa. Chen has reported a variant with mutation in the cytoplasmic domain of GPIIIa, which uncoupled the signal transduction by GPIIb-IIIa.[19]

The management of bleeding episodes in patients with Glanzmann's thrombasthenia may include transfusion of normal platelets. However, to minimize the development of alloantibodies, one should avoid unnecessary transfusion and use single-donor or HLA-matched platelets if possible.

Congenital defects in platelet activation/secretion

As mentioned in the previous section, the platelet activation involves a cascade of signal transduction including G protein-coupled receptors, activation of phospholipases, mobilization of arachidonic acid and formation of thromboxane. Any defect along these pathways can, potentially, lead to platelet dysfunction. Specifically, platelets from patients with familial platelet cyclo-oxygenase deficiency have impaired response to ADP, epinephrine, collagen and arachidonic acid, but normal response to prostaglandins, which are downstream to the action of cyclo-oxygenase in the activation cascade.[20] Deficiency in thromboxane synthetase has also been reported,[21,22] the platelet aggregation is normal to TXA_2, but impaired to prostaglandins.

Congenital storage pool defects

These disorders are heterogeneous and storage pool disorders involve abnormalities with α and δ granules.

α-Granule deficiency (α-storage pool deficiency, gray platelet syndrome)

The gray platelet syndrome was first described in 1971 by Raccuglia.[23] It gained the name due to platelet's gray appearance on Romanowsky stains, which is a result of the absence of normal α-granules in cytoplasm. These patients have a bleeding tendency, mild to moderate thrombocytopenia and giant platelets. α-Granules contain vWF, platelet factor 4, β-thromboglobulin, platelet-derived growth factor (PDGF), thrombospondin, fibrinogen, albumin and factor V. The defect resides in the packaging of these proteins into the α-granules. The plasma membrane of α-granule is present and plasma levels of platelet factor 4 and β-thromboglobulin are increased owing to an inability

of storage. The patients have various degrees of bleeding diathesis, nor are the aggregation abnormalities consistent. The bone marrow has increased reticulin fibers, especially around megakaryocytes, probably because of local release of PDGF by the megakaryocytes. This disorder is inherited in an autosomal pattern, although the molecular defect has not yet been identified. These patients should avoid antiplatelet agents; any hemorrhage is treated with platelet transfusion.

Dense-granule deficiency (δ-storage pool deficiency)

Normally, the dense granules (δ granules) contain ADP, ATP, calcium, serotonin and pyrophosphate, which are secreted upon platelet activation. In δ-storage pool disease, however, the δ-granules are absent while the α-granules are normal. Platelets with δ-storage pool disease thus are unable to secrete the δ-granule contents, of which ADP and serotonin are the most important in response to activation. In platelet aggregation studies, the primary wave may be normal but the secondary wave is absent owing to lack of ADP secretion (see Figure 4.1). The bleeding time is prolonged, but platelet quantity and morphology are usually normal in δ-storage pool disease; patients usually have mild mucocutaneous bleeding.

δ-Storage pool disease is transmitted as autosomal dominant inheritance. It can occur alone as a congenital disorder or be associated with other congenital syndromes, such as Hermansky-Pudlak syndrome,[24] Chediak-Higashi syndrome, *t*hrombocytopenia and *a*bsent *r*adii syndrome (TAR), and Wiskott-Aldrich syndrome.[25] The molecular defect of δ-storage pool disease has not yet been identified. Management is similar to that for gray platelet syndrome, in other words avoiding antiplatelet agents and giving platelet transfusion when needed.

Combined α, δ storage pool deficiency
Patients may have a deficiency of both α- and δ-granules with similar bleeding diathesis.

Disorders of platelet procoagulant activity
The platelet membrane surface is a major site for the hemostatic reaction. During the formation of a fibrin plug, platelets provide a surface for the assembly of several of the enzyme complexes that leads to the generation of thrombin. The plasma membrane of activated platelets is able to bind factor VIIIa through its phospholipid moiety. It then binds factor IXa and X, and also activates factor X (thus called ten*ase* activity). Factor Xa then binds prothrombin and factor Va, and forms the prothrombinase complex, which in turn activates prothrombin to thrombin. The detailed molecular mechanism of this property of platelets, that is, platelet procoagulant activity (previously termed platelet factor 3), has not yet been well defined. It may involve the reorientation and exposure of anionic phospholipid in platelet membrane.

Isolated deficiency of platelet procoagulant activity is extremely rare. Several isolated cases were reported but a unique one has been well documented as the Scott syndrome.[26] This patient presented with prolonged bleeding after surgery, dental extraction, and a spontaneous retroperitoneal hematoma, but had no excessive bleeding from superficial cuts or excessive bruising. Most of the laboratory studies were normal, including bleeding time, prothrombin and partial thromboplastin times, platelet aggregation and secretion studies. However, the patient's platelets were unable to express procoagulant activity. Consistent with a primary platelet defect, excessive postoperative bleeding can be prevented by prophylactic platelet transfusion. It was recently proposed that the Scott syndrome is transmitted as an autosomal recessive trait with the deletion or mutation of a putative outward phosphatidylserine translocase.[27]

Acquired systemic disorders causing platelet dysfunction (Table 4.2)

Uremia
Uremia can affect multiple platelet functions; namely, adhesion, aggregation, together with reactions on the platelet membrane.

Adhesion Platelets of uremic patients have been shown to be defective in adhering to glass beads and subendothelial structures.[28] The vWF antigen level in plasma is normal or increased in these patients. There may be a change in multimer distribution of vWF but this is not consistent. High plasma levels of vWF antigen are reported and may be associated with low ristocetin cofactor activity.[29] The actual cause is not known for certain, but increased vWF levels seem to compensate for the qualitative defect of vWF-platelet interaction.

Activation and secretion Platelets of the uremic patient contain low levels of ADP, serotonin, membrane ATPase and α-granules.[30] Uremic platelets also are defective in their ability to mobilize arachidonic acid in response to thrombin. These platelet storage pool defects may also be the result of platelet activation by dialysis membrane, which leads to depletion of the storage pool.

Aggregation The defects in platelet aggregation of uremic patients are at most mild, if present. In fact, the thrombin- and ristocetin-induced platelet aggregation are normal in most patients.

Platelet membrane The platelet membrane surface is actively involved in the coagulation process, and is a major site for the hemostatic reaction. Platelets provide proximity to coagulation factors and also phospholipid, and, as

Systemic disorders	Uremia
	Cardiopulmonary bypass
	Antiplatelet antibodies
	Chronic liver disease
	Miscellaneous (ARDS, Bartter syndrome, non-thrombocytopenic purpura with eosinophilia)
Hematologic disorders	Chronic myeloproliferative disorders
	Acute leukemias and myelodysplastic syndromes
	Dysproteinemias
	Acquired Bernard-Soulier syndrome and thrombasthenia
Drugs	*See Table 4.3*

Table 4.2
Acquired platelet disorders.

such, 'procoagulant activity'. This platelet procoagulant activity has been shown to be decreased in uremia.[31] How this activity is impaired is still not clear.

Besides causing platelet dysfunction, uremia can affect the vascular endothelium. The vascular endothelial cells normally release certain platelet inhibitory substances and prevent unwanted platelet aggregation. These platelet inhibitory substances include prostacyclin (PGI_2) and nitric oxide, the latter of which has been identified as endothelium-derived relaxing factor (EDRF). The uremic vascular endothelium releases excess PGI_2 and nitric oxide.[32] The anemia of chronic renal failure also contributes to the bleeding diathesis. Correction of the anemia in uremia with recombinant erythropoietin or red cell transfusion can improve the bleeding disorder.

The treatment for uremic bleeding diathesis includes: (a) dialysis; (b) correction of anemia; (c) DDAVP; (d) cryoprecipitate and (e) estrogens. The target hematocrit for correction of

the bleeding times has been determined to be between 27 and 32%,[33] which requires about 150–300 units/kg/week erythropoietin. With the implementation of regular dialysis and erythropoietin injections, most bleeding complications of uremia can be prevented. In the case of acute bleeding, one can administer DDAVP and/or cryoprecipitate. Most uremic patients will respond initially to DDAVP, which induces the release of functional multimeric forms of vWF from the storage pool in the vascular endothelium. Nevertheless, tachyphylaxis, that is acute tolerance, may occur—even after two or three doses. DDAVP is given at 0.3–0.4 µg/kg (i.v. or s.c.) or 2–3 µg/kg by intranasal application with the onset of effect within 1 hour and duration of 4–8 hours. Janson first reported the effectiveness of cryoprecipitate to correct bleeding time in uremic patients,[34] but subsequent studies have indicated the variability in its response and that more than one-half of patients do not respond. Finally, estrogens also have an effect on the hemostatic defect of uremia, especially for bleeding of gastrointestinal telangiectasias. The effect is delayed in onset (days), but persists for 2 weeks. Conjugated estrogen is given at 0.6 mg/kg i.v. daily for 4–5 days. Alternatively, Premarin® can be given p.o. at 50 mg daily.

Cardiopulmonary bypass

Cardiopulmonary bypass can lead to a reduction of plasma level of coagulation factors, increased fibrinolysis and platelet dysfunction. A fall in the platelet count and platelet dysfunction can be seen in most patients undergoing cardiopulmonary bypass with either a bubble or a membrane oxygenator. Patients may also have a prolonged bleeding time, reduced platelet aggregation to several agonists, and decreased storage pools of α- and/or dense-granules. Fortunately, these abnormalities resolve several hours after completion of cardiopulmonary bypass and excessive bleeding occurs only in 5% of patients. The excessive bleeding is detected primarily as an increased blood loss via the chest tube.

Thrombocytopenia induced by cardiopulmonary bypass is caused by a combination of hemodilution, adherence of platelets to the bypass circuit, and sequestration of damaged platelets by the liver. It typically takes a few days for the platelet count to return to normal. The platelet defect is the result of the effects of platelet activation and fragmentation within the extracorporeal circuit. These effects are the consequences of bypass priming solutions, adhesion and aggregation of platelets to fibrinogen from the plasma adsorbed onto the circuit, hypothermia, blood-conservation devices, trace concentration of circulating thrombin and ADP, complement activation, blood–air interface, and mechanical trauma and shear stress, including cardiotomy suction.

Prophylactic platelet transfusions are not indicated routinely for cardiopulmonary bypass surgery. However, patients with excessive bleeding and a prolonged bleeding time in the postoperative period usually benefit from platelet transfusions. In a randomized study, DDAVP has been shown to decrease the amount of postoperative blood loss in patients undergoing bypass for complex cardiovascular surgery.[34] However, trials in uncomplicated cardiac surgery have not shown a beneficial effect using DDAVP.[36–38]

Antiplatelet antibodies

A normal platelet stores IgG in the α-granules. Immunoglobulin molecules can be found on platelet surface from patients with idiopathic thrombocytopenic purpura (ITP), systemic lupus erythematosus and platelet alloimmunization. These antiplatelet antibodies can interfere various membrane receptors and platelet aggregation. They can also induce platelet secretion, deplete granules and lead to acquired storage pool deficiency. Isolated qualitative platelet defect from these antibodies usually does not cause major bleeding problems, unless concomitantly associated with a quantitative platelet disorder.

Chronic liver disease

The bleeding from hepatic failure is multifactorial, and includes anatomic derangement (such as varices), coagulopathy, excessive fibrinolysis, thrombocytopenia and qualitative platelet dysfunction. Thrombocytopenia usually is the result of hypersplenism. Several qualitative platelet disorders are reported but there is no consistent or uniform pattern. These defects include abnormal arachidonic acid metabolism, reduced ATP and serotonin release, inhibition of platelet aggregation, presence of platelet-associated immunoglobulin owing to polyclonal hypergammaglobulinemia, and acquired dysfibrinogenemia, which interferes platelet aggregation. Treatment is usually not very effective. Besides blood component replacement, DDAVP is reported to be helpful in some patients.[39]

Miscellaneous

Bartter syndrome, a disorder of primary renal potassium-wasting and hypokalemic alkalosis can be associated with a prolonged bleeding time and decreased platelet aggregation and secretion in response to epinephrine or ADP.[40] Mild prolongation of the bleeding time and platelet dysfunction are also seen in patients with adult respiratory distress syndrome (ARDS) and non-thrombocytopenic purpura with eosinophilia.

Acquired hematological disorders causing platelet dysfunction

Chronic myeloproliferative disorders and myelodysplastic syndrome

The bone marrow in myelodysplasia or myeloproliferative disorders may release abnormal platelets into the peripheral circulation, probably as a result of dysmegakaryocytopoiesis. Various abnormalities have been noted but a storage pool defect is the most common. Both α- and dense-granule deficiency have been reported. The identification of circulating activated platelets suggests a process of degranulation. In fact, PDGF and transforming growth factor-β, two mitogens secreted from α granules of activated platelets, are implicated in stimulating fibroblast proliferation and, subsequently, causing myelofibrosis in myeloproliferative disorders.[41] The platelet GPIIb-IIIa receptors of patients with myelodysplastic and myeloproliferative disorders may be decreased in number, or be defective in function. Platelet procoagulant activity is defective in some patients with myeloproliferative disorders. Other defects include reduced α-adrenergic receptors, which in theory may lead to bleeding, and reduced PGD_2 receptors or increased Fc receptors, which theoretically could increase the thrombotic tendency; however, clinical correlation has not yet been established. Very recently, the platelets from patients with polycythemia vera and idiopathic myelofibrosis were found to have reduced expression of the thrombopoietin receptor Mpl,[42] although this defect has not been seen in patients with other forms of myeloproliferative disorders or secondary erythrocytosis.

The arachidonic acid metabolism is abnormal in these patients. The defect is mainly a decrease of lipoxygenase activity. Acquired vWD is also reported in patients with myeloproliferative disorders. The laboratory manifestation is usually similar to type II, that is, decreased functional vWF. It has been postulated that abnormal platelets may sequester the high molecular weight form of vWF, although direct evidence is not yet available.

The treatment for this group of patients depends on the clinical manifestation. In general, unless patients have thrombotic symptoms, antiplatelet agents or reduction of platelet count may not be necessary. Recently, anagrelide (Agrylin) has been shown to be very effective in reducing thrombotic events and platelet count in this group of patients.[43]

Dysproteinemias

The monoclonal protein in patients with myeloma, Waldenstrom's macroglobulinemia, or benign monoclonal gammopathy can inhibit all platelet functions, especially when the concentration of plasma paraprotein is high. When clinically significant platelet dysfunction occurs in patients with a high level of myeloma protein, hyperviscosity syndrome may occur and plasmapheresis should be initiated as an emergency to reduce the concentration of myeloma protein. Chemotherapy should also be considered for a more longlasting control.

Agents		Mechanism
β-Lactam antibiotics	Penicillin	Platelet membrane binding and alteration of agonist receptors
	Cephalosporins	
Non-steroidal anti-inflammatory drugs (NSAIDS)	Ibuprofen	Prostaglandin synthesis inhibition
	Indomethacin	
Acetylsalicylic acid (Aspirin)		Cyclo-oxygenase inhibitor
Dipyridamole (Persantine)		Phosphodiesterase inhibitor
Ticlopidine/Clopidogrel		ADP inhibitor
ReoPro		monoclonal antibody against GP IIb/IIIa receptor
Peptide/Peptidomimetic IIb/IIIa blockers		GPIIb/IIIa receptor antagonist
Anticoagulant drugs	Heparin	Membrane binding; inhibit thrombin generation and action
Fibrinolytic agents	Streptokinase	Membrane binding; decrease GPIb
	Urokinase	
	t-PA	
Cardiovascular drugs	Quinidine	Decrease platelet aggregation and secretion
	Calcium-channel blockers	
	Propranolol	
	Nitroprusside	
	Nitroglycerin	
Volume expanders	Dextran	Inhibit platelet aggregation and procoagulant activity
	Hydroxyethyl starch	
Chemotherapeutic drugs	Mithramycin	Inhibit platelet aggregation
	Daunorubicin	
	BCNU	
Psychotropic or anesthetic drugs	Tricyclic antidepressants	Inhibit platelet aggregation
	Phenothiazines	
	Halothane	
Foods and food additives	Ethanol	Inhibit platelet adhesion
	Chinese black-tree fungus	Inhibit arachidonic acid metabolism
	Onion extract	Inhibit fibrinogen binding
	Ajoene (garlic component)	Decrease arachidonic acid
	eicosapentaenoic acid (in fish oils)	Decrease platelet thromboxane production
	Spices (clove, cumin)	

Table 4.3
Drugs affecting platelet function.

Disorder	Inheritance	Platelet function tests	Other findings
I. Macrothrombocytes			
Bernard-Soulier syndrome	AR	↓ agg to ristocetin BT markedly increased	Decreased membrane GPIb-IX (V)
Montreal platelet syndrome	AD	↓ agg to thrombin; normal agg to ristocetin, ADP, collagen	Normal to reduced GPIb
May-Hegglin anomaly	AD	Normal	Dohle bodies in leukocytes
Epstein's syndrome Alport's syndrome	AD	Abnormal agg to ADP, collagen	Renal disease, nerve deafness
(Fechtner variant)		Normal	Leukocyte inclusions
(Sebastian variant)		Normal	Leukocyte inclusions; no associated defect
Gray platelet syndrome	Autosomal	Abnormal agg to ADP, collagen thrombin	↓ α-granules; pale-staining platelets and agranular megakaryocytes
Genetic thrombocytopenia (Najean-Lecompte)	AD	Normal	Normal microscopy and platelet survival
II. Normothrombocytes			
Thrombocytopenia with absent radius (TAR)	AR	↓ agg to L-epi and collagen	↓ megakaryocytes; absent radii, normal thumbs; presentation at birth

Table 4.4
Congenital thrombocytopenias

Disorder	Inheritance	Platelet function tests	Other findings
Chediak-Higashi syndrome	AR	↓ agg to L-epi and collagen	Oculocutaneous albinism, recurrent infections, large abnormal granules in leukocytes, macrophages ↓ platelet survival
Hereditary intrinsic platelet defect (Murphy)	AD	Normal	
Familial platelet disorder (Dowton)	AD	Abnormal agg to L-epi and collagen	Hematologic neoplasms; normal GPs
Pseudo-von Willebrand disease	AD	↓ agg to ristocetin	↓ plt binding of vWf; plt agg with normal plasma; abnormality of GPIb
III. Microthrombocytes			
Wiskott-Aldrich syndrome	X-linked	Abnormal agg to ADP, collagen thrombin	↓ plt survival; eczema, recurrent infections, immune deficiency due to failure of lymphocytes maturation (decreased CD43)

*agg, agglutination; plt, platelet; L-epi, L-epinephrine
Source: adapted from Hathaway WE, Goodnight SH Jr,[4] pp. 79, 80, with permission.

Table 4.4
(continued)

Acquired Bernard-Soulier syndrome and thrombasthenia

If patients develop autoantibodies against the GPIb-IX complex, they can develop a bleeding disorder similar to Bernard-Soulier syndrome known as acquired Bernard-Soulier syndrome. This syndrome has been reported in patients with chronic ITP,[44] in a patient taking procainamide[45] and in a patient with juvenile myelodysplastic syndrome.[46]

The autoantibodies against GPIIb-IIIa can also disturb the function of GPIIb-IIIa function and lead to an acquired form of thrombasthenia.[47] In fact, the majority of autoepitopes implicated in ITP are associated with GPIIb-IIIa complex. Alloantibodies against GPIIb-IIIa can cause post-transfusional purpura (PTP) or neonatal alloimmune thrombocytopenia. Patients with post-transfusional purpura present with an acute onset of severe thrombocytopenia and high titer of platelet-specific alloantibodies about 1 week after receiving a blood transfusion. PI^{A1} (Zw^a) is the alloantigen most frequently associated with PTP. Bak are other alloantigens implicated in PTP. PI^{A1} is associated with GPIIIa and the Bak system is associated with GPIIb. Neonatal alloimmune thrombocytopenia is caused by maternal IgG alloantibodies, which cross the placenta and are directed against paternal-derived alloantigens on neonatal platelets. Most common alloantigens associated with neonatal alloimmune thrombocytopenia are PI^{A1} and Br^a (Zav^a).

Drugs

A variety of drugs can affect platelet function (see Table 4.3), and probably represent the most common cause of platelet dysfunction. The major classes are anti-inflammatory agents, antibiotics and anticoagulants. The effects of antiplatelet agents are discussed extensively in other chapters. The mechanism of action for each class is also tabulated in Table 4.3.

Quantitative platelet disorders

Congenital thrombocytopenia

Hereditary forms of thrombocytopenia are rare but have been reported with increasing frequency. A list of these disorders, their inheritance, and laboratory findings are tabulated in Table 4.4. The diagnosis is suspected when there is a family history of thrombocytopenia of unknown cause or neonatal thrombocytopenia, abnormal platelet morphology, or presence of other developmental anomalies. The management for acute bleeding is platelet transfusion and avoidance of antiplatelet agents.

Acquired thrombocytopenia

The acquired thrombocytopenia is caused by either increased destruction/sequestration or decreased production. These disorders are listed in Table 4.5. A systemic approach including medical history, physical examination, examination of complete blood count and blood smear, is the key to identifying the underlying cause(s). Finally, a bone marrow examination with aspiration and biopsy is often needed for a definitive diagnosis. The management is treatment or elimination of underlying cause(s). For acute bleeding episodes, platelet transfusions can be given. For therapy of immune disorders such as ITP, steroid and/or intravenous immunoglobulin (IVIG) can be given. The detailed discussion about management of ITP is beyond the scope of this chapter.

Increased platelet destruction and/or sequestration

Immune thrombocytopenias
Primary
ITP, posttransfusion purpura
Secondary
Infections: Viral, bacterial, protozoan
Autoimmune disorders (SLE, Evan's syndrome)
Lymphoma
Hodgkin's disease
Carcinomatosis

Drugs: Heparin	Cimetidine
Gold	Digoxin
Quinidine	Valproic acid
Quinine	α-Interferon
Penicillins	

Nonimmune
DIC syndromes
Kasabach-Merritt syndrome
Hemolytic uremic syndrome
Thrombotic thrombocytopenic purpura
Chronic hemolytic anemia and thrombocytopenia
Congenital or acquired heart disease
Hypersplenism
Catheters, protheses, cardiopulmonary bypass
Familial hemophagocytic reticulosis

Decreased platelet production
Aplastic anemia, Fanconi's pancytopenia
Marrow infiltrative processes
Leukemias
Metastatic carcinoma
Myelofibrosis
Multiple myeloma
Histiocytoses
Osteopetrosis
Infections

Megakaryocytic thrombocytopenia
Ethanol abuse
HIV-1
Parvovirus infections
Myelodysplastic syndrome
Antibody and T-cell suppression
Nutritional deficiencies
Iron
Folate
B_{12}
Drug or radiation induced
Ethanol
Phenylbutazone
Chloramphenicol
Chemotherapeutic agents
Paroxysmal nocturnal hemoglobinuria
Cyclic thrombocytopenia (Garcia's disease)

Hereditary thrombocytopenias
(*see Table 4.4*)

Miscellaneous
Liver disease
Uremia, renal diseases, renal transplant rejection
Exchange transfusion, massive transfusions, extracorporeal circulation
Heat or cold injury
Thyroid diseases (hyperthyroidism, hypothyroidism)
Fat embolism
Allogeneic bone marrow transplantation
Graft-versus-host disease

Source: adapted from Hathaway WE, Goodnight SH Jr., pp. 75, 76, with permission.

Table 4.5
Causes of acquired thrombocytopenia.

References

1. Lopez JA, Andrews RK, Afshar-Kharghan V, Berndt MC. Bernard-Soulier syndrome. *Blood* 1998;**91**(12):4397–418.
2. Fox JE. Platelet activation: New aspects. *Haemostasis* 1996;**26**:102–31.
3. Weiss HJ, Turitto VT, Baumgartner HR. Further evidence that glycoprotein IIb-IIIa mediate platelet spreading on subendothelium. *Thromb Haemost* 1991;**65**:202–5.
4. Hathaway WE, Goodnight SH Jr. (eds). Disorders of Hemostasis and Thrombosis (McGraw-Hill, New York, 1993).
5. Hartwig JH, DeSisto M. The cytoskeleton of the resting human blood platelet: structure of the membrane skeleton and its attachment to actin filaments. *J Cell Biol* 1991;**112**:407–25.
6. Bernard J, Soulier JP. Sur une nouvelle variété de dystrophie thrombocytaire-hemorragipare congenitale. *Semin Hop Paris* 1948;**24**:3217.
7. Weiss HJ, Turitto VT, Baumgartner HR. Effect of shear rate on platelet interaction with subendothelium in citrated and native blood. 1. Shear rate-dependent decrease of adhesion in von Willebrand disease and the Bernard-Soulier syndrome. *J Lab Clin Med* 1978;**92**:750–64.
8. Lopez JA, Leung B, Reynolds CC, Li CQ, Fox JEB. Efficient plasma membrane expression of a functional human glycoprotein Ib-IX complex requires the presence of its three subunits. *J Biol Chem* 1992;**267**:12851–9.
9. Miller JL, Lyle VA, Cunningham D. Mutation of leucine-57 to phenylalanine in a platelet glycoprotein Ibα leucine tandem repeat occurring in patients with an autosomal dominant variant of Bernard-Soulier disease. *Blood* 1992;**79**:439–46.
10. Miller JL, Cunningham D, Lyle VA, Finch CN. Mutation in the gene encoding the α-chain of platelet glycoprotein Ib in the platelet type von Willebrand disease. *Proc Natl Acad Sci USA* 1991;**88**:4761–5.
11. Staatz WD, Rajpara SM, Wayner EA, Carter WG, Santoro SA. The membrane glycoprotein Ia-IIa (VLA-2) complex mediates the Mg^{++}-dependent adhesion of platelets to collagen. *J Cell Biol* 1989;**108**:1917–24.
12. Coller BS, Beer JH, Scudder LE, Steinberg MH. Collagen-platelet interactions: evidence for a direct interaction with platelet GP IIb/IIIa mediated by adhesive proteins. *Blood* 1989;**74**:182–92.
13. Nieuwenhuis HK, Akkerman JWN, Houijik WPM, Sixma JJ. Human blood platelets showing no response to collagen fail to express surface glycoprotein Ia. *Nature* 1985;**318**:470–2.
14. Moroi M, Jung SM, Okuma M, Shinmyozu K. A patient with platelets deficient in glycoprotein IV that lack both collagen-induced aggregation and adhesion. *J Clin Invest* 1989;**84**:1440–5.
15. Ryo R, Yoshida A, Sugano W et al. Deficiency of p62, a putative collagen receptor, in platelets from a patient with defective collagen-induced platelet aggregation. *Am J Hematol* 1992;**39**:25–31.
16. George JN, Caen JP, Nurden AT. Glanzmann's thrombasthenia: the spectrum of clinical disease. *Blood* 1990;**75**:1383–95.
17. Caen JP. Glanzmann's thrombasthenia. *Baillières Clin Haematol* 1989;**2**:609–25.
18. Ginsberg MH, Lightsey A, Kunicki TJ, Kaufman A, Marguerie G, Plow EF. Divalent cation regulation of the surface orientation of platelet membrane glycoprotein IIb. Correlation with fibrinogen binding function and definition of a novel variant of Glanzmann's thrombasthenia. *J Clin Invest* 1986;**78**:1103–11.
19. Chen YP, Djaffar I, Pidard D et al. Ser-752-Pro mutation in the cytoplasmic domain of integrin β₃ subunit and defective activation of platelet integrin α$_{IIb}$β$_3$ (glycoprotein IIb-IIIa) in a variant of Glanzmann thrombasthenia. *Proc Natl Acad Sci USA* 1992;**89**:10169–73.
20. Lagande M, Byron PA, Vargaftig BB, Dechavanne M. Impairment of platelet thromboxane A₂ generation and of platelet release reaction in two patients with congenital deficiency of

platelet cyclo-oxygenase. *Br J Haematol* 1978;**38**:251–66.

21. Machin SJ, Carreras LO, Chamone DAF, Defreyn G, Dauden M, Vermylen J. Familial deficiency of thromboxane synthase (abstract). *Br J Haematol* 1981;**47**:629.

22. Mestel F, Oetliker O, Beck E, Felix R, Imbach P, Wagner H-P. Severe bleeding associated with defective thromboxane synthase. *Lancet* 1980;**1**:157.

23. Racculgia G. Gray platelet sundrome—a variety of qualitative platelet disorder. *Am J Med* 1971;**51**:818–28.

24. Gerrard JM, Lint D, Simms PJ et al. Identification of a platelet dense granule membrane protein deficient in a patient with Hermansky-Pudlak syndrome. *Blood* 1991;**77**:101–12.

25. Parkman R, Remmold-O'Donnell E, Kenny DM, Perrines S, Rosen FS. Surface protein abnormalities in lymphocytes and platelets from patients with Wiskott-Aldrich syndrome. *Lancet* 1991;**2**:1387–9.

26. Weiss HJ. Scott syndrome: a disorder of platelet coagulant activity. *Semin Hematol* 1994;**31**:312–19.

27. Toti F, Satta N, Fressinaud E, Meyer D, Freyssinet J-M. Scott syndrome, characterized by impaired transmembrane migration of procoagulant phosphatidylserine and hemorrhagic complications, is an inherited disorder. *Blood* 1996;**84**:1409–15.

28. Moia M, Mannucci PM, Vizzotto L. Improvement in the haemostatic defect of uraemia after treatment with recombinant human erythropoietin. *Lancet* 1987;**8570**:1227–9.

29. Gralnick HP, McKeown LP, Williams SB et al. Plasma and platelet von Willebrand's factor defects in uremia. *Am J Med* 1988;**85**:806–10.

30. Guzzo J, Niewiarowski S, Musial J et al. Secreted platelet proteins with antiheparin and mitogenic activities in chronic renal failure. *J Lab Clin Med* 1980;**96**:102–13.

31. Juberlirer SJ. Hemostatic abnormalities in renal disease. *Am J Kidney Dis* 1985;**V**:219–25.

32. Remuzzi G, Perico N, Zoja C, Corna D, Macconi D, Vigano G. Role of endothelium-derived nitric oxide in the bleeding tendency of uremia. *J Clin Invest* 1990;**86**:1768–71.

33. Vigano G, Benigni A, Mendogni D, Mingardi G, Mecca G, Remuzzi G. Recombinant human erythropoietin to correct uremic bleeding. *Am J Kidney Dis* 1991;**18**:44–9.

34. Janson PA, Jubelier SJ, Weinstein MJ, Deykin D. Treatment of the bleeding tendency in uremia with cryoprecipitate. *N Engl J Med* 1980;**303**:1318–22.

35. Salzman EW, Weinstein MJ, Weintraub RM et al. Treatment with desmopressin acetate to reduce blood loss after cardiac surgery. A double-blind randomized trial. *N Engl J Med* 1986;**314**:1402–6.

36. Rocha E, Llorens R, Paramo JA. Does desmopressin acetate reduce blood loss after surgery in patients on cardiopulmonary bypass? *Circulation* 1988;**77**:1319–23.

37. Hackmann T, Gascoyne RD, Naiman SC et al. A trial of desmopressin (1-desamino-8-D-arginine vasopressin) to reduce blood loss in uncomplicated cardiac surgery. *N Engl J Med* 1989;**321**:1437–43.

38. De Prost D, Barbier-Boehm G, Hazebroucq J et al. Desmopressin has no beneficial effect on excessive postoperative bleeding or blood product requirements associated with cardiopulmonary bypass. *Thromb Haemost* 1992; **68**:106–10.

39. Mannucci PM, Vicente V, Vianello L et al. Controlled trial of desmopressin in liver cirrhosis and other conditions associated with a prolonged bleeding time. *Blood* 1986;**67**:1148–53.

40. Stoff JS, Stemerman M, Steer M et al. A defect in platelet aggregation in Bartter's syndrome. *Am J Med* 1980;**68**:171–80.

41. Roberts AB, Sporn MB, Assoian RK. Transforming growth factor type β: rapid induction of fibrosis and angiogenesis *in vivo* and stimulation of collagen formation *in vitro*. *Proc Natl Acad Sci USA* 1986;**83**:4167–71.

42. Moliterno AR, Hankins WD, Apivak JL. Impaired expression of the thrombopoietin receptor by platelets from patients with polycythemia vera. *N Engl J Med* 1998;**338**: 572–80.

43. Petitt RM, Silverstein MN, Petrone ME. Anagrelide for control of thrombocythemia in polycythemia and other myeloproliferative disorders. *Semin Hematol* 1997;**34**:51–4.

44. Varon D, Gitel SN, Varon N et al. Immune Bernard-Soulier-like syndrome associated with anti-glycoprotein-IX antibody. *Am J Hematol* 1992;**41**:67.

45. Devine DV, Currier MS, Rosse WF, Greenberg CS. Pseudo-Bernard-Soulier syndrome: thrombocytopenia caused by autoantibody to platelet glycoprotein Ib. *Blood* 1987;**70**:428–31.

46. Berndt MC, Kabral A, Grimsley P et al. An acquired Bernard-Soulier like platelet defect associated with juvenile myelodysplastic syndrome. *Br J Haematol* 1988;**68**:97–101.

47. Niessner H, Clemetson KJ, Pamzer S, Mueller-Eckhardt C, Santoso S, Bettelheim P. Acquired thrombasthenia due to GPIIb-IIIa-specific platelet autoantibodies. *Blood* 1986; **68**: 571–6.

5

Overview of antiplatelet agents

Martin Quinn and Desmond Fitzgerald

Introduction

Platelets are known to play an important role in many cardiovascular diseases, accordingly antiplatelet agents have assumed an ever-increasing role in their treatment (Figure 5.1). Aspirin, the prototypic antiplatelet agent, is over 100 years old. Its platelet inhibitory effects were first noted in the early 1970s. It was not until the landmark thrombolytic and unstable angina trials of the 1980s and 1990s, however, that its full potential in the treatment of cardiovascular diseases was realized. In the ISIS-2 trial, aspirin used alone in the early stages of acute myocardial infarction had an equivalent benefit to thrombolytic therapy, producing significant lasting reductions in death, recurrent myocardial infarction and stroke with minimal side-effects.[1] Furthermore, aspirin doubled the benefit seen with streptokinase alone without an increase in complications. Impressive benefits were also seen in the treatment of patients with unstable angina, stable angina, symptomatic cerebrovascular disease, peripheral vascular disease, following coronary artery bypass grafting and in patients undergoing percutaneous coronary interventions.[2–4]

These clinical trials have made the use of an antiplatelet agent mandatory in many cardiovascular conditions. Aspirin is usually the agent of choice as it is cheap and generally well-tolerated. However, aspirin is a fairly weak antiplatelet agent. It inhibits thromboxane A_2 production, but this is only one of the many mediators that can cause platelet activation.[5] Even with complete suppression of thromboxane A_2, other strong agonists, such as thrombin or collagen, can induce full platelet activation and aggregation. Similarly, platelet activation is detectable in vivo and clinical thrombosis may occur while on aspirin.[6,7] Also, while aspirin is generally well-tolerated, side-effects, particularly gastrointestinal, can limit its use.[8]

The appreciation that thrombosis plays a critical role in cardiovascular disease has led to a search for newer and more powerful

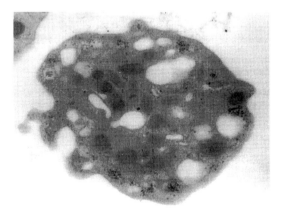

Figure 5.1
Electronmicrograph of a platelet. Note the dense granules and large α-granules.

platelet inhibitors. Our understanding of the underlying processes that mediate platelet activation and the functional role that platelet surface receptors and secreted products play has helped to identify new targets for therapeutic intervention. Several newly developed agents are in clinical use, some with impressive results. Many other agents are in the development phase and are approaching clinical application. In the near future, workers in the cardiovascular field can expect an array of antiplatelet agents at their disposal.

Platelet physiology

Platelets are smooth discoid particles derived from megakaryoctes. They circulate around the body in an inactive state, however in areas of endothelial damage, such as a ruptured coronary plaque, they adhere to exposed subendothelial collagen and von Willebrand factor and activate. Other factors including high fluid shear stress and activation of the coagulation cascade also induce platelet activation. The activated platelet changes shape and releases its cytoplasmic granules, which contain the platelet agonists ADP and serotonin and other vasoactive and mitogenic substances. In additon arachidonic acid is released from the platelet membrane and is converted to thromboxane A_2 a potent platelet agonist, smooth muscle mitogen and vasoconstrictor. The release of thromboxane A_2 and the platelet granules serves to recruit other circulating platelets to the area of platelet activation. Coincident with these changes the platelet fibrinogen receptor glycoprotein (GP) IIb/IIIa undergoes a conformational change, which increases its affinity for fibrinogen. Fibrinogen is a multivalent ligand and can bind to adjacent platelets thus cross-linking them to form an aggregate.

Many different agents have been developed

in order to inhibit the process of platelet activation and subsequent aggregation. Inhibition of thromboxane A_2 production by aspirin or its effects with a TXA_2 receptor antagonist prevents this positive feedback loop of platelet activation. ADP-receptor antagonists prevent the action of released ADP. GPIIb/IIIa receptor antagonists prevent fibrinogen binding to the activated platelet. This chapter provides an overview of the available antiplatelet agents.

Inhibition of thromboxane A_2

Cyclo-oxygenase converts arachidonic into the prostaglandin (PG) endoperoxides, PGG_2 and PGH_2. These are converted into thromboxane $(TX)A_2$ by thromboxane synthase in platelets or into prostacyclin (PGI_2) by prostacyclin synthase in endothelial cells (Figure 5.2). Aspirin inactivates cyclo-oxygenase by acetylating a serine residue at position 529 within the active site of the enzyme, preventing TXA_2 and PGI_2 production.[9-11] The inhibition of platelet cyclo-oxygenase is irreversible and lasts for the life-span of the platelet (7–10 days).[12] Other non-steroidal anti-inflammatory agents (NSAIDS) bind either irreversibly but non-covalently (e.g. indomethacin) or reversibly to the active site of cyclo-oxygenase, such that their antiplatelet actions are of shorter duration. The inhibition of TXA_2 production prevents TXA_2-mediated granule release and aggregation. Nevertheless, aggregation via thromboxane independent mechanisms, such as that induced by thrombin or elevated shear stress, can still occur.

Much evidence supports the use of aspirin in the secondary prevention of cardiovascular disease. Its benefit in treating patients suffering an acute myocardial infarction has been confirmed by the large ISIS-2 trial with over 17 000 patients.[1] Aspirin reduced the com-

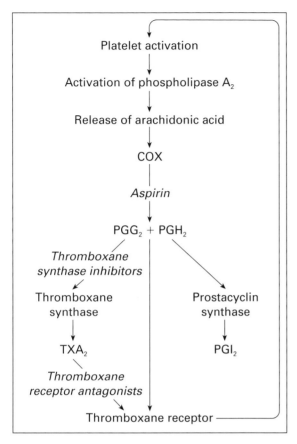

Figure 5.2
Platelet activation results in activation of phospholipase A$_2$. This releases arachidonic acid from the platelet membrane. Cyclo-oxygenase (COX) converts this to prostaglandin (PG)G$_2$ and PGH$_2$. Thromboxane synthase and prostacyclin synthase convert these to thromboxane A$_2$ (TXA$_2$) and prostacyclin (PGI$_2$). TXA$_2$ is released from the platelet and binds to specific membrane receptors causing further platelet activation. The sites of action of the various drugs are indicated.

ity of acute myocardial infarction by 50%. Other trials have demonstrated the benefit of aspirin in the prevention of stroke in patients with a history of transient ischemic attack,[13] in reducing the risk of death or myocardial infarction in unstable angina by anywhere from 37–70%,[14] in the prevention of peri-procedural myocardial infarction or other complications of coronary angioplasty or stent placement,[15] in preserving coronary bypass grafts[16] and in the prevention of hemodialysis shunt thrombosis.[17] A meta-analysis of all trials of antiplatelet therapy by the Antiplatelet Trialists' Collaboration demonstrated the benefits of aspirin, irrespective of the dose in a wide range of vascular diseases.[2,3] Overall, antiplatelet therapy produced a consistent reduction in events in patients at high risk as a result of a history of previous myocardial infarction, unstable angina, transient ischemic attack, or stroke. Non-fatal myocardial infarction or stroke was reduced by one-third and vascular deaths were reduced by one-sixth.

One potential drawback of aspirin is inhibition of endothelial production of PGI$_2$ a potent inhibitor of platelet aggregation. It has been proposed, however, that endothelial cyclo-oxygenase is less sensitive to aspirin at low dose. Platelets are highly sensitive to aspirin as its target, cyclo-oxygenase, turns over slowly. For this reason, it is possible to induce a cumulative inhibition of platelet cyclo-oxygenase using repeated low doses, such as 30–50 mg/day[18,19] (in contrast, maximum inhibition following a single dose of aspirin requires 100 mg).[12] Dose-response data on the effects of aspirin on TXA$_2$ and PGI$_2$ formation in vivo, however, show that, while there is a relative degree of PGI$_2$-sparing at all doses of aspirin, there is no dose that is absolutely specific for TXA$_2$ inhibition. Thus, at all doses that provided near complete inhibition of platelet cyclo-oxygenase and

bined endpoints of death, recurrent myocardial infarction or stroke by one-third. There was also a very impressive interaction with streptokinase in that the combination of aspirin and streptokinase reduced the mortal-

inhibition of TXA_2 there was also inhibition of PGI_2 formation.[20]

Pedersen and FitzGerald noticed that following a single dose of aspirin, platelet cyclo-oxygenase was inhibited prior to the appearance of aspirin in the circulation. This suggested that platelets were inhibited by aspirin in the portal circulation during drug absorption. Moreover, aspirin delivered over hours was more efficient for the inhibition of platelet cyclo-oxygenase than a single oral dose, since aspirin is rapidly hydrolysed to the inactive salicylate with a half-life of 20 minutes.[21] These investigators subsequently reported on an oral-controlled release aspirin preparation of 75 mg where delivery was virtually continuous over 10 hours. Very little drug was detected systemically, yet platelet cyclo-oxygenase was inhibited by over 95%. Moreover, bradykinin-induced PGI_2 formation in vivo was unaffected. In contrast, bradykinin-induced PGI_2 formation was abolished by ingestion of 75 mg of regular aspirin given orally.[22] A second aspirin preparation delivered transdermally was similarly selective for TXA_2, with no detectable effect on PGI_2 formation.[23] Whether these highly selective preparations of aspirin are more effective as antithrombotic agents than regular oral aspirin is unknown.

Selective inhibition of thromboxane synthetase provides an alternative approach.[24] These inhibitors have the theoretical advantage of decreasing TXA_2 production without affecting PGI_2 formation. Moreover, the intermediate PGH_2 may be metabolized to PGI_2 by prostacyclin synthase in contiguous endothelium. Thromboxane synthase inhibitors are, however, weak inhibitors of platelet aggregation since the PGH_2 produced can fully substitute for TXA_2 in activating the thromboxane receptor.[25] Combined TXA_2 synthase and TXA_2 receptor antagonists have been devel-oped to overcome this problem; they suppress TXA_2 formation and enhance PGI_2 biosynthesis while preventing PGH_2-mediated platelet activation.[26,27] Clinical results have not however, been very promising. Coronary artery patency in patients receiving thrombolytic therapy for myocardial infarction was no different in patients treated with aspirin or ridogrel, a combined thromboxane synthase inhibitor and TXA_2 receptor antagonist.[28] Post-hoc analysis revealed a reduction in the combined endpoint of recurrent infarction, ischemic stroke or unstable angina in the rido-grel treated group, without increasing bleeding events;[29] however, such data needs to be interpreted cautiously. A second TXA_2 synthase inhibitor/receptor antagonist, picotamide, has been compared with placebo in 2304 patients with peripheral vascular disease. The incidence of major events (e.g. death, myocardial infarction, stroke or amputation) was unaltered. However, primary events occurred less frequently than expected and reduced the power of the study. Picotamide was marginally better than placebo (p value 0.056) when major and minor events (e.g. angina, probable or possible MI, TIA, minor stroke, deep venous thrombosis or pulmonary embolism, severe renal failure or hypertension and peripheral vascular disease deterioration) were combined, with 10.6% of treated patients experiencing an event compared with 13.1% in the placebo group.[30] These data, and the lack of a dose-dependent response to aspirin, suggest that preservation of PGI_2 formation contributes little to the benefit of TXA_2 inhibition.

Platelet prostaglandin production is also modified by omega-3 fatty acids, particularly eicospentanoiec acid (EPA). These are found in fish oils and prolong bleeding time, reduce platelet aggregation and TXA_2 production.[31] EPA substitutes for arachidonic acid in the platelet membrane and acts as a substrate for cyclo-oxygenase, which converts it to TXA_3, a biological inert form of TXA_2. The corresponding PGI_3 produced by prostacyclin synthase is active. This results in a relative reduction in the balance of proaggregatory TXA_2 to the antiaggregatory and vasodilator PGI_2 and PGI_3. Although EPA in high doses produces a potent antiplatelet effect in some species,[32] the antithrombotic activity is fairly modest in man.[33]

ADP receptor antagonists

ADP has long been known as a platelet agonist and acts as a local mediator at the site of platelet activation where it is released from the platelet dense-granules. Although not so powerful as thrombin or collagen, it can still produce full platelet activation and aggregation. Clopidogrel and ticlopidine are thienopyridine inhibitors of the platelet ADP receptor.[34,35] Both compounds are orally active and are effective in the treatment of patients at risk of platelet-mediated thrombotic disease. Recent studies demonstrating the efficacy of ticlopidine in preventing complications after coronary stent placement have led to an increase in its use. Care is needed, however, since complications are frequent and there have been several reports of treatment-related deaths. Clopidogrel provides an attractive alternative with fewer side-effects. In the CAPRIE study its efficacy, in comparison to aspirin, has been proven in patients at high risk of vascular events. Further study is however, required to define its role in other clinical syndromes.[36] Both agents are inactive in vitro and require metabolism in the liver, via the cytochrome P_{450} system, to acquire activity.[37] Plasma from treated patients results in inhibition of untreated platelets indicating the presence of (an) active metabolite(s); however, these have not been identified.[38] The antiplatelet effects of

the metabolites result from non-competitive and irreversible inhibition of the platelet ADP receptor. Thienopyridines do not prevent ADP-induced platelet shape change or calcium flux; instead, they suppress platelet aggregation and the reduction in cAMP levels induced by ADP. Work with specific antagonists of the platelet ADP receptors indicates that the $P2T_{AC}$ receptor is involved in the inhibition of adenylate cyclase. Inhibition of this receptor results in inhibition of aggregation, but calcium flux or shape change is not altered. Therefore, it is likely that ticlopidine and clopidigrel act through the $P2T_{AC}$ receptor. Both agents inhibit shear-induced platelet aggregation and platelet adherence to endothelial matrix, whereas aspirin has no effect on these parameters. In addition to their antiaggregatory effects, ticlopidine and clopidigrel may influence vascular tone since they reduce serotonin and endothelin-1-induced vasoconstriction in animal models.[39] Clopidigrel also reduces platelet induced-endothelial cell expression of tissue factor, although its not clear whether this contributes to the antithrombotic activity of the drug.[40]

The main indication for ticlopidine is as an antithrombotic in cardiovascular disease and during cardiovascular interventions associated with a risk of platelet clot formation. Care is needed, however, since serious and sometimes fatal side-effects occur. Neutropenia has been reported in 2.4% of treated patients and this can be severe (less than 450 neutrophils/mm^3) in 0.8% of patients. Most cases develop within the first 3 months of therapy and may be clinically silent. Thrombocytopenia and aplastic anemia also occur and there have been reports of thrombotic thrombocytopenic purpura.[41,42] Consequently, frequent full blood counts are mandatory in patients on ticlopidine. Diarrhoea is the main gastrointestinal side-effect and may require discontinuation of the drug.[34,43]

Ticlopidine has been studied in several large randomized trials comparing it to placebo, to aspirin alone or to a combination with aspirin. Balsano et al, in a non-placebo-controlled trial, demonstrated the beneficial effect of ticlopidine in over 600 patients with unstable angina with an absolute reduction in the combined endpoint of vascular death and non-fatal infarction of 6.3% (13.6% reduced to 7.3%).[44] This is similar to the benefit seen with the use of aspirin in unstable angina. No randomized trials have compared the use of ticlopidine and aspirin directly in unstable coronary syndromes. Trials have focused more on the comparison of the combination of ticlopidine and aspirin to either agent alone. Indeed, this combination is now used routinely during coronary stenting, often with ticlopidine started just before the procedure and continued for 2–4 weeks.[15,45–49] However, given the time required for ticlopidine to inhibit platelets (5–7 days), it is difficult to see how ticlopidine is exerting any acute antithrombotic effect. Indeed, studies comparing aspirin alone to aspirin and ticlopidine have yielded conflicting results. The largest to date, the STARS study, had three treatment limbs: aspirin therapy alone; aspirin plus ticlopidine; and aspirin plus warfarin.[50] The primary event rate was lowest in the aspirin plus ticlopidine group (8.2% vs 13.1% for the aspirin alone group and 11.6% for the aspirin plus warfarin group). In accordance with this, combination therapy has been shown to reduce markers of platelet activation compared with therapy with aspirin alone.[51] Smaller trials have failed to demonstrate any benefit of the aspirin plus ticlopidine over aspirin alone, although events were marginally more common with aspirin monotherapy.[52] Recent studies demonstrating that ticlopidine therapy for as short as 10–14 days post-stenting is equivalent to 4 weeks' of treatment with ficlopidine certainly raises

questions as to whether this drug should be used at all.[53] It is worth emphasizing yet again that deaths have arisen from the use of ticlopidine. Finally, although combination therapy produces major reductions in ischemic events in comparison with anticoagulant therapy, it does not alter the incidence of re-stenosis.[54]

Ticlopidine monotherapy has been shown to be effective, in comparison with placebo, in preventing stroke in patients with a history of transient ischaemic attack[55] and may be marginally better than aspirin in this regard.[56] Results in patients with peripheral vascular disease are less impressive. There are conflicting reports of its ability to improve walking distance and prevent progression of the disease process. The largest study to date, the Swedish Ticlopidine Multicenter Trial (STIMS), failed to show a reduction in primary endpoints (MI, stroke or TIA), although there was a significant benefit in overall mortality (18.5% vs 26.1%).[57] Ticlopidine has been shown to improve the long-term patency of lower-limb saphenous vein bypass grafts compared with placebo.[58]

The CAPRIE trial is the largest trial to date to examine the efficacy of clopidogrel in preventing vascular events in patients with a history of ischemic stroke, recent myocardial infarction or symptomatic peripheral vascular disease.[36] The outcome favoured clopidigrel, although the benefit over aspirin was marginal, with only a 0.5% absolute reduction in the combined endpoint of ischemic stroke, myocardial infarction or vascular death in the 19 185 patients enrolled. The relative risk reduction was 8.7% ($p = 0.045$) and this difference persisted for up to 3 years. The benefit was largest in the patients with a history of peripheral vascular disease, with an absolute risk reduction of 1.15% ($p < 0.0028$). In patients enrolled with a history of myocardial infarction, clopidogrel was not superior to aspirin in reducing primary events (5.03% vs 4.84% respectively), although caution is needed when interpreting such subset analyses. The lack of a detectable effect may simply be the result of a lack of power in the study, as the rate of endpoints for this subgroup was far lower than expected. Side-effects were uncommon with both treatments. Importantly, there was no excess of neutropenia in patients treated with clopidogrel (0.1% vs 0.7% for aspirin).

Potent short-acting intravenous ADP receptor antagonists have been developed.[59] These may extend the application of this form of antiplatelet therapy to acute cardiovascular interventions, and further enhance our knowledge of the ADP receptor in platelet physiology.

In summary, ADP antagonists are effective antiplatelet agents and are certainly an alternative to aspirin. It would be of interest to know whether the combination of aspirin and clopidigrel is better than aspirin alone and how it compares with newer, potent agents such as the GPIIb-IIIa antagonists. Clopidigrel certainly has a safer profile than ticlopidine and, in all likelihood, will replace the latter.

Dipyridamole and prostacyclin analogs

Agents that increase platelet cAMP or cGMP have potent antiplatelet effects.[60] Iloprost, a stable PGI_2 analog, increases cAMP levels; however, its vasoactive properties limit its use as an antiplatelet agent.[61] Several attempts have been made to localize PGI_2 effects and minimize its systemic activity. A novel method involves adenoviral-mediated transfer of the cyclo-oxygenase-1 (COX-1) gene to endothelial cells.[62] This results in a five-fold increase in the production of PGI_2 in cultured endothelial cells. Local administration of the vector in an animal model of carotid angioplasty resulted in a four-fold increase in PGI_2 production and inhibited cyclical flow variations and thrombus formation. Another method involves the incorporation of iloprost into platelets by electrical permeablization.[63] When the iloprost-containing platelets were reinfused into an animal angioplasty model, they reduced platelet deposition and prevented re-stenosis in minimally injured arteries.

Dipyridamole has several effects that result in increased platelet (cyclic) cGMP and cAMP, which in turn suppress platelet activation. Dipyridamole inhibits the uptake of adenosine by erythrocytes, thus increasing its availability. The increased adenosine stimulates platelet adenylate cyclase, increasing cAMP levels. Dipyridamole also inhibits cGMP-phosphodiesterase, so preventing the breakdown of cGMP. However, these effects do not occur at the concentrations that are seen in man following standard doses of dipyridamole. Consistent with this, dipyridamole does not prolong the bleeding time or inhibit platelet aggregation at therapeutic doses. Overall, there is no evidence that standard doses of dipyridamole confer any benefit when added to aspirin and dipyridamole has minimal protective effects as monotherapy.[64] Nevertheless, a novel, controlled release preparation of dipyridamole 200 mg given twice daily, was equally effective as aspirin in patients that had suffered a transient ischemic attack (TIA) or recent stroke.[65] In addition, the combination of aspirin and the controlled-release dipyridamole was more effective than either drug alone. The advantage of this preparation is that it avoids the high peak plasma levels of dipyridamole, which are vasoactive and have limited the total dose of the standard preparation. With the controlled-release preparation, a stable, antiplatelet plasma concentration is achieved.

GPIIb/IIIa receptor antagonists

The realization of the central role that the GPIIb-IIIa plays in platelet aggregation has led to the development of several antagonists of this receptor as antiplatelet agents. These include RGD-containing peptides called disintegrins (e.g. eichistatin) from venomous snakes and their analogs, monoclonal antibodies to the GPIIb-IIIa receptor and synthetic peptides (fibatides) and non-peptide (fibans) that mimic the fibrinogen-binding motifs.[66-69] The clinical use of disintegrins is limited by their potential for serious side-effects, including thrombocytopenia, allergic reactions and modulation of the immune system. Abciximab, or 7E3, a monoclonal antibody inhibitor was the first GPIIb-IIIa antagonist to reach clinical use. Two other compounds, the peptide, epifibatide, and the non-peptide, tirofiban, both intravenous agents, have just been approved. Many other peptides and peptide derivatives are in development.

Abciximab is a Fab fragment of a chimeric human/murine monoclonal antibody to the GPIIb-IIIa, and it is modified to limit antigenicity.[70] It is a potent inhibitor of platelet aggregation and its efficacy in the prevention of complications at the time of coronary angioplasty and stent placement has been proven in several large randomized trials.[71-74] It has a prolonged duration of action and can be detected on platelets for up to 14 days after administration.[75] It is estimated that it is used in over 40% of coronary interventions in the USA. While it increases the risk of bleeding, with careful attention to the heparin dosage, the bleeding risk is low. Thrombocytopenia

and allergic reactions occur rarely,[76] although antibodies against abciximab have been detected in 6.5% of patients following a single administration.

In the EPIC trial, abciximab therapy was associated with a lower incidence of elective repeat interventions, suggesting that the initial benefit was maintained over a prolonged period.[72] Although patients were not restudied, one possibility was that the reduction in clinical events resulted from a lower incidence of restenosis. Interestingly, abciximab is not specific for GPIIb-IIIa but also binds to $\alpha_v\beta_3$, an integrin present on vascular smooth muscle cells (VSMC). $\alpha_v\beta_3$ is the receptor for vitronectin and has been implicated in the VSMC proliferation that characterizes arterial restenosis. Recently, Stouffer et al have demonstrated that $\alpha_v\beta_3$ expression is increased in an animal model of balloon injury and that 7E3 partially inhibits thrombospondin and α-thrombin-induced VSMC proliferation, implying that 7E3 may have a role to play in the prevention of restenosis.[76] It has been suggested, therefore, that the lack of integrin specificity displayed by abciximab may be advantageous. However, a more recent study, EPILOG, has failed to confirm the long-term benefit of EPIC.[73] While abciximab has primarily proved effective in reducing thrombotic complications at the time of coronary revascularization, data from the CAPTURE study suggest that it also reduced the risk of acute myocardial infarction in patients with unstable angina awaiting intervention. Therefore, abciximab may prove effective in other settings, including unstable angina or acute myocardial infarction.

Future directions with GPIIb-IIIa antagonists

Many other synthetic peptides and peptide derivatives are being developed. In general, intravenous forms of these agents have not been so effective as abciximab, although dosing may have been suboptimal and, unlike abciximab, the duration of effect is quite short.[78–80] Thrombocytopenia has been seen with all compounds and, although rare (less than 1%), can be very severe. Several of the compounds under development display oral bioavailability, raising the potential for chronic therapy. Several phase III trials with oral agents are underway. Hopefully, these will address the potential of these agents in the secondary or even primary prevention of cardiovascular diseases.

Although GPIIb-IIIa antagonists block fibrinogen binding to platelets, the inhibition of secretion is dependent on the agonist.[81] This may limit the effectiveness of GPIIb-IIIa antagonists since several secreted products are thought to play an important role in restenosis.[82] In vivo, several GPIIb-IIIa antagonists decrease TXA_2 production.[83] However, we have demonstrated continued TXA_2 production in spite of treatment with a GPIIb/IIIa antagonist alone at the time of coronary angioplasty.[84] Thus combination therapy with aspirin may still be required in order to prevent TXA_2 production.

In addition to inhibiting platelet fibrinogen binding, some of GPIIb-IIIa antagonists have been shown to inhibit thrombin production and to prevent tissue-factor-induced thrombosis in animal models.[85] Indeed, the activated clotting time was higher in patients treated with abciximab in the EPIC trial.[86] Thus, some of these compounds may have combined antithrombotic and antiplatelet effects, reducing the need for concomitant anticoagulation.

Monitoring antagonists of the platelet GPIIb-IIIa

Monitoring is not usually required with conventional antiplatelet therapy. The newer agents, however, particularly the potent oral glycoprotein IIb-IIIa receptor antagonists which are aimed at chronic therapy, may require some form of monitoring. Many of these agents have variable inter-individual pharmacokinetic and pharmacodynamic profiles. This may result in fluctuations in their inhibitory effects and alterations in dosage may be required to maintain efficacy or to limit nuisance bleeding side-effects. More importantly, an assessment of bleeding risk may be required at the time of emergency surgery. Although platelet aggregation by lumi-aggregometry is usually the means of monitoring therapy, it requires specialist equipment and has several disadvantages. Platelet aggregation may be affected by several factors such as the agonist used, the platelet count and the use of concurrent medications.[87,88] In addition, the response to the certain GPIIb-IIIa antagonists is dependent on the anticoagulant added to the sample, since the binding affinity is dependent on the concentration of divalent cations.[89,90] Platelet aggregation is dependent on cross-linking of GPIIb-IIIa receptors from adjacent platelets and is unaffected at low levels of receptor occupancy.[91] As receptor occupancy exceeds 80%, aggregation may be completely inhibited, particularly to weak agonists, despite the presence of unoccupied receptors. Inhibition of these residual unoccupied receptors may have functional effects as evidenced by a further increase in bleeding time, with levels of occupancy greater than 80%, which platelet aggregation may fail to detect.[91]

In order to try to overcome some of these difficulties, several alternative techniques are being examined. Monoclonal antibodies to the GPIIb-IIIa receptor that are differentially displaced by different receptor antagonists in a concentration-dependent manner can be used to assess receptor occupancy directly. An alternative technique involves the use of antibodies to epitopes on the receptor that are induced by ligand-binding (anti-LIBS antibodies). Nevertheless, GPIIb-IIIa antagonists vary in their ability to induce LIBS and this method may not be useful in all cases. A bedside device, the Accumetrix™ Rapid Platelet Function Assay (RPFA), is currently being evaluated. RPFA is based on the ability of antagonists to inhibit the agglutination of platelets with fibrinogen-coated beads.[92] All of these methods are being studied in clinical trials, which will provide an indication of the overall need for monitoring during chronic therapy.

Conclusion

Antiplatelet agents play an important role in modern cardiovascular therapy. The physiological processes that control platelet function are complex and there are many different tar-gets for inhibition. GPIIb-IIIa receptor antagonists block fibrinogen binding and thus prevent platelet aggregation to all known agonists. They have produced impressive benefits in addition to aspirin. However, platelet activation and secretion can still occur with these agents and several platelet-secreted products may play an important role in restenosis. Recently, Henn et al have shown that platelets express CD40L on their surface. This is a transmembrane protein structure related to the cytokine TNF-α, which is involved in the regulation of the immune response. Expression of CD40L on platelets is increased with activation and results in the secretion of cytokines and the expression of adhesion molecules by endotheial cells.[93] Thus, platelet activation may play an important role in activation of the immune system at the site of vascular injury and consequently in restenosis and in the pathogenesis of atherosclerosis. Inhibition of activation as well as secretion may be required to prevent this process. Thus, although many advances have been made in the field, there is still some distance to go before we have conquered the platelet in the pathogenesis of atherothrombotic disease.

References

1. ISIS-2 Collaborative Group. Randomized trial of intravenous streptokinase, oral aspirin, both, or neither among 17 187 cases of suspected acute myocardial infarction: ISIS-2. *Lancet* 1988;**2**:349–60.

2. Antiplatelet Trialists' Collaboration. Collaborative overview of randomised trials of antiplatelet therapy—II: Maintenance of vascular graft or arterial patency by antiplatelet therapy. *Br Med J* 1994;**308**:159–68.

3. Antiplatelet Trialists' Collaboration. Collaborative overview of randomised trials of antiplatelet therapy—I: Prevention of death, myocardial infarction, and stroke by prolonged antiplatelet therapy in various categories of patients. *Br Med J* 1994;**308**: 81–106.

4. Antiplatelet Trialists' Collaboration. Collaborative overview of randomised trials of antiplatelet therapy—III: Reduction in venous thrombosis and pulmonary embolism by antiplatelet prophylaxis among surgical and medical patients. *Br Med J* 1994;**308**:235–46.

5. Vane J. Inhibition of prostaglandin biosynthesis as a mechanism of action of aspirin-like drugs. *Nature* 1971;**231**:232–5.

6. Cipollone F, Patrignani P, Greco A, et al. Differential suppression of thromboxane biosynthesis by indobufen and aspirin in patients with unstable angina. *Circulation* 1997;**96**:1109–16.

7. Pengo V, Boschello M, Marzari A, Baca M, Schivazappa L, Dalla Volta S. Adenosine diphosphate (ADP)-induced alpha-granules release from platelets of native whole blood is reduced by ticlopidine but not by aspirin or dipyridamole. *Thromb Haemost* 1986;**56**: 147–50.

8. Roderick PJ, Wilkes HC, Meade TW. The gastrointestinal toxicity of aspirin: an overview of randomised controlled trials. *Br J Clin Pharm* 1993;**35**:219–26.

9. Smith WL, Lands WE. Stimulation and blockade of prostaglandin biosynthesis. *J Biol Chem* 1971;**246**:6700–702.

10. Smith JB, Willis AL. Aspirin selectively inhibits prostaglandin production in human platelets. *Nature* 1971;**231**:235–7.

11. Patrono C. Aspirin as an antiplatelet drug. *N Engl J Med* 1994;**330**:1287–94.

12. Patrignani P, Filabozzi P, Patrono C. Selective cumulative inhibition of platelet thromboxane production by low-dose aspirin in healthy subjects. *J Clin Invest* 1982;**69**:1366–72.

13. Farrell B, Godwin J, Richards S, Warlow C. The United Kingdom transient ischaemic attack (UK-TIA) aspirin trial: final results. *J Neurol Neurosurg Psychiatr* 1991;**54**: 1044–54.

14. The RISC Group. Risk of myocardial infarction and death during treatment with low dose aspirin and intravenous heparin in men with unstable coronary artery disease. *Lancet* 1990;**336**:827–30.

15. Barragan P, Sainsous J, Silvestri M, et al. Coronary artery stenting without anticoagulation, aspirin, ultrasound guidance, or high balloon pressure: prospective study of 1051 consecutive patients. *Cath Cardio Diag* 1997; **42**:367–73.

16. Lorenz RL, Schacky CV, Weber M, et al. Improved aortocoronary bypass patency by low-dose aspirin (100 mg daily). Effects on platelet aggregation and thromboxane formation. *Lancet* 1984;**1**:1261–4.

17. Harter HR, Burch JW, Majerus PW, et al. Prevention of thrombosis in patients on hemodialysis by low-dose aspirin. *N Engl J Med* 1979;**301**:577–9.

18. De Caterina R, Giannessi D, Boem A, et al. Equal antiplatelet effects of aspirin 50 or 324 mg/day in patients after acute myocardial infarction. *Thromb Haemost* 1985;**54**: 528–32.

19. Patrono C, Ciabattoni G, Patrignani P, et al. Clinical pharmacology of platelet cyclooxygenase inhibition. *Circulation* 1985;**72**: 1177–84.

20. FitzGerald GA, Oates JA, Hawiger J, et al.

Endogenous biosynthesis of prostacyclin and thromboxane and platelet function during chronic administration of aspirin in man. *J Clin Invest* 1983;**71**:676–88.

21. Pedersen AK, FitzGerald GA. Dose-related kinetics of aspirin. Presystemic acetylation of platelet cyclo-oxygenase. *N Engl J Med* 1984;**311**:1206–11.

22. Clarke RJ, Mayo G, Price P, FitzGerald GA. Suppression of thromboxane A₂ but not of systemic prostacyclin by controlled-release aspirin. *N Engl J Med* 1991;**325**:1137–41.

23. McAdam B, Keimowitz RM, Maher M, Fitzgerald DJ. Transdermal modification of platelet function: an aspirin patch system results in marked suppression of platelet cyclooxygenase. *J Pharmacol Exp Ther* 1996; **277**:559–64.

24. Vermylen J, Deckmyn H. Thromboxane synthase inhibitors and receptor antagonists. *Cardiovasc Drugs Ther* 1992;**6**:29–33.

25. Fitzgerald DJ, Doran J, Jackson E, FitzGerald GA. Coronary vascular occlusion mediated via thromboxane A₂-prostaglandin endoperoxide receptor activation in vivo. *J Clin Invest* 1986;**77**:496–502.

26. Guth BD, Muller TH. DTTX30, a combined thromboxane receptor antagonist and thromboxane synthetase inhibitor, prevents coronary thrombosis in anesthetized dogs. *Basic Res Cardiol* 1997;**92**:181–90.

27. Brownlie RP, Brownrigg NJ, Butcher HM, et al. ZD9583, an orally effective thromboxane A₂ synthase inhibitor and receptor antagonist with a sustained duration of action in rat and dog. *J Pharm Pharmacol* 1997;**49**:187–94.

28. Tranchesi B, Pileggi F, Vercammen E, Van de Werf F, Verstraete M. Ridogrel does not increase the speed and rate of coronary recanalization in patients with myocardial infarction treated with alteplase and heparin. *Eur Heart J* 1994;**15**:660–4.

29. The Ridogrel Versus Aspirin Patency Trial (RAPT). Randomized trial of ridogrel, a combined thromboxane A₂ synthase inhibitor and thromboxane A₂ prostaglandin endoperoxide receptor antagonist, versus aspirin as adjunct to thrombolysis in patients with acute myocardial infarction. *Circulation* 1994; **89**:588–95.

30. Balsano F, Violi F. Effect of picotamide on the clinical progression of peripheral vascular disease. A double-blind placebo-controlled study. *Circulation* 1993;**87**:1563–9.

31. von Schacky C, Fischer S, Weber PC. Long-term effects of dietary marine omega-3 fatty acids upon plasma and cellular lipids, platelet function, and eicosanoid formation in humans. *J Clin Invest* 1985;**76**:1626–31.

32. Catella F, Lawson J, Braden G, Fitzgerald DJ, Shipp E, FitzGerald GA. Biosynthesis of P_{450} products of arachidonic acid in humans: increased formation in cardiovascular disease. *Adv Prost Thromb Leuk Res* 1991; **21A**:193–6.

33. Stone NJ. Fish consumption, fish oil, lipids, and coronary heart disease. *Circulation* 1996;**94**:2337–40.

34. Saltiel E, Ward A. Ticlopidine. A review of its pharmacodynamic and pharmacokinetic properties, and therapeutic efficacy in platelet-dependent disease states. *Drugs* 1987;**34**:222–62.

35. Boneu B, Destelle G. Platelet anti-aggregating activity and tolerance of clopidogrel in atherosclerotic patients. *Thromb Haemost* 1996; **76**:939–43.

36. CAPRIE Investigators. A randomized, blinded, trial of clopidogrel versus aspirin in patients at risk of ischaemic events (CAPRIE). *Lancet* 1996; **348**:1329–39.

37. Savi P, Combalbert J, Gaich C, et al. The anti-aggregating activity of clopidogrel is due to a metabolic activation by the hepatic cytochrome P_{450}-1A. *Thromb Haemost* 1994;**72**:313–17.

38. Bruno JJ. The mechanisms of action of ticlopidine. *Thromb Res* 1983;**4**:59–67.

39. Yang LH, Fareed J. Vasomodulatory action of clopidogrel and ticlopidine. *Thromb Res* 1997;**86**:479–91.

40. Savi P, Bernat A, Dumas A, Ait-Chek L, Herbert JM. Effect of aspirin and clopidogrel on platelet-dependent tissue factor expression in endothelial cells. *Thromb Res* 1994;**73**: 117–24.

41. Page Y, Tardy B, Zeni F, Comtet C, Terrana R, Bertrand J. Thrombotic thrombocytopenic purpura related to ticlopidine. *Lancet* 1991;**337**:774–6.

42. Kupfer Y, Tessler S. Ticlopidine and thrombotic thrombocytopenic purpura. *N Engl J Med* 1997;**337**:1245.

43. McTavish D, Faulds D, Goa KL. Ticlopidine. An updated review of its pharmacology and therapeutic use in platelet-dependent disorders. *Drugs* 1990;**40**:238–59.

44. FitzGerald GA. Ticlopidine in unstable angina. A more expensive aspirin? *Circulation* 1990;**82**:296–8.

45. Albiero R, Hall P, Itoh A, et al. Results of a consecutive series of patients receiving only antiplatelet therapy after optimized stent implantation. Comparison of aspirin alone versus combined ticlopidine and aspirin therapy. *Circulation* 1997;**95**:1145–56.

46. Goods CM, Al-Shaibi KF, Yadav SS, et al. Utilization of the coronary balloon-expandable coil stent without anticoagulation or intravascular ultrasound. *Circulation* 1996;**93**:1803–8.

47. MATTIS Investigators. Multicenter aspirin and ticlopidine trial after intracoronary stenting in high risk patients. *J Am Coll Cardiol* 1998;**31**:397A [Abstract].

48. Karrillon GJ, Morice MC, Benveniste E, et al. Intracoronary stent implantation without ultrasound guidance and with replacement of conventional anticoagulation by antiplatelet therapy. 30-day clinical outcome of the French Multicenter Registry. *Circulation* 1996;**94**:1519–27.

49. Schomig A, Neumann FJ, Kastrati A, et al. A randomized comparison of antiplatelet and anticoagulant therapy after the placement of coronary-artery stents. *N Engl J Med* 1996;**334**:1084–9.

50. STARS Investigators. Late clinical results of Stent Anticoagulation Regimen Study (STARS). *Circulation* 1997;**96**:3317 [Abstract].

51. Rupprecht H, Darius H, Borkowski U, et al. Comparison of antiplatelet effects of aspirin, ticlopidine, or their combination after stent implantation. *Circulation* 1998;**97**:1046–52.

52. Hall P, Nakamura S, Maiello L, et al. A randomized comparison of combined ticlopidine and aspirin therapy versus aspirin therapy alone after successful intravascular ultrasound-guided stent implantation. *Circulation* 1996;**93**:215–22.

53. Szto G, Linnemeier T, Lewis S, et al. Safety of 10 days of ticlopidine after coronary stenting—a randomised comparison with 30 days. Strategic Alternatives with Ticlopidine in Stenting study (SALTS). *J Am Coll Cardiol* 1998;**31**:352A [Abstract].

54. Kastrati A, Schuhlen H, Hausleiter J, et al. Restenosis after coronary stent placement and randomization to a 4-week combined antiplatelet or anticoagulant therapy: six-month angiographic follow-up of the Intracoronary Stenting and Antithrombotic Regimen (ISAR) Trial. *Circulation* 1997;**96**: 462–7.

55. Gent M, Blakely JA, Easton JD, et al. The Canadian American Ticlopidine Study (CATS) in thromboembolic stroke. *Lancet* 1989;**1**: 1215–20.

56. Hass WK, Easton JD, Adams HP, Jr., et al. A randomized trial comparing ticlopidine hydrochloride with aspirin for the prevention of stroke in high-risk patients. Ticlopidine Aspirin Stroke Study Group. *N Engl J Med* 1989;**321**:501–7.

57. Janzon L, Bergqvist D, Boberg J, et al. Prevention of myocardial infarction and stroke in patients with intermittent claudication; effects of ticlopidine. Results from STIMS, the Swedish Ticlopidine Multicentre Study. *J Int Med* 1990;**227**:301–8.

58. Becquemin JP. Effect of ticlopidine on the long-term patency of saphenous-vein bypass grafts in the legs. Etude de la Ticlopidine apres Pontage Femoro-Poplite and the Association Universitaire de Récherche en Chirurgie. *N Engl J Med* 1997;**337**:1726–31.

59. Humphries RG, Robertson MJ, Leff P. A novel series of P2T purinoceptor antagonists: definition of the role of ADP in arterial thrombosis. *Trends Pharmacol Sci* 1995; **16**:179–81.

60. Yu SM, Tsai SY, Kuo SC, Ou JT. Inhibition of platelet function by A02131-1, a novel inhibitor of cGMP-specific phosphodiesterase, in vitro and in vivo. *Blood* 1996;**87**:3758–67.

61. Grant SM, Goa KL. Iloprost. A review of its pharmacodynamic and pharmacokinetic properties, and therapeutic potential in peripheral vascular disease, myocardial ischaemia and extracorporeal circulation procedures. *Drugs* 1992;**43**:889–924.

62. Zoldhelyi P, McNatt J, Xu XM, et al. Prevention of arterial thrombosis by adenovirus-mediated transfer of cyclo-oxygenase gene. *Circulation* 1996;**93**:10–17.

63. Banning A, Brewer L, Wendt M, et al. Local delivery of platelets with encapsulated iloprost to balloon injured pig carotid arteries: effect on platelet deposition and neointima formation. *Thromb Haemost* 1997;**77**:190–6.

64. FitzGerald GA. Dipyridamole. *N Engl J Med* 1987;**316**:1247–57.

65. Diener HC, Cunha L, Forbes C, Sivenius J, Smets P, Lowenthal A. European Stroke Prevention Study. 2. Dipyridamole and acetylsalicylic acid in the secondary prevention of stroke. *J Neur Sci* 1996;**143**:1–13.

66. Trikha M, Rote WE, Manley PJ, Lucchesi BR, Markland FS. Purification and characterization of platelet aggregation inhibitors from snake venoms. *Thromb Res* 1994;**73**:39–52.

67. Huang TF, Liu CZ, Ouyang CH, Teng CM. Halysin, an antiplatelet Arg-Gly-Asp-containing snake venom peptide, as fibrinogen receptor antagonist. *Biochem Pharmacol* 1991;**42**:1209–19.

68. Zabloki JA, Miyano M, Garland RB, et al. Potent in vitro and in vivo inhibitors of platelet aggregation based upon the arg-gly-asp-phe sequence of fibrinogen. A proposal on the nature of the binding interaction between the arg-guanidine of RGDX mimetics and the platelet GPIIb-IIIa receptor. *J Med Chem* 1993;**36**:1811–19.

69. Liu CZ, Peng HC, Huang TF. Crotavirin, a potent platelet aggregation inhibitor purified from the venom of the snake *Crotalus viridis*. *Toxicon* 1995;**33**:1289–98.

70. Knight DM, Wagner C, Jordan R, et al. The immunogenicity of the 7E3 murine monoclonal Fab antibody fragment variable region is dramatically reduced in humans by substitution of human for murine constant regions. *Molec Immunol* 1995;**32**:1271–81.

71. The CAPTURE Investigators. Randomised placebo-controlled trial of abciximab before and during coronary intervention in refractory unstable angina: the CAPTURE Study. *Lancet* 1997;**349**:1429–35.

72. The EPIC Investigators. Use of a monoclonal antibody directed against the platelet glycoprotein IIb/IIIa receptor in high-risk coronary angioplasty. The EPIC Investigation. *N Engl J Med* 1994;**330**:956–61.

73. The EPILOG Investigators. Platelet glycoprotein IIb/IIIa receptor blockade and low-dose heparin during percutaneous coronary revascularization. The EPILOG Investigators. *N Engl J Med* 1997;**336**:1689–96.

74. Simoons ML, de Boer MJ, van den Brand MJ, et al. Randomized trial of a GPIIb/IIIa platelet receptor blocker in refractory unstable angina. European Cooperative Study Group. *Circulation* 1994;**89**:596–603.

75. Mascelli M, Lance E, Wagner CL. Abciximab (7E3) pharmacodynamics demonstrates an extended and gradual recovery from GPIIb/IIIa blockade. *Circulation* 1996;**94**:I-513 [Abstract].

76. Berkowitz SD, Harrington RA, Rund MM, Tcheng JE. Acute profound thrombocytopenia after C7E3 Fab (abciximab) therapy. *Circulation* 1997;**95**:809–13.

77. Stouffer G, Hu Z, Sajiid M, et al. β3 integrins are upregulated after vascular injury and modulate thrombospondin- and thrombin-induced proliferation of cultured smooth muscle cells. *Circulation* 1998;**97**:907–15.

78. Simpfendorfer C, Kottke-Marchant K, Lowrie M, et al. First chronic platelet glycoprotein IIb/IIIa integrin blockade. A randomized, placebo-controlled pilot study of xemilofiban in unstable angina with percutaneous coronary interventions. *Circulation* 1997;**96**:76–81.

79. IMPACT Investigators. Randomised placebo-controlled trial of effect of eptifibatide on complications of percutaneous coronary intervention: IMPACT-II. Integrilin to Minimise Platelet Aggregation and Coronary Thrombosis-II. *Lancet* 1997;**349**:1422–8.

80. Theroux P, Kouz S, Roy L, et al. Platelet membrane receptor glycoprotein IIb/IIIa antagonism in unstable angina. The Canadian Lamifiban Study. *Circulation* 1996;**94**:899–905.

81. Nobiletti J, Morse E, Sophia P, et al. Inhibition of platelet aggregation and release in vitro by GPIIb/IIIa receptor antagonists. *Circulation* 1997;**96**:I-721 [Abstract].

82. Pakala R, Willerson JT, Benedict CR. Effect of serotonin, thromboxane A$_2$, and specific receptor antagonists on vascular smooth muscle cell proliferation. *Circulation* 1997;**96**: 2280–6.

83. Murphy NP, Practico D, Fitzgerald DJ. Functional relevance of the expression of ligand induced binding sites in the response to platelet

GPIIb/IIIa antagonists in vivo. *J Pharmacol Exp Ther* 1998;**273**:20317–22.

84. Byrne A, Moran N, Maher M, Walsh N, Crean P, Fitzgerald DJ. Continued thromboxane A₂ formation despite administration of a platelet glycoprotein IIb/IIIa antagonist in patients undergoing coronary angioplasty. *Arterioscler Thromb Vasc Biol* 1997;**17**:3224–9.

85. Reverter JC, Beguin S, Kessels H, Kumar R, Hemker HC, Coller BS. Inhibition of platelet-mediated, tissue factor-induced thrombin generation by the mouse/human chimeric 7E3 antibody. Potential implications for the effect of c7E3 Fab treatment on acute thrombosis and 'clinical restenosis'. *J Clin Invest* 1996;**98**:863–74.

86. Ammar T, Scudder LE, Coller BS. In vitro effects of the platelet glycoprotein IIb/IIIa receptor antagonist c7E3 Fab on the activated clotting time. *Circulation* 1997;**95**:614–17.

87. Kereiakes DJ, Runyon JP, Kleiman NS, et al. Differential dose-response to oral xemilofiban after antecedent intravenous abciximab. Administration for complex coronary intervention. *Circulation* 1996;**94**:906–10.

88. Umemura K, Kondo K, Ikeda Y, Nakashima M. Enhancement by ticlopidine of the inhibitory effect on in vitro platelet aggregation of the glycoprotein IIb/IIIa inhibitor tirofiban. *Thromb Haemost* 1997;**78**:1381–4.

89. Phillips DR, Teng W, Arfsten A, et al. Effect of Ca²⁺ on GP IIb-IIIa interactions with integrilin: enhanced GP IIb-IIIa binding and inhibition of platelet aggregation by reductions in the concentration of ionized calcium in plasma anticoagulated with citrate. *Circulation* 1997;**96**:1488–94.

90. Wallen NH, Ladjevardi M, Albert J, Broijersen A. Influence of different anticoagulants on platelet aggregation in whole blood; a comparison between citrate, low molecular mass heparin and hirudin. *Thromb Res* 1997;**87**:151–7.

91. Coller BS, Folts JD, Smith SR, Scudder LE, Jordan R. Abolition of in vivo platelet thrombus formation in primates with monoclonal antibodies to the platelet GPIIb/IIIa receptor. Correlation with bleeding time, platelet aggregation, and blockade of GPIIb/IIIa receptors. *Circulation* 1989;**80**:1766–74.

92. Coller BS, Lang D, Scudder LE. Rapid and simple platelet function assay to assess glycoprotein IIb/IIIa receptor blockade. *Circulation* 1997;**95**:860–7.

93. Henn V, Slupsky JR, Grafe M, et al. CD40 ligand on activated platelets triggers an inflammatory reaction of endothelial cells. *Nature* 1998;**391**:591–4.

Section II:

Antiplatelet agents

6

Aspirin and dipyridamole

Freek WA Verheugt

Introduction

Thrombosis plays a major role in the patho-genesis of cardiovascular diseases. Throm-boses in both coronary and cerebral arteries are complications of atherosclerosis, the most important single cause of mortality in the Western world. Both myocardial and cerebral infarction cause impressive mortality and mor-bidity in millions of patients each year. Not only arterial thrombosis but also thrombosis in the heart cavities is responsible for the major morbidity and mortality of cardiovascu-lar disease. Intracardiac thrombosis can be seen in atrial fibrillation, in patients with arti-ficial valves and in those with left ventricular aneurysms.

From the 1950s antithrombotic therapy has been applied with large success to prevent these frequently fatal thrombotic complica-tions. Anticoagulants (heparin and coumadin) were the first antithrombotic agents used in the prevention and treatment of arterial thrombosis. In the 1970s agents interfering with platelet function were introduced and found to be effective in the prevention and treatment of arterial thrombosis. Males and females benefit equally from antiplatelet ther-apy in the secondary prevention of cardiovas-cular disease.[1] In hypertensive patients, the efficacy of antiplatelet agents is similar to that in normotensives and in diabetes antiplatelet therapy is as effective as in non-diabetics.[1]

The most regularly used antiplatelet agents in cardiovascular disease are aspirin (acetylsal-icylic acid) and dipyridamole (Persantin).[1]

Pharmacology of aspirin and Persantin

Pharmacology of aspirin

The effect of aspirin on haemostasis has been recognized for several decades. The second step of the aggregation of blood platelets by ADP is almost completely blocked by the drug.

Platelet aggregation is one of the pathways through which clots are formed on damaged arterial wall. Platelets can aggregate under sev-eral stimuli, one of which is mediated through thromboxane A_2 a platelet specific pros-taglandin that can only be generated in the presence of cyclo-oxygenase. Cyclo-oxygenase production is regulated in the cell nucleus. Aspirin inactivates cyclo-oxygenase. Since platelets lack nuclei, cyclo-oxygenase is inacti-vated irreversibly by aspirin during the life of the platelet. Therefore, one dose of aspirin blocks, almost completely, and for several days the platelet's ability to aggregate via the thromboxane pathway and produce further thromboxane (Figure 6.1). Thromboxane promotes platelet aggregation and also vaso-constriction. Each active mechanism in nature is counterbalanced: in this case, platelet

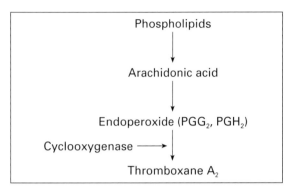

Figure 6.1
Platelet prostaglandin metabolism

thromboxane production and aggregation is opposed by the endothelial generation of prostaglandin I$_2$ (PGI$_2$ prostacyclin), which inhibits platelet aggregation and which also dilates blood vessels. Prostacyclin production is also mediated by cyclo-oxygenase and therefore is also inhibited by aspirin (Figure 6.2). However, the nucleated endothelial cell generates cyclo-oxygenase in large quantities and the aspirin-induced inhibition is short-lived. These mechanisms explain the effect of aspirin

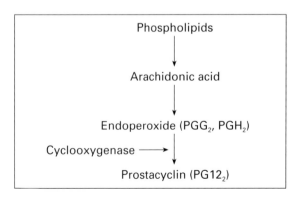

Figure 6.2
Endothelial prostaglandin metabolism

on the platelet–vessel wall interaction and thus its long-standing effect on haemostasis.

Oral aspirin blocks venous thromboxane within 5 minutes following ingestion, which suggests the presystemic acetylation of cyclo-oxygenase.[2] Antithrombotic tolerance of aspirin is highly unlikely.[2] In the 1970s aspirin was found to have a paradoxical effect on bleeding time. Bleeding time is still the best in vivo parameter of platelet activity. The inverse dose–response curve is due to the fact, that high dosages of aspirin block completely both thromboxane and prostacyclin production, while ultra low dosages (10 mg per day) block thromboxane production by only 50% leaving endothelial prostacyclin production intact.[3]

Recently, two isoforms of cyclo-oxygenase have been identified: COX-1, the ubiquitous constitutive cyclo-oxygenase; and COX-2, which is inducible by cytokines and growth factors and can be found in smooth muscle cells, monocytes, proliferating vascular smooth muscle cells and dysfunctioning endothelium (Table 6.1). Both forms mediate the formation of prostaglandins and, thus of thromboxane A$_2$ from arachidonic acid. Acetylsalicylic acid (aspirin) fits like a key in COX-1 and inactivates it almost completely, but leaves COX-2 relatively intact at the current antithrombotic dose.[4] Non-steroidal anti-inflammatory drugs (NSAIDS) other than aspirin inhibit both COX-1 and COX-2. In 1990, it was detected that, in some patients with unstable angina, thromboxane biosynthesis persisted despite aspirin therapy. Two theories were proposed to explain this:

(1) Prostaglandin precursors (endoperoxides) formed in atheromatous cells in a COX-2 environment switch over to platelets that have adhered locally and which can produce TXA$_2$ from these 'imported' endoperoxides; or

	COX-1	COX-2
Expression	Constitutive	Inducible by growth factors and cytokines, for example
Prevalence	Ubiquitous	Monocytes, macrophages, proliferating vascular smooth muscle cells, dysfunctioning endothelium
Product	Prostaglandin endoperoxides	Prostaglandin endoperoxides
Major inhibitor(s)	Low-dose aspirin, ibuprofen	High-dose aspirin, ibuprofen

Table 6.1
Biological properties of the cyclo-oxygenase (COX) isoforms.

(2) Monocytes, which are almost always involved in unstable atheromatous plaques, produce TXA_2 themselves and that this reaction is catalysed by COX-2 and COX-1 after aspirin clearance, since monocytes are nucleated.

It should be noted that ibuprofen suppresses the apparently extraplatelet TXA_2 production better than aspirin at the normal antithrombotic dose.[5]

These observations cast a new light on the strong preventative effects of aspirin in cardiovascular disease. Platelet activation on the one hand, and platelet inhibition on the other, are major players in the acute thrombotic syndromes such as unstable angina, acute myocardial infarction and stroke. Aspirin, although effective[1] and extremely cost-effective,[6] is a relatively weak platelet inhibitor. This makes it a safe and widely applicable agent but its protective mechanism may go far behind thromboxane-dependent platelet-aggregation inhibition. Therefore, trial regimens comparing a new platelet inhibitor to aspirin should include aspirin because of its, thus far, poorly understood protective mechanisms. A classic example of this is the outcome of the CAPRIE trial, in which the strong platelet inhibitor clopidogrel alone was compared with aspirin alone. In the 6000 post-myocardial infarction patients there was no benefit of clopidogrel, since it was not show to inhibit platelets more strongly than aspirin.[7] Nevertheless, there are still some new antiplatelet drug trials running with one or more treatment arms without aspirin.

Dose of aspirin

The most widely used and effective dosage of aspirin in cardiovascular disease is between 50 mg and 325 mg daily. Usually life-long administration of aspirin is recommended in cardiovascular patients. Since the 1980s low-dose aspirin has been introduced and found to be equally effective as high-dose aspirin when compared with placebo or control treatment.[1] Comparative trials on aspirin dosing have been conducted in stroke patients[8,9] and in those with peripheral vascular disease.[10] Although the number of direct comparison trials is small and only less than 5000 patients have been studied, the outcome of these trials is interesting not only in terms of side-effects but also efficacy. Overall prevention of cardiovascular death, myocardial infarction and stroke was similar with high- or low-dose aspirin; however, non-fatal myocardial infarction was consistently better prevented with the higher dose in the trials.[11] This may suggest that, besides its antiplatelet effect, aspirin has also other actions, such as antiphlogistic activity, which may interfere with the inflammatory processes underlying the acute complications of atherosclerosis. Interestingly, in carotid atherosclerosis detected using ultrasonography, aspirin in a dose of 900 mg daily seems to lead to disease regression, while a daily dose of 50 mg leads to disease progression.[12] Recently, high-dose intravenous aspirin showed to improve acutely endothelial dysfunction in the femoral arteries of coronary patients.[13] Apparently cyclo-oxygenase-dependent endothelium-driven vasomotion exists in man. These observations suggest that, in cardiovascular patients, aspirin has a greater effect than platelet inhibition alone. This may have implications for the eternal search for the optimal aspirin dose.

There is probably no 'highest' dose of aspirin, where the inhibition of prostacyclin overrules its antiplatelet effect, although more research is clearly needed in this field.

Side-effects of aspirin

Aspirin causes gastrointestinal ulceration and subsequent bleeding. Gastric discomfort is also a common side-effect of aspirin. These adverse effects are clearly dose-related and their incidence declines with lowering the aspirin dose. Allergy and bronchospasm are extremely rare side-effects.

Pharmacology of dipyridamole

Dipyridamole (2,6-bis-diethanolamino-4,8-dipiperidinopyrimido-5,4-d-pyrimidine) is derived from the papaverine family. It interferes with adenosine uptake in many cells, including red blood cells and vascular smooth muscle cells. Owing to its vasodilating properties, it was introduced as an antianginal agent, but has been found to induce myocardial ischaemia. Its intravenous formulation is now used solely for the diagnostic induction of stress-induced myocardial ischaemia, for example, instead of thallium scintigraphy in patients unable to exercise physically. Dipyridamole also inhibits adenosine uptake in the platelet and, therefore, diminishes platelet adhesion and possibly subsequent aggregation.

Its clinical efficacy as a single agent is, however, questionable,[1] as such it is almost uniformly used in combination with aspirin. The benefit of combination therapy with aspirin is also debatable, however.[1] Recently, one large placebo-controlled study in over 6600 patients, who had suffered a transient ischemic attack or minor stroke, dipyridamole provided secondary prevention of stroke or death with the same magnitude as low dose aspirin alone[14] suggesting that the drug has a place as monotherapy in cerebrovascular disease: RR reduction with aspirin alone 13% ($p = 0.016$), with dipyridamole alone 15% ($p = 0.015$) and with aspirin and dipyridamole 24% ($p < 0.001$). This may be of interest to patients who do not tolerate aspirin.

Dose of dipyridamole

The usual dosage of dipyridamole is

75–100 mg three times daily. Recently a slow-release formulation of 200 mg to be given twice daily has become available.

Side-effects of dipyridamole

Owing to its vasodilating properties, dipyridamole may induce headache and vertigo; sometimes flushing is noted. Nausea, vomiting and diarrhoea are rare side-effects. These adverse effects usually disappear rapidly following drug withdrawal.

Conclusions

Both aspirin and Persantin (dipyridamole) are well-tolerated antiplatelet agents. Although aspirin is a relatively weak platelet inhibitor, its efficacy and safety is overwhelming and its cost-effectiveness in the management of cardiovascular disease unparalleled. Aspirin in its usual low-dose formulation irreversibly blocks platelet cyclo-oxygenase, but not extraplatelet prostaglandin production by, for example, macrophages and proliferating smooth muscle cells. Persantin is an antiplatelet agent with a questionable efficacy. Although it is probably safe, its main use is as an intravenous drug to precipitate myocardial ischaemia for diagnostic purposes.

References

1. Antiplatelet Trialists' Collaboration. Collaborative overview of randomised trials of antiplatelet therapy I: prevention of death, myocardial infarction, and stroke by prolonged antiplatelet therapy in various categories of patients. *Br Med J* 1994;**308**:81–106.
2. Pedersen AK, Fitzgerald GA. Dose-related kinetics of aspirin. Presystemic acetylation of platelet cyclo-oxygenase. *N Engl J Med* 1984;**311**:1206–11.
3. Toivanen J, Ylikorkala O, Viinikka L. One milligramme of acetylsalicylic acid daily inhibits platelet thromboxane A_2 production. *Thromb Res* 1984;**35**:681–7.
4. Schror K. Aspirin and platelets: the antiplatelet action of aspirin and its role in thrombosis treatment and prophylaxis. *Sem Thrombos Hemostas* 1997;**23**:349–55.
5. Cipollone F, Patrignani P, Greco A, Panara MR, Padavano R, Cuccurullo F, et al. Differential suppression of thromboxane biosynthesis by indobufen and aspirin in patients with unstable angina. *Circulation* 1997;**96**:1109–16.
6. Verheugt FWA. Aspirin, the poor man's statin? *Lancet* 1998;**351**:227–8.
7. CAPRIE Steering Committee. A randomised, blinded, trial of clopidogrel versus aspirin in patients at risk of ischaemic events (CAPRIE). *Lancet* 1996;**349**:1329–39.
8. Farrell B, Godwin J, Richards S, Warlow C. United Kingdom transient ischaemic attack (UK-TIA) aspirin trial: final results. *J Neurol Neurosurg Psychiatry* 1991;**54**:1044–54.
9. Van Gijn J, Algra A, Kappelle J, Koudstaal PJ, Van Latum A. A comparison of two doses of aspirin (30 vs 383 mg a day) in patients after a transient ischemic attack or minor stroke. *N Engl J Med* 1991;**325**:1261–6.
10. Heiss HW, Just H, Middleton D, Deichsel G. Reocclusion prophylaxis with dipyridamole combined with acetyl salicylic acid following PTA. *Angiology* 1990;**41**:263–9.
11. Verheugt FWA. Differential dose effect of aspirin in the primary prevention of myocardial infarction. *J Am Coll Cardiol* 1998;**31**(**Suppl. A**):352A.
12. Ranke C, Hecker H, Creutzig A, Alexander K. Dose-dependent effect of aspirin on carotid atherosclerosis. *Circulation* 1993;**87**:1873–9.
13. Husain S, Andrews NP, Mulcahy D, Panza JA, Quyyumi A. Aspirin improves endothelial dysfunction in atherosclerosis. *Circulation* 1998;**97**:716–20.
14. Diener HC, Cunha L, Forbes C, Silvenius J, Smets P, Lowenthal A. European Stroke Prevention Study 2. Dipyridamole and acetylsalicylic acid in the secondary prevention of stroke. *J Neurol Sciences* 1996;**143**:1–13.

7

Ticlopidine and clopidogrel

Karsten Schrör

Introduction

Ticlopidine and clopidogrel are two structurally related thienopyridines without any structural relationship to other antiplatelet agents (Figure 7.1). The first report on the antiplatelet effects of oral ticlopidine in man was published more than 20 years ago.[1] The inhibition of platelet function by this compound appeared to be specific for ADP. Maximum effects were observed after 5–6 days of treatment and antiplatelet effects persisted for several days after drug withdrawal. Similar data were reported a few years later for the more potent analog clopidogrel (PCR 4099).[2,3] The oral activity and the apparent irreversibility of antiplatelet actions of ticlopidine and clopidogrel resembled the antiplatelet actions of aspirin. However, it was obvious that its mechanism of action could not be the same because the thienopyridines did not interfere with the arachidonic acid metabolism, that is, platelet-dependent thromboxane formation. This paper summarizes the pharmacology and clinical pharmacology of these two compounds.

Pharmacology

Inhibition of ADP-induced platelet activation

Ticlopidine and clopidogrel exclusively inhibit ADP-induced platelet activation. This involves both platelet-derived ADP, that is, ADP released from the platelet dense granules[4] as well as ADP from non-platelet sources, such as red blood cells. Regarding the mechanism of action, the following steps of ADP-induced platelet aggregation are possible targets of thienopyridines:

(1) Platelet ADP-receptors;
(2) Phospholipase C (PLC) and a subsequent increase in cytosolic Ca^{2+};
(3) Adenylate cyclase and an increase in cAMP; and
(4) Mobilization of the GPIIb-IIIa complex, with subsequent clustering and binding of soluble fibrinogen, in other words platelet aggregation.

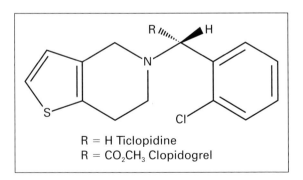

R = H Ticlopidine
R = CO_2CH_3 Clopidogrel

Figure 7.1
Chemical structure of ticlopidine and clopidogrel.

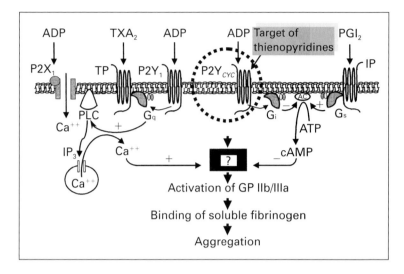

Figure 7.2

Signal transduction pathways for ADP-induced platelet activation and possible targets of clopidogrel and ticlopidine. (After Schrör, 1998,[5] modified with permission.)

ADP receptors

Platelets contain at least three subsets of ADP receptors that are involved in ADP-induced platelet activation and these are probably coupled to different signal transduction pathways, namely, P2X1, $P2Y_{CYC}$ (or P2T) and P2Y1.[6–8] The exact molecular nature of the interactions between ADP and its platelet receptors and the modification of these interactions by thienopyridines is not, however, completely understood.[9,10] The initial, ADP-induced stimulation of the rapid Ca^{2+} entry from the extracellular space is mediated via the P2X1 receptor. This receptor is coupled to an ionic channel and is not a target for the thienopyridines.[8] The two G-protein-coupled receptors $P2Y_{CYC}$ and P2Y1 are connected to the inhibition of adenylate cyclase by ADP via the G-protein G_i and stimulation of PLC and Ca^{2+} entry via the G-

protein G_q. It is not entirely clear, however, whether these two G-protein-coupled receptors are structurally distinct.[6,11] What is known, however, is that, thienopyridines reduce ADP binding to G-protein-coupled platelet receptors by 60–70%.[9,12–14] Nevertheless the rationale behind this is unknown: structural and/or functional changes of the receptor(s) that result in reduced ADP-binding might occur at the level of the platelet or the megakaryocyte, or an irreversible binding of the thienopyridines to the ADP receptor(s) might occur, thus preventing access of the agonist. The affinity of the receptors to ADP remains unchanged, however. The inhibition is nevertheless apparently irreversible, that is non-competitive, and, therefore, cannot be antagonized by increasing the concentration of the agonist ADP. There is also evidence for an impaired G-protein coupling and interruption of further signal transduction.[15] About 20–30% of receptors remain unchanged. Since neither clopidogrel nor ticlopidine affect platelet shape change, it was suggested that this population of receptors, possibly connected to the P2Y1-ADP-receptor subtype, might cause platelet shape change.[8]

ADP-induced activation of PLC and cytosolic Ca^{2+}

Platelet P2Y1 receptors are coupled to PLC via G_q and mediate the increase in cytosolic Ca^{2+} after stimulation by ADP.[6,10] The significance of these receptors for ADP-induced platelet aggregation is demonstrated by the failure of platelets of G_q-knock-out mice to aggregate in response to ADP.[16] However, these receptors are pharmacologically distinct from the $P2Y_{CYC}$ receptor.[6] Neither ticlopidine[17] nor clopidogrel[18] cause any changes of ADP-induced stimulation of cytosolic Ca^{2+} levels in human platelets ex vivo, suggesting that the antiplatelet effects of thienopyridines in man do not involve changes in cytosolic Ca^{2+} levels.

ADP-induced inhibition of adenylate cyclase activity

Stimulation of platelets by ADP inhibits adenylate cyclase activity and reduces (stimulated) cAMP levels.[19] Although several studies have suggested that ticlopidine and clopidogrel suppress this ADP-mediated inhibition of the adenylate cyclase,[13,17,20] several others were unable to confirm this.[21–23] Available evidence suggests that thienopyridines antagonize the ADP-induced decrease in platelet cAMP, and that this effect is possibly significant in vivo,[9] for example under conditions of locally elevated prostacyclin levels.

GPIIb-IIIa complex

The common final step of platelet activation is the mobilization of GPIIb-IIIa with subsequent conformational changes, enabling the complex to bind soluble fibrinogen, that is, to form platelet aggregates. Thienopyridines inhibit the ADP-induced conformational changes in the GPIIb-IIIa complex and the subsequent aggregate formation.[18,24] The ADP-induced fibrinogen binding to the GPIIb-IIIa receptor is reduced by about 70%.[18,25,26] These actions of thienopyridines are not caused by structural changes of the GPIIb-IIIa complex, that is the platelet fibrinogen receptor itself[3,27] but rather to an earlier event that is associated with the ADP-receptor stimulation.[18] The fibrinogen binding after stimulation by other agonists (e.g. thrombin, thromboxane mimetics) is also diminished. All of these inhibitory actions are abolished by ADP scavengers, such as apyrase, suggesting that they are ADP-mediated.

Another consequence of reduced fibrinogen binding is that there are more loosely packed platelet aggregates and reduced platelet secretion, including surface expression of P-selectin.[4,18,27–29] This might facilitate deaggregation after stimulation by different agonists and results clinically in a facilitated resolution of platelet thrombi.

Active principle(s) of thienopyridines

Ticlopidine and clopidogrel do not inhibit ADP-induced platelet aggregation in platelet-rich plasma in vitro but do so after oral administration ex vivo. This and other findings, such as the biotransformation of thienopyridines by the hepatic CYP450 system,[30–32] have led to the conclusion that thienopyridines have to undergo a bioactivation in vivo, eventually resulting in generation of active metabolite(s). These yet unidentified active metabolite(s), generated by the liver, are thought to be the active principle that alters certain platelet purinergic receptors in a way that prevents binding of ADP and inhibits further signaling.[9,33] It has also been suggested

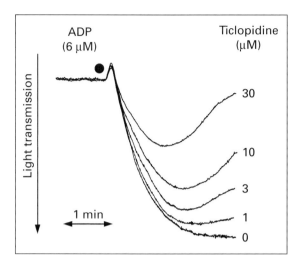

Figure 7.3
Concentration-dependent inhibition of ADP-induced platelet aggregation by ticlopidine in vitro. (After Weber et al, unpublished results.[35])

that the antiplatelet effects of ticlopidine and clopidogrel are not mediated by metabolites detectable in the plasma but are related to a permanent alteration of platelet ADP receptor(s).[21,34]

Recent studies have challenged some of these concepts. Weber and colleagues[23] have demonstrated that both clopidogrel and ticlopidine selectively block ADP-induced aggregation of washed human platelets in vitro (Figure 7.3). No such effect was seen in the presence of plasma or albumin, thus excluding hepatic biotransformation as an essential step for antiplatelet activity. The anti-aggregatory effects of clopidogrel were unchanged when the compound was removed from the platelet suspension buffer, confirming that the active principle is bound to the platelet. Thus, thienopyridines might not be able to bind in

sufficient amounts to the platelets because of a higher affinity binding to plasma albumin, being partially irreversible.[26] DiPerri and colleagues[36] had already shown that the time-course of inhibition of platelet aggregation by ticlopidine ex vivo paralleled that of the platelet-bound unchanged compound. These data do not exclude the possibility of additional effects of metabolites generated by hepatic biotransformation. However, none of the at least 13 structurally identified metabolites of ticlopidine was found to be active in vitro and hepatic biotransformation of thienopyridines was studied mainly in laboratory animals, receiving 10–50-fold higher doses of ticlopidine on a weight basis than that administered to man.

Pharmacokinetic aspects of antiplatelet action

After oral administration, ticlopidine is almost completely (90%) absorbed and subject to intensive hepatic biotransformation. Only 1% of the drug is excreted unchanged in the urine.[32,33] Similar results might be expected for clopidogrel. Only trace level (1–2 ng/ml) of the unchanged compound were detected in human plasma after 16 days of treatment.[31] Regular daily intake of ticlopidine over 3 weeks is associated with a prolongation of its half-life from 7–8 hours to about 4 days (Table 7.1). This is associated with a maximum 3–7-fold increase in the AUC and a 2–3-fold increase in C_{max}.[37,38] The plasma levels of ticlopidine are twice as much in the elderly (mean age 70 years) compared with younger people (mean age 29 years) (see Table 7.1), and in patients with impaired renal function (glomerular filtration rate—GFR: 10–30 ml/min) compared with healthy controls.[38] The fractional increase in unchanged ticlopidine after multiple dosing suggests saturation of the metabolism.[32]

Parameter	Day 1		Day 21	
	Young	Elderly	Young	Elderly
C_{max} [µg/ml]	0.41	0.70*	0.89	1.42*
t_{max} [h]	2.0	2.0	1.0	2.0
$t_{1/2}$ [h]	7.9	12.7*	98	91*
AUC [µg.h/ml]	1.4	2.8	3.6	8.3*
C_{AV} [µg/ml]	–	–	0.30	0.69*

*Significant difference by comparison with Day 1; n = 11–13.

†Abbreviations: C_{max}, maximum plasma concentration; t_{max}, time of maximum plasma concentration; $t_{1/2}$, plasma elimination half-life; AUC, total area under the plasma concentration-time-curve; C_{AV}: average steady-state plasma concentration (AUC/12 [dosing interval in hours]).

‡Reproduced from Shah et al. 1991,[37] with permission.

Table 7.1
Pharmacokinetic parameters of oral ticlopidine (250 mg) once (day 1) or twice daily for 21 days (day 21) in young (mean 29 years) and elderly (mean 70 years) subjects.

An antiplatelet effect of ticlopidine can be detected 2–3 hours after oral administration. However, a clinically relevant effect requires treatment for 2–3 days and a maximum inhibition of platelet function is seen after about 1 week.[39] The reasons for this slow-onset reaction are under discussion. One possibility is the time-dependent generation of an active metabolite, another the saturation of a deep compartment with the active compound.[36] The half-life of the antiplatelet activity is about 5 days and platelet function fully recovers after about 1 week,[39] suggesting normalization of platelet function according to platelet turnover. Similar data have been reported for clopidogrel.[13,31,40] Administration of a loading dose of clopidogrel (375 mg) resulted in 80% inhibition of ADP-induced platelet aggregation after 5 hours while a maximal (about 2-fold) prolongation in bleeding time was seen after 3 days.[41]

No differences in inhibition of platelet function or prolongation of bleeding time were seen between 1 week and 3 months of continuous administration of clopidogrel (75 mg/day) compared with steady state inhibition at 8–12 days.[42,43] There appear also to be no differences in the antiplatelet activity between young and elderly patients and between patients with and without atherosclerosis.[44] These data suggest that the prolonged half-life of ticlopidine and clopidogrel metabolites after a regular daily intake is not transferred into any potentiation of antiplatelet effects or prolongation of bleeding time. Clearly, these findings are also compatible with the view that the antiplatelet effect of thienopyridines is caused by the compounds themselves and is independent of any hepatic biotransformation that possibly generates products that do not affect platelet function.

Antiplatelet and antithrombotic effects of ticlopidine and clopidogrel in vivo

There are numerous sources of adenine nucleotides, including ADP, in vivo, for example erythrocytes. ATP in whole blood can be dephosphorylated to ADP.[45] In endothelial injury, the ADPase activity of the endothelium may, however, be reduced,[46] eventually resulting in higher local levels of ADP at a site of endothelial dysfunction, which will be further elevated in adhering platelet thrombi. In platelet aggregates, local extracellular nucleotide concentrations might temporarily exceed 100 µM.[45] Thus, ADP from platelet and non-platelet sources is an important platelet agonist in vivo, particularly at sites of vessel injury.[47]

Shear-stress-induced platelet aggregation, which is largely mediated by ADP,[48,49] is only modestly sensitive to aspirin.[50-52] Conversely, platelets from ticlopidine-treated volunteers exhibit reduced aggregation and reduced deposition to the subendothelium under shear-stress conditions.[53-55] Inhibition of platelet adhesion was also demonstrated for clopidogrel.[56] Consequently, the thienopyridines may become most valuable agents to prevent the consequences of ADP accumulation for local thrombus formation. In addition, both ADP and TXA_2 have a synergistic effect in the hemostatic process, providing the background for the combined use of thienopyridines and aspirin (cf. Figure 7.1).

Prevention of atherothrombotic vessel occlusion in patients at elevated vascular risk

Oral long-term prevention

Several controlled clinical trials have shown that oral administration of ticlopidine or clopidogrel has a protective effect with regard to acute thromboembolic arterial occlusion, that is myocardial infarction and stroke, in patients at elevated vascular risk. The CATS trial[57] studied the action of ticlopidine in 1053 patients with ischemic stroke (no cardioembolic strokes). Treatment was started within 1 week to 4 months (average 6 weeks) after the acute event. Patients received either ticlopidine (250 mg b.i.d.) or placebo in a double-blind randomized order for about 2 years. The combined primary endpoint was the occurrence of a new vascular event (e.g. myocardial infarction, stroke, vascular death). The incidence was 15.3% in the placebo group and 10.8% in the ticlopidine group, which was equivalent to a relative risk reduction by 30.2% ($P = 0.006$).

The TASS trial[58] compared ticlopidine (250 mg b.i.d.) with aspirin (650 mg b.i.d.) in 3069 patients with cerebral ischemia (those with transient ischemic attacks—TIA, amaurosis fugax, minor stroke with at least 80% recovery within 3 weeks) but without preceding major stroke. The qualifying event occurred within the last 3 months prior to entry into the trial, the observation period was between 2 and 6 years, the mean duration of treatment was 2–2.5 years. The primary endpoint was non-lethal stroke or death, independent of the cause. The combined risk at 3 years was 17% for ticlopidine and 19% for aspirin. This was equivalent to a 12% relative-risk reduction. The combined risk of lethal and non-lethal stroke was 10% for ticlopidine and 13% for aspirin. This was equivalent to a relative risk reduction of 21% ($P = 0.024$). The maximum therapeutic benefit was obtained after 1 year and remained unchanged thereafter.

The STIMS-trial[59] investigated the effects of ticlopidine on ischemic events in 687 patients with intermittent claudication in a placebo-controlled double-blind trial. Exclusion criteria were recent myocardial infarction (less than 3 months) and insulin-dependent diabetes mellitus. The mean duration of treatment was 5.6 years. Ticlopidine (250 mg b.i.d.) reduced total mortality by 29% ($P = 0.015$), mainly from a reduction of myocardial infarctions.

There is only one large-scale clinical study of clopidogrel, the CAPRIE trial. Gent et al[60] compared clopidogrel (75 mg/day) with aspirin (325 mg/day) in 19 185 patients with previous myocardial infarction, stroke or advanced peripheral arterial disease. Treatment was for 1–3 years, with a median 1.9 years. The primary endpoint events (new myocardial infarction, ischemic stroke or cardiac death) were reduced from 5.8% in the aspirin group to 5.3% in the clopidogrel group, which was equivalent to a relative-risk reduction of 8.7% ($P = 0.043$) for the combined endpoint in favour of clopidogrel.

These and several smaller studies[26] indicate that ticlopidine and clopidogrel are effective antithrombotic compounds in patients at high vascular risk of atherothrombotic vessel occlusion. Both compounds were slightly but significantly (by about 10%) more effective than aspirin in the TASS and CAPRIE trial. In addition to the different mode of action of aspirin and thienopyridines, the different spectrum of side-effects (see later discussion) is also of considerable interest and forms the background for alternative or combined use of these antiplatelet agents.

PTCA *and stenting*

The most common area of application for thienopyridines in cardiology is following stent placement, as described in Chapter 15. PTCA and coronary stenting is associated with a significant platelet activation (assessed in terms of expression of platelet adhesion molecules) which is not antagonized by conventional anticoagulant treatment with aspirin, heparin and coumadin. The platelet activation, determined by measuring activated platelet fibrinogen receptors (LIBS), was prevented by combined treatment with ticlopidine and aspirin.[61] Platelet-derived ADP is an important determinant for cyclic flow variations in stenosed arteries. Yao et al,[62] using the model of coronary artery injury/stenosis-induced cyclic flow variations in dogs, have shown that clopidogrel prevents the reoccurrence of cyclic flow reductions, being comparable to the combination of apyrase and thromboxane receptor blockade (SQ 29548). Similar results were obtained in pigs with injury/stenosis-induced injury of the femoral artery.[63] This suggests that the combined inhibition of thromboxane- and ADP-induced platelet activation may provide supraadditive protection from shear-stress-induced platelet activation at a site of endothelial injury. Rupprecht and colleagues reported that combined use of ticlopidine and aspirin was superior to either compound alone with respect to inhibition of platelet activation after stent implantation.[64] Aspirin alone (300 mg/day) did not affect ADP-induced platelet aggregation, expression of GP IIb/IIIa receptors or fibrinogen binding but enhanced the antiplatelet responses to ticlopidine (250 mg b.i.d.) (Table 7.2). In agreement with experimental studies, it was found that ticlopidine had to be administered at least 3 days before the acute intervention to be fully active.[65] Several controlled clinical trials also

Parameter	A		B		C	
	d1	d14	d1	d14	d1	d14
Platelet aggregation	75±1	55±3*	72±3	53±4*	73±2	72±2
CD62p expression	68±3	41±3*	65±3	39±4*	66±3	63±2
Fibrinogen binding	61±4	36±4*	58±2	39±3*	59±4	57±4

*Significant difference at Day 1.

[†]All patients were on heparin (d1) and were pretreated with 100 mg/day aspirin until the day of PTCA (d 1). The patients were then randomly assigned to one of the following groups: A, aspirin (300 mg/day) + ticlopidine (250 mg b.i.d.); B, ticlopidine (250 mg b.i.d.); C, aspirin (300 mg/day).

Data are mean ± SEM in percent of the respective control after stimulation by ADP.

[‡]After Rupprecht et al,[66] with permission.

Table 7.2
Time-dependent antiplatelet effects of aspirin, ticlopidine or their combination in 61 patients, subjected to PTCA and stent implantation.

indicate that the combined use of ticlopidine and aspirin is more effective and has less side effects than conventional therapy with anticoagulants.[66–73] Similar beneficial results were obtained in a prospective study in 529 patients who received stents as a bail-out procedure for failed angioplasty or suboptimum result of PTCA.[74] The beneficial effects of ticlopidine on acute stented vessel occlusion, i.e. recurrent myocardial infarction, were maintained at 6 months but no effect on restenosis was observed[67] confirming earlier data in patients after angioplasty.[75,76] This issue has not been studied so far with clopidogrel.

In clinical practice, ticlopidine plus aspirin has supplanted chronic coumadin anticoagulation in stent patients, based on the data from clinical studies,[66–68] STARS,[69] ISAR,[70,71] FAN-TASTIC[72] and MATTIS.[73] Ticlopidine has been customarily administered in stent patients for 2–4 weeks following coronary

intervention. A recent study[77] suggested that only 2 weeks of post-stent ticlopidine therapy is necessary to prevent the vast majority of thrombotic complications. The major factor limiting the use of ticlopidine for longer periods of time has been the issues related to its side effects of neutropenia and TTP, and the need for hematologic monitoring. Given the favourable safety profile of clopidogrel over ticlopidine,[60] it is a logical potential substitute for ticlopidine in these circumstances, and may be given safely for longer periods of time.

A number of retrospective, historically controlled studies have suggested that clopidogrel can be safely substituted for ticlopidine in patients undergoing coronary stent placement, without compromising clinical efficacy.[78–81] The only available randomized data currently available on the use of clopidogrel vs ticlopidine in patients undergoing stenting come from the recently-reported CLASSICS trial, involving 1020 patients undergoing elective stenting.[82]

The CLASSICS trial was a multicenter, randomized controlled trial of clopidogrel plus aspirin versus ticlopidine plus aspirin in 1020 patients undergoing coronary stent implantation at 48 European centers. The three treatment groups included aspirin (325 mg qd) plus ticlopidine (250 mg b.i.d.; $n = 340$), aspirin plus clopidogrel (75 mg qd; $n = 335$), or aspirin plus front-loaded clopidogrel (300 mg on day, followed by 75 mg qd; $n = 345$). Therapy was initiated within 6 hours of the stent procedure, and continued for 28 days afterward. The trial was primarily designed as a safety study. Patients requiring the use of IIb/IIIa antagonists were excluded from the study. The primary endpoint of the study was the composite of bleeding, neutropenia, thrombocytopenia and early drug discontinuation for non-cardiac adverse events. A secondary endpoint was clinical efficacy, assessed as the composite of cardiovascular death, myocardial infarction, and target vessel revascularization at 30 days. The primary safety endpoint was significantly reduced with clopidogrel occurring in 9.1% of the ticlopidine group, 6.3% of the 75 mg clopidogrel group, 2.9% of the 300/75 mg clopidogrel group, and 4.6% in the two clopidogrel groups combined. There were no instances of thrombocytopenia with clopidogrel. The major contribution to the primary endpoint came from a much higher percentage of early drug discontinuation for non-cardiac adverse events (primarily allergic reactions, GI disorders, and skin rashes) with ticlopidine (8.2% compared to 5.1% in the 75 mg clopidogrel group, 20% in the 300/75 mg clopidogrel group, and 3.5% in the two clopidogrel groups combined. The secondary endpoint of composite adverse cardiac events was not significantly different among the groups (0.9%, 1.5%, 1.2% in the respec-

tive treatment arms) 1.3% in the two clopidogrel groups combined.

The forthcoming CREDO trial will examine the potential advantages of acute procedural loading and long-vs-short-term therapy in a factorially designed trial.

Side effects of ticlopidine and clopidogrel and drug interactions

Side-effects

The most frequent side-effects of ticlopidine are skin rash and gastrointestinal symptoms but not gastrointestinal bleeding (Table 7.3). The most severe side-effects of ticlopidine are those affecting the hemostatic and hematopoetic system.[26,32,83] Neutropenia (neutrophil count less than 1200/µl) occurred in 2.4% of patients in the CATS and TASS trials with ticlopidine. Severe neutropenia occurred at about 1% in the CATS, TASS[58] and STIMS[59] trials. All severe cases occurred within the first 3 months of treatment (specifically days 26–62). A regular monitoring of the white blood cell count (WBC) is mandatory for patients receiving ticlopidine treatment. Other very rare but serious hematologic complications of ticlopidine are aplastic anemias[84] and thrombotic thrombocytopenic purpura. A recent review reported 60 cases, 33% of them died.[85] Ono et al[86] have suggested that these actions may be explained by bone marrow toxicity of ticlopidine; however, the mechanism is unknown. Clopidogrel did not exhibit these severe side-effects in the CAPRIE study at incidences higher than aspirin. So far there is no evidence for bone marrow toxicity of clopidogrel.

Another very rare complication of ticlopidine is liver toxicity (e.g. cholestatic jaundice or drug-induced hepatitis). No signs of liver toxicity were reported for clopidogrel in the CAPRIE trial.

Side effect	TASS trial (2–6 years) ≈ 3 years"		CAPRIE trial (1–3 years) ≈ 2 years¶	
	Ticlopidine 500	ASA 1300	Clopidogrel 75	ASA 325
Diarrhoea	20.4	9.8*	4.5	3.4*
Rash	11.9	5.2*	6.0	4.6*
Abn. liver function	—	—	3.0	3.2*
Cholesterol ↑				
Any bleeding	9.0	10.0	9.3	9.3
GI-bleeding	0.5	1.4*	2.0	2.7*

* Significant.

† Not all side-effects included.

‡ ASA intolerance excluded.

§ No event rates given, increase in total cholesterol 9% (Ticlo) vs 2% (ASA) 'no liver dysfunction'.

¶ No evidence of any unusual findings of adverse effects in either treatment group'.

" At 3 year event calculation, treatment shorter and highly variable: 778 ± 603 days (ticlopidine) vs 858±582 days (ASA).

Table 7.3
Side-effects of ticlopidine (Ticlo), aspirin (ASA) and clopidogrel in the TASS[58,†] and CAPRIE[60,†] trials.

Drug interactions

The (elderly) patient population for clopidogrel and ticlopidine is likely to take additional medications. Therefore, the possible interactions of the compounds with the kinetics of other (hepatically-inactivated) drugs is of considerable interest. In addition, the combined use of different antiplatelet agents might be associated with an increased risk of bleeding.

As discussed before, animal experiments (using rats) have shown that ticlopidine interacts with at least two components of the hepatic CYP-450 system;[87] however there are no detailed studies in man. Several reports indicate that ticlopidine might interfere with the metabolism of other compounds being subject of significant hepatic clearance, such as phenytoin,[88–90] theophylline and antipyrine[26,32,91,92] as well as warfarin[93] with

the risk of acute toxicity[88] because of increased plasma levels of the compound. For example, there was a 2-fold increase in theophylline plasma level by ticlopidine.[94]

According to preliminary data, clopidogrel (75 mg/day for 10 days to healthy volunteers) did not change the half-life of antipyrine. There was also no change in γ-glutamate transferase (γ-GT) and cortisol levels in these volunteers. This led the authors to conclude that clopidogrel, under the conditions of this study, did not cause hepatic enzyme induction or modify the activities of hepatic oxidative enzyme systems in man.[95] No liver dysfunction was reported with ticlopidine in the TASS trial[58] and a similar conclusion was made from data obtained in the CAPRIE trial with clopidogrel.[60]

The percentage of patients who stopped

Compound	Aspirin	Clopidogrel
Mechanism of antiplatelet action	Inhibition of TX generation	Inhibition of ADP action via G-protein coupled receptor(s)
Specific for platelets	No	(Yes)
Active in vitro	Yes	(Yes)
Action reversible	No	No
Significant side-effects	Bleeding Gastrointestinal-intolerance	Bleeding Gastrointestinal-intolerance Rash

*Other effects might contribute to its clinical efficacy.
†From Schrör,[100] with permission.

Table 7.4
Some pharmacological properties of aspirin and clopidogrel (thienopyridine) with respect to platelet function.[*†]

treatment early because of adverse events in the CAPRIE trial was similar between aspirin- and clopidogrel-treated subjects;[60] however, the spectrum of side-effects was different. The most frequent side-effect with clopidogrel was diarrhea and rash, as previously also noted for ticlopidine (see Table 7.3) while gastro-intestinal-intolerance and bleeding were more frequent with aspirin. Nevertheless, it should be considered that the CAPRIE trial was a phase III study with numerous exclusion criteria for patient selection, including a history of drug-induced hepatic abnormalities. A more complete overview of side-effects of ticlopidine is published elsewhere.[26,32] No pharmacological interactions were described or coadministration of clopidogrel and aspirin,[96] digoxin,[97] heparin,[98] atenolol or nifedipine.[99]

Thienopyridines versus aspirin and GPIIb-IIIa inhibitors

A brief overview regarding some important pharmacological properties of these antiplatelet agents is summarized in Table 7.4.

Clopidogrel/Ticlopidine versus aspirin

Aspirin does not affect primary ADP-induced platelet aggregation or aggregation at physiological Ca^{2+} levels[101] or ADP-induced exposure of the fibrinogen receptor.[21] Aspirin acts exclusively on thromboxane-dependent platelet activation, while thienopyridines do not affect the arachidonic acid metabolism.[21,102–104] This is the background for the combined use of both agents, for example in PTCA and stenting.

Antiplatelet therapy with both ticlopidine and aspirin has been suggested to significantly enhance as well as to extend the therapeutic efficacy.[105,106] Combined use of ticlopidine and aspirin was found to be superior to either treatment alone in preventing acute cardiac events in patients with prior myocardial infarction.[107] In addition, aspirin resistance or contraindications against aspirin use, including aspirin sensitivity, are indications for thienopyridines.

Clopidogrel/Ticlopidine versus GPIIb/IIIa antagonists

GPIIb-IIIa antagonists antagonize platelet aggregation in response to all physiological stimuli, that is the formation of platelet aggregates after binding of fibrinogen to the activated GPIIb-IIIa complex[108] (cf. Figure 7.1). In contrast to thienopyridines, selective GPIIb-IIIa antagonists, such as integrelin or tirofiban, bind directly to this platelet integrin and prevent the access of ligands, such as soluble fibrinogen to the activated GPIIb-IIIa, by a competitive mode of action. The benefits of antibody-type GPIIb-IIIa antagonists, such as abciximab, are obvious and discussed in another chapter of this book and other reviews.[109] The issue to be discussed here, is the question of whether or not orally active GPIIb-IIIa antagonists, such as xemilofibane, sibrafibane and others, are competitors for thienopyridines in oral long-term treatment, since thienopyridines suppress ADP-induced activation of GPIIb-IIIa by about 70%. The published antagonists have a largely variable half-life and cross placental blood–brain barrier because of their lipophilicity. All known compounds are prodrugs and require metabolic conversion into the active agent, pointing to a crucial role for the liver. The systemic bioavailability of the more advanced compounds is in the range of 30%.[100] It is not entirely clear to what degree of GPIIb-IIIa receptor occupation has to be obtained and maintained for a clinically relevant inhibition of platelet function, but 70–80% may be necessary, suggesting a narrow therapeutic window. It should also be considered that these compounds, in contrast with thienopyridines, are competitive inhibitors of the GPIIb-IIIa receptor, in other words their efficacy is determined by the amount of the active compound or metabolite, respectively. Thus, the finding of an optimal chronic dose for an oral agent might be difficult.[108] There is also little information about side-effects. So far, no studies comparing orally active GPIIb-IIIa antagonists with thienopyridines have been published.

Current clinical role of clopidogrel

Given the favorable safety profile of clopidogrel, and the large scale clinical data from CAPRIE, there are a number of clinical scenarios where clopidogrel can be very useful. First of all, clopidogrel can serve as a substitute for aspirin in aspirin-allergic or aspirin-intolerant patients, or patients with significant gastrointestinal pathology in which aspirin may be relatively contraindicated. Secondly, clopidogrel can be used as a general substitute for ticlopidine in patients who require new thienopyridine therapy (such as stent patients). Clopidogrel is better tolerated, has a faster onset of action, is a once-a-day drug, does not require hematologic monitoring, and (in the US) is actually cheaper than ticlopidine. All of this strongly points to clopidogrel as a fairly broad replacement for ticlopidine in clinical practice. A more difficult question is whether patients who are already on chronic ticlopidine therapy and tolerating it well should be switched to clopidogrel. Since most of the risk for blood dyscrasias with ticlopidine come in the first 6 months, a switch after this time may not be absolutely necessary. The third general area of potential clinical application is in patients who present with new cardiovascular events while already on aspirin therapy. In this circumstance consideration could be given to adding a thienopyridine to aspirin, in case this recurrent event were a manifestation of aspirin failure. In fact, given the recent awareness of a substantial group of patients in whom aspirin therapy may not provide adequate antiplatelet protection, clopidogrel could be considered as adjunctive therapy in this group of patients as a whole. A fourth group of patients who might benefit from clopidogrel therapy are those patients felt to be at high risk for recurrent events, such as patients with a previous MI, stroke, or TIA. Again, in these patients, consideration could be given to combining clopidogrel therapy with aspirin. Finally, on the basis of the strongly favorable outcomes in CAPRIE, clopidogrel could be considered as potential monotherapy (a *replacement* for aspirin) in patients with PAD or patients with double bed vascular disease (coronary artery disease plus PAD or cerebrovascular disease).

In the US marketplace, clopidogrel has largely displaced ticlopidine, on the basis of its superior safety profile. The role of combination therapy with aspirin plus clopidogrel for non-stent coronary interventions remains unclear. Without the complications of neutropenia and TTP, clopidogrel is being utilized in more non-stent interventions, although there are, as yet, no prospective data to support this use. The combination of clopidogrel with aspirin in the broader treatment of patients with atherosclerotic disease has tremendous potential as a multi-targeted approach to antiplatelet therapy, but it will require much more clinical evaluation before it could be viewed as the 'standard of care'. Clopidogrel is a substantial addition to our antiplatelet armamentarium, but it is not an out-and-out widespread substitute for aspirin therapy except in a few well-defined (and well documented) circumstances. Its role as an add-on to aspirin therapy, while mechanistically very exciting, will need to be documented in further prospective randomized, well-designed clinical trials.

Future clinical trials

As previously mentioned, the CREDO trial will examine further refinements of the use of aspirin plus clopidogrel in patients undergoing stent placement. The CURE/OASIS 4 trial is a large-scale randomized study comparing aspirin versus aspirin plus clopidogrel in patients with acute coronary syndromes (excluding those going to early intervention). Other future studies include WATCH (a 3-arm study in the US, UK and Canada of aspirin vs. clopidogrel vs. coumadin in patients with heart failure), CCS II (a large-scale study in China comparing aspirin versus aspirin plus clopidogrel in patients with acute myocardial infarction), and the VA hemodialysis study (evaluating the utility of aspirin plus Plavix in preserving dialysis shunt access). Trials of combined aspirin/clopidogrel therapy in patients with atrial fibrillation and in patients with documented peripheral vascular disease are also being considered.

Acknowledgments

The author is grateful to Dr Artur-Aron Weber and Dr Marina Braun for critical reading of the manuscript and the helpful criticism, and to Erika Lohmann for competent secretarial assistance.

References

1. Thebault JJ, Blatrix CE, Blanchard JF, Panak EA. Effects of ticlopidine, a new platelet aggregation inhibitor in man. *Clin Pharmacol Ther* 1975;**18**:485–90.

2. Maffrand JP, Vallee E, Bernat A, et al. Animal pharmacology of PCR 4099, a new thienopyridine compound. *Thromb Haemost* 1985;**54**:133 [Abstract].

3. Gachet C, Stierle A, Cazenave JP, et al. The thienopyridine PCR 4099 selectively inhibits ADP-induced platelet aggregation and fibrinogen binding without modifying the membrane glycoprotein IIb/IIIa complex in rat and man. *Biochem Pharmacol* 1990a;**40**:229–38.

4. Féliste R, Delebassee D, Simon MF, et al. Broad-spectrum anti-platelet activity of ticlopidine and PCR 4099 involves the suppression of the effects of released ADP. *Thromb Res* 1987;**48**:403–15.

5. Schrör K. Clinical pharmacology of the adenosine diphosphate (ADP) receptor antagonist, clopidogrel. *Vasc Med* 1998;**3**:247–51.

6. Fagura MS, Dainty IA, McKay GD, et al. P2Y$_1$-receptors in human platelets which are pharmacologically distinct from P2Y$_{ADP}$ receptors. *Br J Pharmacol* 1998;**124**:157–64.

7. Geiger J, Hönig-Liedl P, Schanzenbächer P, Walter U. Ligand specificity and ticlopidine effects distinguish three human platelet ADP receptors. *Eur J Pharmacol* 1998;**351**:235–46.

8. Savi P, Beauverger P, Labouret C, et al. Role of P2Y1 purinoceptors in ADP-induced platelet activation. *FEBS Lett* 1998;**422**:291–5.

9. Mills DC. ADP receptors on platelets. *Thromb Haemost* 1996;**76**:835–55.

10. Boarder MR, Hourani SMO. The regulation of vascular function by P2 receptors: multiple sites and multiple receptors. *Trends in Pharmacol Sci* 1998;**19**:99–107.

11. Léon C, Hechler B, Vial C, Leray C, Cazenave J-P, Gachet C. The P2Y$_1$ receptor is an ADP receptor antagonized by ATP and expressed in platelets and megakaryoblastic cells. *FEBS Lett* 1997;**403**:26–30.

12. Lips JPM, Sixma JJ, Schiphorst ME. The effect of ticlopidine administration to humans on the binding of adenosine diphosphate to blood platelets. *Thromb Res* 1980;**17**:19–27.

13. Mills DCB, Puri RN, Hu CJ, et al. Clopidogrel inhibits the binding of ADP analogues to the receptor mediating inhibition of platelet adenylate cyclase. *Arterioscl Thromb* 1992;**12**:430–6.

14. Gachet C, Cattaneo M, Ohlmann PO, et al. Purinoceptors on blood platelets: further pharmacological and clinical evidence to suggest the presence of two ADP receptors. *Br J Haematol* 1995;**91**:434–44.

15. Gachet Ch, Cazenave J-P, Ohlmann P, Hilf G, Wieland Th, Jakobs KH, ADP receptor-induced activation of guanine-nucleotide-binding proteins in human platelet membranes. *Eur J Biochem* 1992;**207**:259–63.

16. Offermans S, Toombs CF, Hu Y-H, Simon MI, Defective platelet activation in G alpha (q) deficient mice. *Nature* 1997;**389**:183–6.

17. Gachet C, Cazenave J-P, Ohlmann P, et al. The thienopyridine ticlopidine selectively prevents the inhibitory effects of ADP but not of adrenaline on cAMP levels raised by stimulation of the adenylate cyclase of human platelets by PGE$_1$. *Biochem Pharmacol* 1990b;**40**:2683–7.

18. Humbert M, Nurden P, Bihour C, et al. Ultrastructural studies of platelet aggregates from human subjects receiving clopidogrel and from a patient with an inherited defect of an ADP-dependent pathway of platelet activation. *Arterioscl Thromb Vasc Biol* 1996;**16**:1532–43.

19. Cooper DMF, Rodbell M. ADP is a potent inhibitor of human platelet plasma membrane adenylate cyclase. *Nature* 1979;**282**:517–18.

20. Defreyn G, Gachet C, Savi P, Driot F, Cazenave JP, Maffrand JP. Ticlopidine and clopidogrel (SR 25990C) selectively neutralize ADP inhibition of PGE$_1$-activated platelet adenylate cyclase in rats and rabbits. *Thromb Haemost* 1991;**65**:186–90.

21. Harker LA, Bruno JJ, Ticlopidine's mechanism of action on human platelets. In: Hass WK, Easton JD, eds, *Ticlopidine, Platelets and Vascular Disease* (Springer-Verlag, New York, 1993) 41–59.

22. Savi P, Pflieger AMN, Herbért J-M. cAMP is not an important messenger for ADP induced platelet aggregation. *Blood Coagul Fibrinol* 1996;7:249–52.

23. Weber A-A, Reimann S, Schrör K. Specific inhibition of ADP-induced platelet aggregation by clopidogrel in vitro. *Br J Pharmacol* 1999;**126**:415–20.

24. Nurden AT. New thoughts on strategies for modulating platelet function through the inhibition of surface receptors. *Haemostasis* 1996;**26 (suppl 4)**:78–88.

25. Bruno JF. The mechanism of action of ticlopidine. *Thromb Res* 1983;(**Suppl IV**):59–67.

26. Harbison JW, Ticlopidine hydrochloride. In: Messerli FH (ed.), *Cardiovascular Drug Therapy*, 2nd edn (WB Saunders, Philadelphia, 1996) 1465–73.

27. Hardisty RM, Powling MJ, Nokes TJC. The action of ticlopidine on human platelets: Studies on aggregation, secretion, calcium mobilization and membrane glycoproteins. *Thromb Haemost* 1990;**64**:150–5.

28. Pengo V, Boschello M, Marzari A, Baca M, Schivazappa L, Dalla Volta S, Adenosine diphosphate (ADP) induced α-granules release from platelets of native whole blood is reduced by ticlopidine but not by aspirin or dipyridamole. *Thromb Haemost* 1986;**56**:147–50.

29. Cattaneo M, Akkawar B, Kinlough-Rathbone RL, Packham MA, Cimminiello C, Mannucci PM. Ticlopidine facilitates the deaggregation of human platelets aggregated by thrombin. *Thromb Haemost* 1994;**71**:91–4.

30. Savi P, Herbért J-M, Pflieger AM, et al. Importance of hepatic metabolism in the antiaggregating activity of the thienopyridine clopidogrel. *Biochem Pharmacol* 1992;**44**:527–32.

31. Herbért JM, Frekel D, Vallee E, et al. Clopidogrel, a novel antiplatelet and antithrombotic agent. *Cardiovasc Drug Rev* 1993a;**11**:180–98.

32. Teitelbaum P. Pharmacodynamics and pharmacokinetics of ticlopidine. In: Hass WK, Easton JD (eds), *Ticlopidine, Platelets and Vascular Disease* (Springer-Verlag, Heidelberg, 1993) 27–40.

33. Defreyn G, Bernat A, Delebassée D, Maffrand JP. Pharmacology of ticlopidine: a review. *Semin Thromb Hemost* 1989;**15**:159–66.

34. Di Minno G, Cerbone AM, Mattioli PL, Turco S, Iovine C, Mancini M. Functionally thrombasthenic state in normal platelets following the administration of ticlopidine. *J Clin Invest* 1985;**75**:328–38.

35. Weber et al unpublished results

36. DiPerri T, Pasini FL, Frigerio C, et al. Pharmacodynamics of ticlopidine in man in relation to plasma and blood cell concentration. *Eur J Clin Pharmacol* 1991;**41**:429–34.

37. Shah J, Teitelbaum P, Molony M, Gabuzda T, Massey I, Single and multiple dose pharmacokinetics of ticlopidine in young and elderly subjects. *Br J Clin Pharmacol* 1991;**32**:761–4.

38. Buur T, Larsson R, Berglund U, Donat F, Tronquet C. Pharmacokinetics and effect of ticlopidine on platelet aggregation in subjects with normal and impaired renal function. *J Clin Pharmacol* 1997;**37**:108–15.

39. Kuzniar J, Splawinska B, Malinga K, Mazurek AP, Splawinski J. Pharmacodynamics of ticlopidine: relation between dose and time to administration to platelet inhibition. *Int J Clin Pharmacol Ther* 1996;**34**:357–61.

40. Caplain H, Kieffer G, Thiercelin JF, Thebault JJ. Tolerance and clinical pharmacology of repeated administration of clopidogrel (SR 25990 C), a new antiplatelet agent, at three dose levels in normal healthy volunteers. *Thromb Haemost* 1989;**62**:410 [Abstract].

41. Bachmann F, Savcic M, Hauert J, Geudelin B, Kieffer G, Cariou R. Rapid onset of inhibition of ADP-induced platelet aggregation by a loading dose of clopidogrel. *Eur Heart J* 1996;**17**(Suppl):263.

42. Boneu B, Destelle G, Platelet anti-aggregating activity and tolerance of clopidogrel in atherosclerotic patients. *Thromb Haemost* 1996;**76**:939–43.

43. D'Honneur GD, Caplain H, Cariou R, Serres-Lacroix E, De La Forest Divonne N. Clinical tolerance and pharmacological activity of long-term administration of clopidogrel in young healthy volunteers. *Haemostasis* 1996b;**26** (Suppl 3):555.

44. Guillin M-C, Bonnet G, Sissmann J, Necciari J, Dickinson JP. Pharmacodynamics and pharmacokinetics of the novel anti-platelet agent, clopidogrel, in the young and the elderly with and without symptomatic atherosclerosis. *Eur Heart J* 1996;17(**Suppl.**):161.

45. Coade SB, Pearson JD. Metabolism of adenine nucleotides in human blood. *Circ Res* 1989; 65:531–7.

46. Marcus AJ, Safier LB, Hajjar KA, et al. Inhibition of platelet function by an aspirin-insensitive endothelial cell ADPase. Thromboregulation by endothelial cells. *J Clin Invest* 1991;88:1690–6.

47. Born GVR. Adenosine diphosphate is a mediator of platelet aggregation in vivo. An editorial view. *Circulation* 1985;72:741–6.

48. Moritz MW, Reimers RC, Baker RK, Sutera SP, Joist JH. Role of cytoplasmic and releasable ADP in platelet aggregation induced by laminar shear stress. *J Lab Clin Med* 1983;101:537–44.

49. Rajagopalan S, McIntyre LV, Hall ER, Wu KK. The stimulation of arachidonic acid metabolism in human platelets by hydrodynamic forces. *Biochim Biophys Acta* 1988; 958:108–15.

50. Moake JL, Turner NA, Stathopoulos NA, Nolasco L, Hellums JD. Shear-induced platelet aggregation can be mediated by vWF released from platelets, as well as by exogenous large or unusually large vWF multimers, requires adenosine-diphosphate, and is resistant to aspirin. *Blood* 1988;71:1366–74.

51. Ratnatunga CP, Edmondson SF, Rees GM, Kovacs IB. High-dose aspirin inhibits shear-induced platelet reaction involving thrombin generation. *Circulation* 1992;85:1077–82.

52. Maalej N, Folts JD. Increased shear stress overcomes the antithrombotic platelet inhibitory effect of aspirin in stenosed dog coronary arteries. *Circulation* 1996;93: 1201–5.

53. Escolar G, Bastida E, Castillo R, Ordinas A. Ticlopidine inhibits platelet thrombus formation studied in a flowing system. *Thromb Res* 1987;45:561–71.

54. Orlando E, Cortelazzo S, Nosari I, et al. Inhibition by ticlopidine of platelet adhesion to human venous subendothelium in patients with diabetes. *J Lab Clin Med* 1988;112:583–8.

55. Cattaneo M, Lombardi R, Bettega D, Lecchi A, Mannucci PM, Shear-induced platelet aggregation is potentiated by desmopressin and inhibited by ticlopidine. *Arteriosl Thromb* 1993;13:393–7.

56. Herbért JM, Tissinier A, Defreyn G, Maffrand JP. Inhibitory effect of clopidogrel on platelet adhesion and intimal proliferation after arterial injury in rabbits. *Arteriosl Thromb* 1993b; 13:1171–9.

57. Gent M, Blakeley JA, Easton JD, et al and CATS group. The Canadian American Ticlopidine Study (CATS) in thromboembolic stroke. *Lancet* 1989;1:1215–20.

58. Hass WK, Easton JD, Adams HP Jr., et al. for the Ticlopidine Aspirin Stroke Study Group: a randomized trial comparing ticlopidine hydrochloride with aspirin for the prevention of stroke in high-risk patients. *N Engl J Med* 1989;321:501–7.

59. Janzon L, Bergqvist D, Boberg J, et al. Prevention of myocardial infarction and stroke in patients with intermittent claudication; effects of ticlopidine. Results from STIMS, the Swedish Ticlopidine Multicenter Study. *J Int Med* 1990;227:301–8.

60. Gent M and CAPRIE Steering Committee. A randomised, blinded trial of clopidogrel versus aspirin in patients at risk of ischaemic events (CAPRIE). *Lancet* 1996;348:1329–39.

61. Gawaz M, Neumann F-J, Ott I, May A, Schömig A. Platelet activation and coronary stent implantation. Effect of antithrombotic therapy. *Circulation* 1996;94:179–285.

62. Yao S-K, Ober JC, McNatt J, et al. ADP plays an important role in mediating platelet aggregation and cyclic-flow variations in vivo in stenosed and endothelium-injured canine coronary arteries. *Circ Res* 1992;70:39–48.

63. Samama ChM, Bonnin Ph, Bonneau M, et al. Comparative arterial antithrombotic activity of clopidogrel and acetylsalicylic acid in the pig. *Thromb Haemost* 1992;68:500–5.

64. Rupprecht HJ, Darius H, Borkowski U, et al. Comparison of antiplatelet effects of aspirin, ticlopidine, or their combination after stent implantation. *Circulation* 1998;97:1046–52.

65. Gregorini L, Marco J, Fajadet J, et al. Ticlopidine and aspirin pretreatment reduces coagulation and platelet activation during coronary

dilation procedures. *J Am Coll Cardiol* 1997;**29**:13–20.

66. Schömig A, Neumann F-J, Kastrati A, et al. A randomized comparison of antiplatelet and anticoagulant therapy after the placement of coronary-artery stents. *N Engl J Med* 1996;**334**:1084–9.

67. Schömig A, Neumann F-J, Walter A, et al. Coronary stent placement in patients with acute myocardial infarction: Comparison of clinical and angiographical outcome after randomization to antiplatelet or anticoagulant therapy. *J Am Coll Cardiol* 1997;**29**:28–34.

68. Albiero R, Hall P, Itoh A, Blengino S, Nakamura S, Martini G, et al. Results of a consecutive series of patients receiving only antiplatelet therapy after optimized stent implantation. Comparison of aspirin alone versus combined ticlopidine and aspirin therapy. *Circulation* 1997;**95**:1145–56.

69. Leon MB, Baim DS, Popma JJ, et al, for the Stent Anticoagulation Restenosis Study Investigators. A clinical trial comparing three antithrombotic-drug regimens after coronary-artery stenting. *N Engl J Med* 1998;**339**: 1665–71.

70. Kastrati A, Schülen H, Hausleiter J, et al. Restenosis after coronary stent placement and randomization to a 4-week combined antiplatelet or anticoagulant therapy. Six month angiographic follow-up of the Intracoronary Stenting and Antithrombotic Regimen (ISAR) trial. *Circulation* 1997;**96**:462–7.

71. Schühlen H, Hadamitzky M, Walter H, Ulm K, Schömig A. Major benefit from antiplatelet therapy for patients at high risk for adverse cardiac events after coronary Palmaz-Schatz stent placement. Analysis of a prospective risk stratification protocol in the Intracoronary Stenting and Antithrombotic Regimen (ISAR) trial. *Circulation* 1997;**95**:2015–21.

72. Bertrand ME, Legrand V, Boland J, et al. Randomized multicenter comparison of conventional anticoagulation versus antiplatelet therapy in unplanned and elective coronary stenting. The Full Anticoagulation Versus Aspirin and Ticlopidine (FANTASTIC) Study. *Circulation* 1998;**98**:1597–603.

73. Urban P, Macaya C, Rupprecht H-J, et al. for the MATTIS Investigators. Randomized evaluation of anticoagulation versus antiplatelet therapy after coronary stent implantation in high-risk patients. The Multicenter Aspirin and Ticlopidine Trial after Intracoronary Stenting (MATTIS). *Circulation* 1998;**98**:2126–32.

74. Lablanche J-M, McFadden EP, Bonnet J-L, et al. Combined antiplatelet therapy with ticlopidine and aspirin. A simplified approach on intracoronary stent management. *Eur Heart J* 1996;**17**:1373–80.

75. White CW, Knudson M, Schmidt D, et al. Neither ticlopidine nor aspirin-dipyridamole prevents restenosis post PTCA: results from a randomized placebo-controlled multicenter trial. *Circulation* 1987;**76**:IV-213.

76. Bertrand ME, Allain H, La Blanche JM, et al. Results of a randomized trial of ticlopidine versus placebo for prevention of acute closure and restenosis after coronary angioplasty (PTCA). The TACT study. *XII. Congress of the European Society of Cardiology*, 1990;[Abstract Suppl.]:2022.

77. Berger PB, Malcolm RB, David H, et al. Safety and efficacy of Ticlopidine for only 2 weeks after successful Intracoronary stent placement. *Circulation* 1999;**99**:248–53.

78. Berger PB, Bellot V, Melby S, et al. Adjuncts for coronary stenting. Can we possibly make stenting better? *J Am Coll Cardiol* 1999; **33**:34A (abstract).

79. Mischkel GJ, Lucore CL, Ligon RW, Trokey J. Clopidogrel for the prevention of stent thrombosis. *J Am Coll Cardiol* 1999;**33**:34A (abstract).

80. Moussa I, Oetgen M, Roubin G, et al. Effectiveness of clopidogrel and aspirin versus ticlopidine and aspirin in preventing stent thrombosis after coronary stent implantation. *Circulation* 1999;**99**:2364–6.

81. Jauher. Poster presentation. TCT 1998.

82. Bertrand ME. Oral presentation. ACC 1999.

83. Wysowski DK, Bacsanyi J. Blood dyscrasias and hematologic reactions in ticlopidine users [Letter]. *J Am Med Assoc* 1996;**276**:952.

84. Yeh SP, Hsueh EJ, Wu H, Wang YC. Ticlopidine-associated aplastic anemia. *Ann Hematol* 1998;**76**:87–90.

85. Bennett CL, Weinberg PD, Rozenberg-Ben-Dror K, Yarnold PR, Kwaan HC, Green D. Thrombotic thrombocytopenic purpura

associated with ticlopidine. *Ann Intern Med* 1998;**128**:541–4.

86. Ono K, Kurohura K, Yochihara M, Shimamoto Y, Yamaguchi M. Agranulozytosis caused by ticlopidine and its mechanism. *Am J Hematol* 1991;**37**:239–42.

87. Savi P, Combalbert J, Graich C, et al. The antiaggregating activity of clopidogrel is due to metabolic activation by the hepatic cytochrome P450-1A. *Thromb Haemost* 1994;**72**:313–17.

88. Privitera M. Acute phenytoin toxicity followed by seizure breakthrough from a ticlopidine-phenytoin interaction. *Arch Neurol* 1996; **53**:1191–2.

89. Riva R, Ticlopidine impairs phenytoin clearance: a case report. *Neurology* 1996;**46**:1172–3.

90. Donahue SR, Flockhart DA, Abernethy DR, Ko J-W. Ticlipidine inhibition of phenytoin metabolism mediated by potent inhibition of CYP2C19. *Clin Pharmacol Ther* 1997;**62**:572–7.

91. Thebault JJ, Blatrix CE, Blanchard JF, Panak EA. Effect of ticlopidine treatment on liver metabolizing enzymes in man. *Br J Clin Pharmacol* 1980;**10**:311–13.

92. Knudsen JB, Bastain W, Sefton CM, Allen JG, Dickinson JP. Pharmacokinetics of ticlopidine during chronic oral administration to healthy volunteers and its effect on antipyrine pharmacokinetics. *Xenobiotica* 1992;**22**:579–89.

93. Giddal BE, Sorkness CA, McGill KA, Larson R, Levine RR. Evaluation of a potential enantioselective interaction between ticlopidine and warfarin in chronically anticoagulated patients. *Ther Drug Monit* 1995;**17**:33–8.

94. Colli A, Buccino G, Cocciolo M, Parravicini R, Elli GM, Scaltrini G. Ticlopidine-theophylline interaction. *Clin Pharmacol Ther* 1987; **41**: 358–62.

95. Pierce CH, Houle J-M, Kieffer G, Dickinson JP. Absence of effect of clopidogrel on human hepatic P-450 activities. *Eur Heart J* 1996; **17**(Suppl.):160.

96. Caplain H, D'Honneur G, Cariou R. Lack of interaction of aspirin (100 mg) with chronic clopidogrel in volunteers. *Haemostasis* 1996; **26**(Suppl. 3):557.

97. Peeters PAM, Crijns WJ, Tamminga WJ, et al. Absence of pharmacokinetic interaction between the novel antiplatelet agent, clopidogrel, and digoxin. *Eur Heart J* 1996;**17**(Abstract Suppl):160, P913.

98. D'Honneur G, Caplain H, Cariou R, Brouard R. Interaction study between clopidogrel and prolonged intravenous heparin administration in young healthy volunteers. *Haemostasis* 1996a;**26**(Suppl. 3):554.

99. Forbes CD, Belch JJ, Bridges AB, et al. Pharmacodynamic compatibility of clopidogrel with atenolol and nifedipine co-medication in patients with atherosclerotic disease. *Eur Heart J* 1996;**17**(Abstract Suppl.):160.

100. Schrör K. Comparative pharmacology of antiplatelet agents. *Drugs* 1995;**50**:7–28.

101. Packham MA, Bryant NL, Guccione MA, Kinlough-Rathbone RL, Mustard JF. Effect of the concentration of Ca^{2+} in the suspending medium on the responses of human and rabbit platelets to aggregating agents. *Thromb Haemost* 1989;**62**:968–76.

102. Rotondo S, Tascione E, Cerletti C, de Gaetano G. Ticlopidine does not reduce in vivo platelet thromboxane biosynthesis and metabolism in diabetic patients. *Platelets* 1993;**4**:97–100.

103. Schrör K. The basic pharmacology of ticlopidine and clopidogrel. *Platelets* 1993;**4**:252–61.

104. Heptinstall S, May JA, Glenn JR, Sanderson HM, Dickinson JP, Wilcox RG. Effects of ticlopidine to healthy volunteers on platelet function in whole blood. *Thromb Haemost* 1995;**74**:1310–15.

105. De Caterina R, Sicari R, Bernini W, Lazzerini G, Dtrata GB, Gianessi D. Benefit/risk profile of combined antiplatelet therapy with ticlopidine and aspirin. *Thromb Haemost* 1991; **65**:504–10.

106. Splawinska B, Kuzniar J, Malinga K, Mazurek AP, Splawinski J. The efficacy and potency of antiplatelet activity of ticlopidine is increased by aspirin. *Int J Clin Pharmacol Ther* 1996;**34**:352–6.

107. Ishikawa K, Kanamasa K, Hama J, et al. Aspirin plus either dipyridamole or ticlopidine is effective in preventing recurrent myocardial infarction. *Jap Circ J* 1997;**61**:38–45.

108. Coller BS. Platelet GPIIb/IIIa antagonists: the first anti-integrin receptor therapeutics. *J Clin Invest* 1997;**99**:1467–71.

109. Tcheng JE. Platelet glycoprotein IIb/IIIa integrin blockade: recent clinical trials in interventional cardiology. *Thromb Haemost* 1997;**78**: 205–9.

8

Abciximab

James J Ferguson and Paul Kim

Introduction

The purpose of this chapter is to summarize the currently available clinical data on abciximab (c7E3 Fab, ReoPro), a chimeric monoclonal antibody directed at platelet glycoprotein (GP) IIb/IIIa. Since its commercial release in January 1995, there has been considerable controversy about the appropriate clinical role for this potent form of antiplatelet therapy. This chapter provides background information on the development of abciximab, data from recent randomized clinical trials presents some areas of current clinical controversy, and explores some of the potential future applications of abciximab.

Background/development

Platelet glycoprotein IIb/IIIa antagonists are a novel class of therapeutic compounds that inhibit platelets by blocking the final common pathway of platelet aggregation. A variety of antibody, peptide, and nonpeptide compounds have been developed. Several of these agents have been studied in recent clinical trials; the most extensively investigated and the first to enter the commercial marketplace in the USA is abciximab, a chimeric human murine antibody Fab fragment.

Coller was the first to describe the use of a murine monoclonal antibody (m7E3) directed against glycoprotein IIb/IIIa.[1,2] Subsequent studies[3–10] utilized the Fab fragment of this antibody, in the hope that removing the Fc region would reduce the potential for complement activation and decrease the accompanying risk of thrombocytopenia resulting from clearance of antibody-coated platelets by the reticuloendothelial system. However, both the murine antibody and the murine Fab fragment were associated with a high incidence of development of human antimurine antibodies. To reduce the potential immunogenicity of this form of IIb/IIIa-targeted therapy, the DNA sequences for the constant domains of the murine antibody were replaced with corresponding human DNA sequences, leaving intact variable-region murine sequences.[11] The resulting chimeric compound, abciximab, contains approximately 50% human sequences (Figure 8.1).

The Investigational New Drug application for abciximab was filed in February 1990. Phase I dose-escalation trials in normal volunteers were conducted later that year. This was followed in February 1991 by Phase II trials in high-risk patients undergoing percutaneous transluminal coronary angioplasty (PTCA). The pivotal Phase III study, EPIC, was initiated in November 1991, and the results were first presented at the American College of Cardiology Scientific Sessions in March 1993. The commercial product (ReoPro, Centocor and

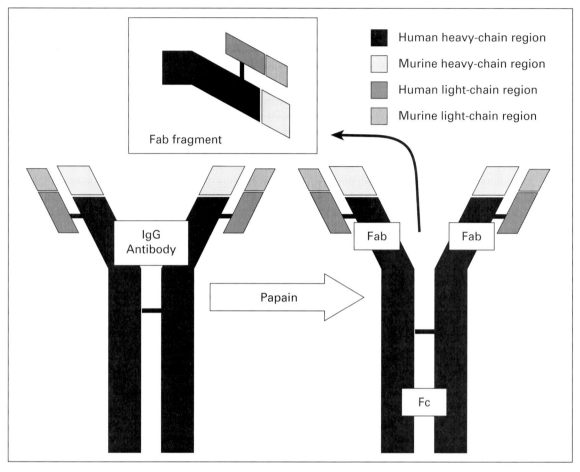

Figure 8.1
The derivation of the Fab fragment of a chimeric human-murine antibody directed at platelet GPIIb/IIIa.

Eli Lilly & Co.) was launched after FDA approval in early 1995.[12] Subsequent large clinical trials (described later) included EPILOG[13], CAPTURE[14], RAPPORT[15], ERASER[16], and EPISTENT[17]. Commercial acceptance of the product was initially guarded, with enthusiastic use at some centers and more gradual incorporation of the new agent into clinical practice in others. With time, however, the clinical uptake and use of abciximab has continued to grow. At the beginning of 1999, ReoPro was used in approximately 45% of coronary interventions performed in the USA.

Pharmacokinetics and pharmacodynamics

The pharmacokinetics of abciximab have been described in some detail.[12] Free drug is cleared rapidly from the plasma, with an initial phase half-life of less than 10 min; there is also a second clearance phase, with a half-life of approximately 30 min. No more than 5% of the drug remains in the plasma 2 h after intravenous bolus therapy (0.15–0.30 mg/kg).[18] However, the drug is avidly bound to platelets; within 30 min of treatment, platelets are coated uniformly with the drug; platelet survival remained normal.

In patients receiving only a bolus of abciximab (0.25 mg/kg), receptor blockade decreased to 50% at 24 h post-infusion. Platelet aggregation in the presence of ADP and the 11-amino acid thrombin receptor-activating peptide (TRAP) was inhibited by 73% and 53% at 2 hours, respectively and by 27% and 30% at 24 hours, respectively. Additional abciximab treatment led to more complete inhibition in the presence of TRAP, supporting the existence of an internal pool of GPIIb/IIIa.[19]

In another study continuous intravenous infusion of abciximab resulted in maximal GPIIb/IIIa blockade of 93%. Median GPIIb/IIIa blockade fell to 68% 12 h after cessation of the infusion. Platelet function recovered gradually over approximately 48 h following completion of abciximab therapy. Flow cytometric analyses at 8 and 15 days, beyond the normal circulating platelet lifespan, showed 29% and 13% GPIIb/IIIa blockade, suggesting that abciximab was transferred to newly released platelets.[20] A similar transfer phenomenon is noted when treated platelets are mixed with untreated platelets.[21]

The actions of the abciximab are not restricted to the GPIIb/IIIa. It also cross-reacts with $\alpha_v\beta_3$ the vitronectin receptor, which is present to a limited extent on platelets but is more prominent on endothelial and smooth muscle cells and is involved in the regulation of cell adhesion, migration, and proliferation.

A recent study[21] has shown redistribution of abciximab between GPIIb/IIIa and $\alpha_v\beta_3$. Abciximab may also cross-react with the MAC-1 receptor or endothelial cells. Whether this cross-reactivity has clinical relevance with respect to neointimal hyperplasia and restenosis is unknown.[22]

Clinical trials of abciximab

The clinical trials of abciximab are summarized in Table 8.1.

EPIC study

The EPIC (Evaluation of 7E3 in Preventing Ischemic Complications) trial[23] was a randomized, controlled trial of abciximab in patients undergoing high-risk angioplasty or atherectomy. 'High-risk' was defined as unstable angina (in 23% of the patients in the study), acute myocardial infarction (MI) (in 3% of the patients), or high-risk lesion morphology (in 74% of the patients). A total of 2099 patients at 56 clinical sites were randomized to one of three treatment arms (Figure 8.2):

(1) A bolus of abciximab (0.25 mg/kg) plus a 12-h abciximab infusion (10 µg/min);
(2) A bolus of abciximab and placebo infusion; or
(3) A placebo bolus and a placebo infusion.

The bolus was administered 10 min before the revascularization procedure. The primary endpoint was the composite incidence of death, non-fatal myocardial infarction (MI), and urgent intervention at 30 days. In addition to standard aspirin pretreatment, patients also received intra- and post-procedure administration of heparin at the discretion of the operator. At 30 days, the composite primary endpoint occurred in 12.8% of the placebo group, compared with 11.5% in the group taking the abciximab bolus alone and 8.3% in

Study	Clinical setting	Endpoint
EPIC[23] (*n* = 2099)	High risk coronary angioplasty or atherectomy	Death, MI, urgent revascularization
PROLOG (*n* = 103)	Coronary intervention (pilot study)	Bleeding complications
EPILOG[13] (*n* = 2792)	Coronary intervention	Death, MI, or urgent revascularization
CAPTURE[14] (*n* = 1265)	Refractory unstable angina undergoing intervention	Death, MI, or urgent revascularization
EPISTENT[17] (*n* = 2399)	Stent-eligible coronary intervention	Death, MI, or urgent revascularization
ERASER[16] (*n* = 225)	Elective stents	In-stent restenosis (IVUS volumetric analysis
RAPPORT[15] (*n* = 483)	Acute MI undergoing primary PTCA	Death, MI, or any revascularization
ADMIRAL (*n* = 299)	Acute MI undergoing intervention (primarily stenting)	Death, MI, ischemia-driven revascularization
TAMI-8 (*n* = 70)	Acute MI (with t-PA) [Using murine m7E3]	Rest angina with ECG changes, reinfarction, the need for urgent revascularization or revascularization and death
TIMI 14[79] (*n* = 888)	Acute MI (with SK or t-PA)	TIMI grade-3 flow at 90 minutes
GRAPE[78] (*n* = 60)	Acute MI	Angiographic TIMI flow grade (median time of 45 minutes)
SPEED[80] (*n* = 305)	Acute MI (with r-PA)	Angiographic TIMI flow grade (median time of 60 minutes)
GUSTO 4 – AMI (*n* = 16 600) [ongoing]	Acute MI (with $\frac{1}{2}$ dose r-PA vs. r-PA alone)	Mortality at 30 days
GUSTO 4 – ACS (*n* = 4500) [ongoing]	Acute coronary syndromes (Placebo vs. 24 hr Rx vs. 48 hr Rx)	Death or MI at 48 hours

Table 8.1
Clinical trials of abciximab.

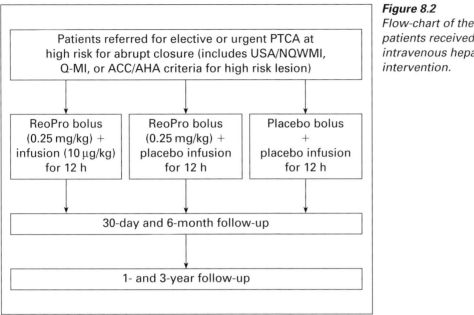

Figure 8.2
Flow-chart of the EPIC study. All patients received aspirin and intravenous heparin prior to intervention.

the abciximab bolus/infusion group. Major bleeding complications were significantly increased with abciximab, occurring in 14% of the abciximab bolus/infusion group, compared with 7% in the placebo group. At 6-month follow-up in the EPIC cohort, the abciximab bolus/infusion group had significantly fewer death/MI/revascularization events (27%) compared with 35.1% in the placebo group.[24] This favorable outcome was due primarily to a decrease in the need for bypass surgery or repeat angioplasty in patients with an initially successful procedure. Continued blinded follow-up throughout an additional 2.5 years was obtained in 93% of the 2099 original EPIC patients.[25] Bolus plus infusion abciximab therapy was associated with a 20% relative improvement at 3 years in composite events, 41.7% versus 47.2% with placebo (Figure 8.3). In the highest risk subgroup of

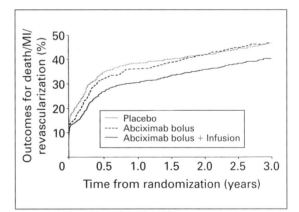

Figure 8.3
Event-free survival up to 3 years in the EPIC treatment arms. The initial benefits achieved in the bolus/infusion abciximab group are sustained, while those in the bolus-alone group are not. Adapted from Topol et al.[25]

patients (those with unstable angina or acute MI) there was a dramatic improvement in the incidence of death (5.1% versus 12.7% with placebo), MI (6.9% versus 14.7% with placebo), revascularization (34% versus 41.1% with placebo) and combined events (39.2% versus 51% with placebo). For every thousand patients treated with a bolus plus infusion of abciximab in EPIC, at 3 years, there were 29 fewer MIs, 54 fewer revascularizations and 18 fewer deaths.

EPIC substudies

Several retrospective substudy analyses have addressed specific patient groups within the overall EPIC study cohort.

Unstable angina

In patients with documented unstable angina ($n = 489$), the 30-day composite endpoint of death, MI, or urgent intervention in the unstable angina population treated with a bolus plus infusion of abciximab was reduced from 12.8% to 4.8%, compared with the overall cohort in which composite events were reduced from 12.8% to 8.3%.[26] At 6-months follow-up, there was an even more dramatic effect of abciximab bolus plus infusion on the incidence of death (1.8% versus 6.6%) and MI (2.4% versus 11.1%). Overall, in the unstable angina population, there was a 94% relative reduction in the incidence of death or MI at 30 days and an 88% relative reduction of the same events over 6 months. However, in contrast to the overall EPIC cohort, abciximab had no effect on the incidence of revascularization in this subgroup.

Acute MI

Within the cohort of patients who underwent angioplasty within 12 h of the onset of a MI ($n = 64$), 42 underwent direct PTCA and 22 had rescue PTCA after failed thrombolysis.[27]

Treatment with bolus plus infusion abciximab was associated with a 91% decrease in 6-month composite endpoints (4.5% versus 47.8% in the placebo group; $p = 0.002$) and a trend toward lower 30-day endpoints (4.5% versus 26.1%; $p = 0.058$).

Directional atherectomy

As in previous studies,[28,29] placebo-treated directional atherectomy (DCA) patients, in this case 197 patients, had an incidence of non-Q-wave MI that was approximately twice that found in the PTCA population (9.6% versus 4.9%, $p = 0.006$).[30] In contrast, the incidence of non-Q-wave MI in abciximab-treated (bolus plus infusion) DCA patients showed a substantial decrease from 15.4% in the placebo arm compared with 4.5% in abciximab-treated (bolus plus infusion) patients ($p = 0.046$). Thus treatment with abciximab reduced the risk of DCA-related non-Q wave MI.

Restenotic lesions

In patients in EPIC with restenotic lesions ($n = 237$),[31] treatment with abciximab bolus/infusion showed substantial benefit in both 30-day composite events (2.9% with abciximab, 14.1% with placebo) and 6-month composite events (26% with abciximab, 39.4% with placebo). Procedure-associated MI tended to be lower with abciximab, and urgent interventions were reduced from 14.1% with placebo to 0% with bolus/infusion abciximab.

Vein graft lesions

There were 126 lesions in 101 patients in EPIC who underwent treatment of saphenous vein-graft lesions.[32] Bolus/infusion treatment with abciximab was associated with an 87% reduction in distal embolization (3.0% versus 21.0% with placebo, $p = 0.037$). Additionally, at 30 days there was a reduction in the incidence of large (CK more than 5 times normal) non-Q-wave MIs (3% versus 14% with placebo). There was, however, no significant overall reduction in composite 30-day or 6-month clinical events.

Diabetes

In a study of 506 patients in EPIC with diabetes, at 6-month follow-up, 40% of patients with diabetes who received placebo developed clinical restenosis, compared with 36% in patients who received bolus/infusion abciximab.[33] In contrast, non-diabetic/placebo patients had a 33% incidence of clinical restenosis, compared with 24% in non-diabetic/abciximab bolus/infusion patients.

Effect of abciximab on activated coagulation times

One surprising finding in EPIC was that abciximab had an independent effect of prolonging procedural activated coagulation times (ACTs).[34] Despite receiving less procedural heparin, and with fewer patients requiring high (more than 14 000 U) heparin doses, abciximab-treated patients had higher mean procedural ACTs (401 s versus 367 s), even after correcting for body weight. Thus, on average, abciximab therapy was associated with an independent 34-s increase in the ACT. Similar, although smaller, increases have been noted with the cyclic heptapeptide integrilin.[35] Additionally, in vitro studies have shown that the prolongation of the ACT was due to GPIIb/IIIa blockade, that was independent of platelet factor 4.[36] The theoretical mechanism for this is, as yet, unclear. While platelets (specifically, the activated platelet membrane) play a key role in the process of coagulation, it is not immediately clear how the inhibition of platelet aggregation might affect ex-vivo coagulation of whole blood in a test tube. Nevertheless blockade of the GPIIb/IIIa receptor appears to prolong coagulation times significantly. Moliterno et al[34] have speculated that as thrombin activity is antagonized by high-dose heparin, coagulation times may become more dependent on platelet function.

Abciximab and bypass surgery

In a study of abciximab in 58 bypass surgery patients, forty-six patients required surgery within 24 h of randomization.[37] All-cause 30-day mortality was not significantly different between groups, although there was an adverse trend with bolus/infusion abciximab (8.0% with placebo, 7.1% with bolus alone abciximab, and 29.4% with bolus/infusion abciximab; $p = 0.28$). Of the 17 emergency surgery patients who had received bolus/infusion abciximab, 5 died; 1 never actually received the drug, and of the remaining 4 patients, none died during surgery or as a direct result of hemorrhage. Major blood loss (>5 g/dL decrease in Hgb) was common in all three groups (72% with placebo, 100% with bolus abciximab, 76% with bolus/infusion abciximab). There was a tendency toward more frequent RBC, whole blood, and platelet transfusions in abciximab-treated patients, although this did not achieve statistical significance. Interestingly, postsurgical thrombocytopenia was significantly less frequent after abciximab therapy.

Economic substudy

As part of the EPIC trial, economic data were collected prospectively on 2045 of the 2099 total patients in the trial.[38] Baseline and follow-up hospital costs and resource utilization were tabulated from the time of randomization through 6 months of follow-up. Cost data were obtained by converting charges using data from each participating hospitals'

Medicare Cost Report and a 'cost-effectiveness ratio', to the incremental cost of achieving one incremental patient free from major adverse outcome events at 6 months of death, myocardial infarction, or repeat revascularization was calculated. Importantly, the cost of the drug was not accounted for in the analyses. Although there was an initial potential in-hospital savings of $539 with bolus/infusion abciximab therapy, this was offset by an increase in the costs associated with bleeding events ($502), so that the mean baseline medical costs (hospital and physician, exclusive of the drug) were $13 565 with abciximab, versus $13 588 for placebo. The median hospital stay in those patients with major bleeding was 7 days compared with 3 days in those without that complication.

With a 22% decrease in repeat hospitalizations and a 26% decrease in repeat revascularizations, abciximab patients, had significantly lower follow-up costs ($3291 versus $4362 with placebo). For every 100 patients treated with abciximab, there were an additional 8 patients with uncomplicated PTCA (free from death, MI and urgent revascularization). Although at the time the study was performed, the cost of abciximab was not known, the current average cost to treat an average-sized patient is approximately $1350. Therefore, the incremental cost per patient treated (incorporating drug costs) is $251, and the cost-effectiveness ratio is $3137 per uncomplicated patient. This cost study, however, is not entirely applicable to other established cost-effectiveness ratios (which are usually expressed in terms of dollar per life year added).

PROLOG study

The PROLOG (Precursor to EPILOG) study[39] was a multicenter pilot trial evaluating the safety and efficacy of weight-adjusted heparin dosing and early sheath removal in PTCA patients treated using abciximab. A total of 103 patients undergoing PTCA were randomized to one of two possible heparin regimens—either 'standard-dose' weight-adjusted heparin (100 U/kg bolus, titrated to an ACT of 300–350 s) or 'low-dose' weight-adjusted heparin (70 U/kg bolus, without ACT-guided titration). Patients were also randomized to one of two possible sheath-removal strategies:

(1) Early (immediately after procedural heparin had worn off); or
(2) 12 h after the procedure.

All patients received uniform abciximab therapy (0.25 mg/kg per bolus followed by a 12-h infusion at 10 (µg/min). The median preinflation ACT in the standard-dose heparin arm was 336 s, and 257 s in the low-dose heparin arm. Hematoma formation and transfusion requirements were significantly lower in the low-dose heparin group, and all bleeding complications were significantly reduced in the early sheath-removal group. There was no increase in ischemic complications in the low-dose heparin group. These pilot safety data set the stage for the subsequent EPILOG trial.

EPILOG trial

The prior EPIC study has demonstrated the efficacy of abciximab in reducing adverse events in high-risk patients undergoing PTCA. There was, however, a high incidence of bleeding in this first major trial. The EPILOG (Evaluation of PTCA to Improve Long-term Outcomes by c7E3 Glycoprotein IIb/IIIa receptor blockade) study[13] sought to:

(1) Evaluate the efficacy of abciximab in both low- and high-risk patients undergoing PTCA; and
(2) Determine whether a reduction in heparin dosing could reduce hemorrhagic compli-

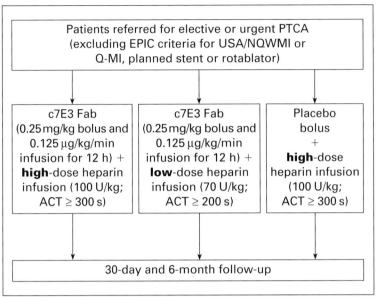

Figure 8.4
Flow-chart of the EPILOG study.

cations without compromising clinical efficacy.

Both low- and medium-risk patients were randomized to receive:

(1) Standard-dose heparin (100 U/kg bolus, titrated to ACT of less than 300 s) plus placebo;

(2) Standard-dose heparin plus abciximab (0.25 mg/kg bolus, 0.125 µg/kg/min (upto 10 µg/kg/min), infusion for 12 h); or

(3) Low-dose heparin (70 U/kg, ACT greater than 200 s) and abciximab (Figure 8.4). The primary endpoint of the study was the 30-day combined incidence of death, MI, or urgent revascularization.

The trial was originally designed to include 4800 patients but was terminated prematurely on the recommendation of the DSMB (Data Safety Monitoring Board) because of an interim analysis (of the first 1500 patients), which demonstrated beneficial effects of 7E3 Fab that exceeded prespecified criteria for discontinuation of the trial. At the time the trial was stopped, 2792 patients had been enrolled. In the EPILOG study cohort, the combined incidence of death and MI (creatine kinase elevation of at least three times baseline) at 30 days was 11.7% in the standard heparin plus placebo group, 5.4% in the standard heparin plus abciximab group, and 5.2% in the low-dose heparin plus abciximab group. This relative decrease of 56% in adverse events in both low- and medium-risk patients was almost twice the benefit shown in the previous EPIC study, which included only higher-risk patients. At 6 months, the incidence of the primary endpoint of death, MI, or any additional revascularization was 25.8% with placebo,

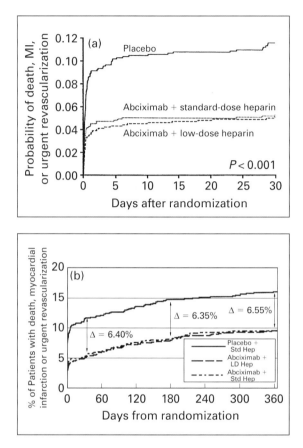

Figure 8.5
(a) Cumulative 30-day events in the EPILOG study: Kaplan-Meier estimate of the probability of death, myocardial infarction (MI), or urgent repeat vascularization. Adapted from Ref 13.
(b) Cumulative 1-year event. From Ref 42.

among the groups at 6 months. The significant clinical benefit associated with abciximab was present in both stable angina and unstable angina patients. Additionally, bleeding complications were greatly reduced in comparison to the EPIC trial. Major bleeding was 3.1% in the standard heparin plus placebo group, 3.5% in the standard heparin plus abciximab group, and 2.0% in the low-dose heparin plus abciximab group ($p = $ NS). Minor bleeding complications, however, were more common in the abciximab plus standard-dose heparin arm (7.4%) compared with the abciximab plus low-dose heparin arm (4.0%), and the placebo arm (3.7%).

EPILOG substudies

Diabetic patients
An EPILOG substudy examined the 638 (23%) diabetic patients in the trial.[40] Both diabetic patients and non-diabetic patients demonstrated an improvement in the composite of death, MI, and urgent intervention. There appeared to be somewhat of a disparity between the two heparin dose arms with abciximab (an effect not noted in the non-diabetic patients). At 6 months, target vessel revascularization in diabetics was not reduced with abciximab, and was even slightly, (but not significantly), worse with abciximab, particularly when low-dose heparin was used. At 6 months, endpoint events occurred in 23.1% of the diabetic patients receiving abciximab and standard dose heparin compared with 31.4% in the abciximab low-dose heparin group.

Unplanned stenting
Kereiakes et al.[41] reported on the subgroup of 326 patients (12%) of the overall EPILOG cohort who had unplanned or bailout stent placement. Patients who received stents were not distinguished by clinical factors although they did tend to have more complex coronary

22.3% with standard heparin plus abciximab, and 22.8% with low-dose heparin plus abciximab (Figure 8.5). The incidence of MI (9.9%, 5.3%, and 5.0%, respectively) and urgent revascularization (6.7%, 3.5%, and 3.1%, respectively) accounted for much of the differences between the treatment arms. There were no significant differences in elective revascularization or target vessel revascularization

lesions (by American College of Cardiology (ACC) criteria), with longer, more eccentric, more irregular, and bifurcation lesions. Patients undergoing unplanned stent placement had a significantly higher incidence of the composite endpoint of death, MI, or urgent intervention (14.4% versus 6.3% in patients not receiving stents). Unplanned stents were required less often in abciximab patients who received low-dose heparin (9.0% versus 13.7% with heparin alone) but not in abciximab patients treated with standard dose heparin (13.6%). Abciximab usage was associated with fewer adverse events at 30 days and 6 months. The incidence of the composite endpoint in stent patients at 30 days was 22.6% in the heparin alone group, 8.6% in the abciximab/low-dose heparin group, and 9.9% in the abciximab/high-dose heparin group. Composite outcome events at 6 months in the respective groups were 24.2%, 11.1%, and 12.5% respectively. In stent patients in EPILOG, abciximab did not increase major and minor bleeding complications; major bleeding events actually tended to be lower in the abciximab groups.

1-Year outcomes

Lincoff et al.[42] recently reported on long-term outcomes (up to 1 year) in the EPILOG cohort. Follow-up at 1 year was 99% complete for survival status and 97% complete for other endpoints. At 1 year, the composite incidence of death, MI, or urgent revascularization was 16.1% in the placebo group, 9.6% in the abciximab/low-dose heparin group, and 9.5% in the abciximab/standard-dose heparin group (Figure 8.5b). Non-urgent revascularization and target vessel revascularization rates were not significantly different between groups.

CAPTURE study

The third major trial of abciximab was a European multicenter randomized study, known as CAPTURE (c7E3 Antiplatelet Therapy in Unstable Refractory Angina), which studied the effect of abciximab on patients with refractory unstable angina undergoing coronary intervention.[14] This study was conducted at the same time as the EPILOG study. Patients were randomized to receive 18–24 h of pretreatment with either abciximab (0.25 mg/kg bolus followed by 10 µg/kg/min infusion) or placebo before undergoing PTCA. Treatment was extended for only 1 h after the interventional procedure, in contrast to EPIC and EPILOG, in which patients received abciximab only at the time of the interventional procedure, and treatment was continued for 12 h afterwards (Figure 8.6). CAPTURE was originally designed to include 1400 patients but was, like EPILOG, stopped prematurely after an interim analysis of 1050 patients demonstrated significant clinical benefit that exceeded prespecified stopping criteria. The primary endpoint of the study was the 30-day combined incidence of death, MI, and urgent intervention. At the time the trial was stopped, 1266 patients had been enrolled. At 30 days, the primary combined endpoint was reduced from 15.9% in the placebo group to 11.3% in the treatment arm; death and MI alone were similarly reduced from 9.0% to 4.8%. All of the individual events that comprised the primary endpoint were also reduced (death, from 1.3% to 1.0%; MI, from 8.2% to 4.1%; and urgent intervention, from 10.9% to 7.8%). Major bleeding complications remained more common in the abciximab-treated group (3.8% versus 1.9% in the placebo group), but at a level much lower than in the earlier EPIC study. However, unlike the EPIC and EPILOG studies, the benefits of the CAPTURE dosing regimen of abciximab were lost at 6 months

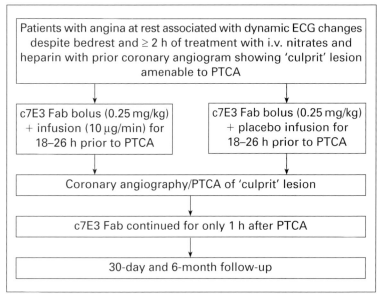

Figure 8.6
Flow-chart of the CAPTURE study.

The flow-chart contains the following boxes:

- Patients with angina at rest associated with dynamic ECG changes despite bedrest and ≥ 2 h of treatment with i.v. nitrates and heparin with prior coronary angiogram showing 'culprit' lesion amenable to PTCA
- c7E3 Fab bolus (0.25 mg/kg) + infusion (10 µg/min) for 18–26 h prior to PTCA
- c7E3 Fab bolus (0.25 mg/kg) + placebo infusion for 18–26 h prior to PTCA
- Coronary angiography/PTCA of 'culprit' lesion
- c7E3 Fab continued for only 1 h after PTCA
- 30-day and 6-month follow-up

(Figure 8.7). There was a 31.0% incidence of the combined clinical endpoint in the abciximab arm compared with 30.8% in the placebo group. These findings strongly suggest that a 12-h post-procedure infusion (as employed in the EPIC and EPILOG studies) is important to achieve a sustained clinical benefit.

CAPTURE substudies

Recurrent ischemia

One substudy of CAPTURE[43] focused on the incidence of recurrent ischemia and overall ischemic burden. A subset of 332 patients (26% of the overall cohort) underwent continuous vector-derived 12-lead ischemia monitoring, beginning no later than 1 h after enrollment, and continuing for at least 24–36 h, including 6 h after the PTCA procedure. There were fewer ischemic episodes detected in abciximab patients (31/169 or 18% vs. 37/163 or 23% with placebo); this difference did not achieve statistical signifi-

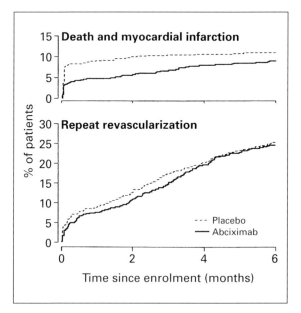

Figure 8.7
Cumulative events of death and myocardial infarction (above) and repeat revascularization (below) in the CAPTURE study. The initial benefits are not sustained at the 6-month follow-up. Adapted from Ref 14.

cance. Significantly fewer abciximab patients had less than two ischemic episodes, however (5% versus 14%; $p < 0.01$). Total ischemic burden was also significantly reduced with abciximab, calculated as either total duration of ischemia, the area under the curve of the ST-segment magnitude, or the sum of the area under the curves of the 12 leads. Furthermore, the presence of both symptomatic and asymptomatic ST-segment episodes during monitoring in the whole population was associated with a much higher likelihood of developing a myocardial infarction or dying.

Troponin T

Recently presented data from CAPTURE have focused on a subpopulation of patients (1088 out of 1265 total in the study) from whom blood samples were obtained at random to measure troponin T by quantitative enzyme immunoassay.[44] Patients with a recent (less than 2 weeks) myocardial infarction were excluded because of the potential confounding influence of the recent cardiac event. Positive (more than 0.2 ng/ml) values of troponin T were noted in 204 patients (23%). During subsequent follow-up there were 17 deaths (0.5) and 79 MIs (8.9%); the likelihood of death or MI was significantly related to the level of troponin T.

There was a dramatic effect of abciximab therapy in improving outcomes in troponin T-positive patients. The 6-month death/MI rate in troponin T-positive patients in the placebo group was 26.3%; compared with 9.5% in troponin T-positive patients in the abciximab group. The salutory effects of abciximab were evident very early in the course of therapy. In troponin T-positive patients, the incidence of death/MI before PTCA was 6.1% with placebo and 0% with abciximab; at 48 h the incidence of death/MI was 17.2% with placebo and 1.9% with abciximab. On the other hand, abciximab had no significant effect in the troponin T-negative patients: the 6-month rate of death/MI was 9.7% in the placebo group and 8.3% in the abciximab group.

Troponin T and recurrent ischemia

A recent report went on to examine the relationship between troponin T and the incidence of recurrent ischemia in the CAPTURE study.[45] In troponin T-negative patients, 19% of the abciximab group and 17% of the placebo group developed recurrent symptoms, with no difference in the number of episodes per patient (1.1 with abciximab, 1.2 with placebo) and necessity for early PTCA (1.4% with abciximab, 1.8% with placebo). Conversely, in the troponin T-positive patients, 21% of the abciximab group compared with 45% of the placebo group developed recurrent symptoms. The abciximab group also tended to have fewer episodes per patient (1.3 versus 2.1 with placebo), and a lower necessity for early PTCA (2.0% versus 6.8% with placebo).

RAPPORT study

The RAPPORT (ReoPro in Acute MI and Primary PTCA Organization and Randomized Trial) trial examined the efficacy of abciximab in the setting of primary PTCA for acute myocardial infarction.[15] In this study, 483 patients presenting within 12 h of an acute MI and deemed to be candidates for primary PTCA, were randomized to receive either an abciximab bolus plus a 12-h infusion ($n = 241$) or placebo ($n = 242$). Early drug administration (more than 30 min before initial balloon inflation) occurred in 19% of the placebo patients and 21% of the abciximab patients. All patients received aspirin. Heparin was administered to all patients as a 100 U/kg bolus (with ACTs titrated to more than 300 s) and could be continued for up to 48 h after the procedure. The primary endpoint of the study was the composite incidence of death, reinfarction, or any (urgent or elective) target vessel revascularization at 6 months. Although there was no significant difference in the primary endpoint at 6 months (28.1% placebo versus 28.2% abciximab using intention-to-treat (ITT) analysis), abciximab significantly reduced the combined incidence of death, reinfarction and urgent target vessel revascularization (TVR) at all time points: 9.9% versus 3.3% at 7 days; 11.2% versus 5.8% at 30 days, and 17.8% versus 11.6% at 6 months. There were a relatively large number of patients ($n = 74$) who did not actually receive per-protocol therapy, usually (in 54 patients) because a PTCA was not actually performed. The need for unplanned, or 'bailout' stenting was also significantly reduced, from 20.4% with placebo to 11.9% with abciximab. There was a significant increase in major bleeding with abciximab (rising from 9.5% to 16.6%); the most frequent site of bleeding being the arterial access site.

ERASER study

Previous data from EPIC (though not EPILOG) had suggested that abciximab might reduce the incidence of recurrent clinical events (i.e. clinical restenosis) following coronary intervention. To examine this further and assess whether abciximab was of value in preventing intimal hyperplasia following stenting, the ERASER trial was undertaken.[16] This was a prospective, randomized, placebo-controlled, multicenter study in 225 patients undergoing elective coronary stent placement, who were randomized to receive either placebo, a bolus and 12-h infusion of abciximab, or a bolus and 24-h infusion of abciximab. The primary endpoint of the study was the percent volume obstruction by IVUS at 6-month follow-up catheterization; 152 patients underwent 6-month follow-up IVUS examination. At 6 month follow-up, the mean IVUS percent volume obstruction was 32.4% in the placebo group, 32.7% in the 12-h abciximab group, and 34.2% in the 24-h abciximab group. The incidence of death, MI, and target vessel revascularization at 6 months was 25.4% in the placebo group, 20.3% in the 12-h abciximab group, and 22.7% in the 24-h abciximab group. Thus, treatment with abciximab did not result in a significant decrease in intimal hyperplasia after intracoronary stent placement.

EPISTENT study

The previous EPIC, EPILOG, and CAPTURE trials had not included patients undergoing elective stent placement. ERASER had suggested no benefit of abciximab in reducing clinical restenosis, but was not adequately powered to assess acute clinical benefit. In the EPISTENT trial,[17] a total of 2399 patients eligible for elective stenting were randomized to one of three groups:

(1) Stent plus placebo;
(2) Stent plus abciximab; and
(3) PTCA plus abciximab (Figure 8.8).

In the stent alone group, heparin was given as a 100 U/kg bolus, and ACTs were titrated to 300–350 s. In the two abciximab groups, low-dose heparin was employed; patients received a 70 U/kg bolus, and ACTs were titrated to over 200 s. The primary composite endpoint of death, MI, or urgent revascularization at 30 days after the intervention was 5.3% in the stent plus abciximab group, 6.9% in the PTCA plus abciximab group, and 10.8% in the group receiving stent with placebo (Figure 8.9). The incidence of death or MI at 30 days (Q-wave MI or CK/CKMB elevation more than five times the control) was also significantly reduced with abciximab; being 3.0% in

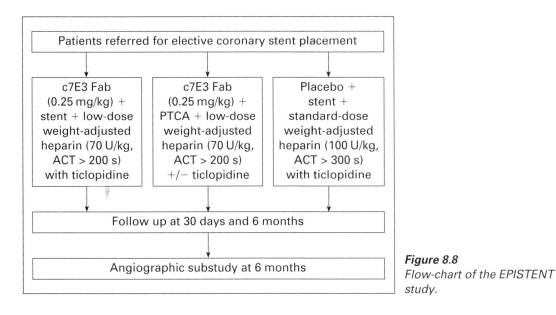

```
┌─────────────────────────────────────────────────────────────┐
│  ┌─────────────────────────────────────────────────────────┐  │
│  │     Patients referred for elective coronary stent placement │  │
│  └─────────────────────────────────────────────────────────┘  │
│         ↓                    ↓                    ↓             │
│  ┌──────────────┐   ┌──────────────┐   ┌──────────────┐      │
│  │  c7E3 Fab    │   │  c7E3 Fab    │   │  Placebo +   │      │
│  │ (0.25 mg/kg)+│   │ (0.25 mg/kg)+│   │   stent +    │      │
│  │ stent + low- │   │ PTCA + low-  │   │ standard-dose│      │
│  │ dose weight- │   │ dose weight- │   │ weight-      │      │
│  │ adjusted     │   │ adjusted     │   │ adjusted     │      │
│  │ heparin      │   │ heparin      │   │ heparin      │      │
│  │ (70 U/kg,    │   │ (70 U/kg,    │   │ (100 U/kg,   │      │
│  │ ACT > 200 s) │   │ ACT > 200 s) │   │ ACT > 300 s) │      │
│  │ with         │   │ +/- ticlo-   │   │ with         │      │
│  │ ticlopidine  │   │ pidine       │   │ ticlopidine  │      │
│  └──────────────┘   └──────────────┘   └──────────────┘      │
│         ↓                    ↓                    ↓             │
│  ┌─────────────────────────────────────────────────────────┐  │
│  │          Follow up at 30 days and 6 months              │  │
│  └─────────────────────────────────────────────────────────┘  │
│                            ↓                                   │
│  ┌─────────────────────────────────────────────────────────┐  │
│  │          Angiographic substudy at 6 months             │  │
│  └─────────────────────────────────────────────────────────┘  │
└─────────────────────────────────────────────────────────────┘
```

Figure 8.8
Flow-chart of the EPISTENT study.

the stent plus abciximab group, 4.7% in the PTCA plus abciximab group and 7.8% in the stent alone group. A major contributing component of these composite endpoints was the difference observed in the incidence of large non-Q myocardial infarction (defined as a CK MB increase of more than five times the control); this was 2.0% in the stent plus abciximab group, compared with 2.6% in the PTCA plus abciximab group and 5.8% in the stent alone group. It was noted that 77% of patients with an early post-procedural MI endpoint event had evidence of other ECG charges or documented clinical symptoms of ischemia. Major bleeding complications were noted in 1.5% of the stent plus abciximab group, in 1.4% of the balloon plus abciximab group and in 2.2% of the stent plus placebo group.

At 6 months follow-up, the combined incidence of death, MI and revascularization (total) was 13.0% in the stent plus abciximab group, 20.5% in the PTCA plus abciximab group and 18.3% in the stent alone group.[46] The respective 6-month rates for death, MI, or urgent revascularization were 12.1%, 9.2%, 6.4% respectively, and for the combined incidence of death or MI at 6 months were 5.6%, 7.8% and 11.4% respectively. Recent longer-term follow-up has also shown a significant 1-year mortality benefit associated with adjunctive abciximab.[47] One-year mortality (intention-to-treat) was 2.4% in the stent alone group, 1.0% in the stent/abciximab group and 2.1% in the PTCA/abciximab group.

Diabetic subgroup

There appeared to be particular benefit in reducing 6-month composite events (death/MI/TVR) in the diabetic cohort within the EPISTENT study.[46] In diabetic patients, 6-month composite events occurred in 25.2% of the stent alone group, 13.0% of the stent/abciximab group, and 23.4% of the PTCA/abciximab group. Comparable events in

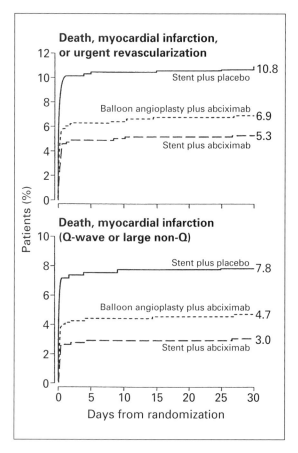

Figure 8.9
Cumulative events in the EPI-STENT study for the first 30 days. The addition of abciximab to stenting or angioplasty was superior to stenting alone. Adapted from Ref 44.

the non-diabetic cohort were 16.5%, 13.0%, and 19.9% respectively. Focusing on TVR alone, the event rates were 16.6%, 8.1% and 18.4% in the respective diabetic groups, and 9.0%, 8.8%, and 14.6% of the respective non-diabetic groups.

Angiographic substudy
Six-month angiographic data from EPISTENT (*n* = 899) have also recently been presented.[48] Overall, the initial gain was 1.53 mm in the stent alone group, 1.60 mm in the stent/abciximab group, and 1.09 mm in the PTCA/abciximab group. Late loss was 0.79 mm, 0.73 mm, and 0.46 mm, respectively; net gain (initial gain minus late loss) was 0.73 mm, 0.86 mm, 0.62 mm, respectively. The respective late loss indices were 0.60 mm, 0.41 mm, and 0.48 mm. In the subgroup of diabetic patients, the net gain at 6 months was 0.55 mm in the stent alone group, 0.88 mm in the stent/abciximab group, and 0.43 mm in the PTCA/abciximab group. The net gains in the comparable non-diabetic groups were 0.78 mm, 0.86 mm, and 0.67 mm. Respective minimum lumen diameters (MLDs) were 1.48 mm, 1.66 mm, and 1.28 mm in the diabetic groups and 1.63 mm, 1.66 mm, and 1.51 mm in the non-diabetic groups.

Abciximab/stenting for acute myocardial infarction
In 1998, Newmann and co-workers reported the results of a prospective, randomized trial of abciximab in patients undergoing stent placement for acute MI.[49] In this study, 200 consecutive MI patients presenting within 48 h after the onset of symptoms and undergoing stent placement were randomized to receive either standard-dose heparin (*n* = 98; total of 15 000 U heparin for the procedure, infusion for 12 h after sheath removal), or abciximab plus low-dose heparin (*n* = 102; abciximab 0.25 mg/g bolus, 10 µg/min infusion for 12 h; total heparin 7500 U. Flow velocity (versus Doppler wire) was assessed immediately following stent placement and at 14-day angiographic follow-up. A total of 152 paired studies were obtained. Papaverine-induced peak flow velocities improved more in the

abciximab group than in patients on heparin alone (18.1 cm/s versus 10.4 cm/s), as did wall motion index measurements (0.44 SD/chord versus 0.15 SD/chord).

At follow-up, the global left ventricular ejection fraction (LVEF) was significantly greater in the abciximab group than the heparin alone group (62% versus 56%). Target lesion reintervention occurred in 4 patients in the control group. During 30-day clinical follow-up after the procedure, 2 patients in the abciximab group and 9 patients in the heparin alone group had adverse clinical events of death, MI and target lesion reintervention.

The ADMIRAL study was a randomized, placebo-controlled trial of abciximab in patients treated with primary interventional therapy for acute MI (48A). Patients presenting within 12 hours of the onset of symptoms were randomized to abciximab ($n = 149$) or placebo ($n = 150$) prior to intervention. All patients were treated with aspirin, heparin, and ticlopidine. Patients with cardiogenic shock were excluded from the study. Stents were utilized in approximately 85% of patients; approximately 30% of patients received ≥ 2 stents. Study drug therapy was initiated prior to arrival in the catheterization laboratory in approximately 25% of patients. Angiography was repeated 24 hours after the interventional procedure. The 30-day primary composite clinical endpoint (death, MI, and ischemia-driven target vessel revascularization) was significantly reduced in the abciximab group (10.7% vs. 20% with placebo). Abciximab patients had a significantly higher incidence of TIMI grade III flow prior to intervention (21% vs. 10.3% with placebo); and at 24 hours following the procedure (85.6% vs. 78.4% with placebo. Major bleeding was slightly, but not significantly, higher in the abcciximab group (4.0% vs. 2.6% with placebo). Minor bleeding was more frequent with abciximab.

Clinical issues relating to interventional applications

Bleeding

One clear message that has emerged from the clinical trials to date is that the high incidence of bleeding complications seen in the EPIC study can be reduced significantly. The PRO-LOG, EPILOG, and EPI-STENT studies have highlighted the importance of reducing the heparin doses used for interventional procedures, and the importance of early sheath removal as a major factor in the reducing local site complications. In much the same way that the initial high incidence of site-related bleeding complications in aggressively anticoagulated coronary stent patients could be reduced, accumulated experience with abciximab therapy has optimized management. Studies such as EPILOG and CAPTURE noted a slight increase in bleeding complications but this problem is clearly not so worrisome as was initially thought. In the more recent EPISTENT study, major bleeding complications actually tended to be less frequent in the abciximab groups (with concomitant low-dose heparin). Currently the recommendation for procedural heparin if abciximab is utilized is 70 U/kg; some investigators are currently evaluating the possibility of utilizing even lower doses, for example 50 U/kg. Other strategies for reducing procedure-associated bleeding complications are outlined in Table 8.2.[50,51]

Coronary artery bypass surgery

Another potential safety issue is the risk of bleeding associated with emergency coronary artery bypass graft (CABG), if required, in the setting of near-complete GPIIb/IIIa receptor

1. Give bolus dosage of abciximab 0.25 mg/kg at least 10 min but less than 1 h prior to intervention.
2. Begin infusion of abciximab 10 µg/min immediately after bolus dose. Consider weight-adjusted dose of 0.125 µg/kg/min up to a maximum of 10 µg/min.
3. Give weight-adjusted heparin bolus of 70 U/kg before intervention; target ACT to be greater than 200 s (measured after both heparin and abciximab have been administered); consider higher heparin doses (100 U/kg; ACT target over 300 s) only in patients at higher risk for thrombosis.
4. Give no postprocedural heparin unless there is evidence of intraprocedural ongoing thrombosis; if heparin is felt to be necessary, use an infusion of 7 U/kg/h.
5. Remove sheath as soon as ACT is less than 175 s or aPTT is less than 50 s (or per usual institutional standard); do not stop abciximab during sheath removal.
6. Use single wall punctures for vascular access; do not try to access recently instrumented sites; Avoid routine venous sheaths.
7. Use adequate patient sedation and immobilization during bedrest.
8. Use Femostop after sheath removal in situations where there is a higher risk of femoral access-site bleeding.

Modified from Lincoff,[50] 1996.

Table 8.2
Strategies to minimize bleeding with abciximab.

blockade. As previously mentioned, in the EPIC study, the incidence of major bleeding was not significantly different between groups, and post-CABG thrombocytopenia in the EPIC study was actually significantly less prominent with abciximab than with placebo.[37] The surgical literature contains several reports[52,53] citing the potential risks of perioperative bleeding, although in these studies conventional doses of heparin (300 U/kg) are usually given prior to surgery. Another report[54] examined the outcome of emergency CABG in the more recent EPILOG and EPISTENT studies. Of the 5191 patients in these two trials, 42 (0.8%) required emergency CABG within 7 days of the interventional procedure: these were 22/1748 (1.3%) placebo patients and 20/3443 (0.6%) abciximab patients. Approximately one-half to two-thirds of patients underwent surgery within 6 h of discontinuation of the study drug. There were no significant differences in the incidence of major bleeding (Hgb decrease $\geqslant 5$ g or intracranial hemorrage (ICH)) or blood transfusion. There was a higher incidence of platelet transfusion in the abciximab group (64% versus 41% with placebo) Blood loss was comparable between groups; although abciximab patients had a somewhat higher incidence of re-exploration for bleeding (12.8% versus 3.6% with placebo). Peak procedural ACTs tended to be higher in the abciximab group (711 s versus 600 s with placebo).

In view of the bleeding risks incurred when

high-dose heparin is used with abciximab in patients undergoing PTCA, it would be prudent to consider more controlled heparin dosing in patients undergoing CABG. One potential strategy might be to more carefully titrate heparin to the usual institutional standard (frequently 450 s) rather than using routine administration of high-dose heparin (300 U/kg, or more, in some centers). Abciximab independently prolongs the ACT, and many of the previously observed bleeding complication appear related more to high doses of heparin than necessarily to abciximab therapy per se.

Platelet transfusions should also be considered strongly in patients requiring emergency surgery; this is because abciximab is rapidly cleared from the plasma and all the drug is on the surface of the platelets, not sequestered elsewhere in the body. Thus the pharmacodynamic effects of abciximab are theoretically reversible with platelet transfusions, which reduce the drug's receptor occupancy on platelet surfaces to less than the critical 50% threshold associated with prolongation of bleeding time. This may be particularly important in the setting of patients who require emergency bypass surgery. Routine platelet transfusions prior to surgery are at the discretion of the operator. It will take up to about 3 h for the complete redistribution of drug to the newly transfused platelets. If it is possible to delay surgery (preferably for at least 12–24 h), aggressive platelet transfusions can essentially reverse the hemostatic defect prior to surgery. If patients require surgery more urgently, aggressive platelet transfusions after surgery can reduce the risk of postoperative bleeding. Clinicians should be aware of the other attendant bleeding risks in patients transferred for emergency surgery. Many of these patients are in cardiogenic shock and have received multiple anticoagulant,

antiplatelet, and even fibrinolytic agents. Postoperative coagulopathies are frequently encountered in these patients. Although adjunctive abciximab may increase the bleeding risks of emergency bypass surgery, in experienced hands, with controlled heparinization, and with aggressive platelet transfusions before **and** after cardiopulmonary bypass, the bleeding risks are certainly manageable.

Stents

Upwards two-thirds to three-quarters of coronary interventions in the USA now involve the use of coronary stents. Until recently, there were no clinical data on the use of abciximab for elective stenting; however, with the recent publication of the EPISTENT data, the concerns about stenting have for the most part, been put to rest. As already mentioned, there are substantial acute benefits associated with the use of adjunctive GPIIb/IIIa targeted therapy with stenting. These acute benefits are durable, and appear to extend the potential application of stents. Furthermore, the recent data on the significant 1-year mortality benefit of adjunctive abciximab are fairly compelling. Given the clinical benefits seen in the EPISTENT study, one could argue that adjunctive GPIIb/IIIa targeted therapy ought at least to be considered in all patients undergoing stent implantation, particularly in higher-risk clinical situations, such as acute coronary syndromes, vein grafts, small vessels, multiple overlapping stents, thrombus-containing lesions, and in diabetic patients.

Whether abciximab will be truly cost effective in low-risk patients undergoing stent implantation remains controversial, but on the strength of the EPISTENT data, treatment of not-low-risk patients is probably warranted.

Treatment of thrombus

In many centers, abciximab has replaced intracoronary thrombolytic agent administration as first-line therapy for the treatment of intra-coronary thrombus. There have also been pre-liminary reports of the conjunctive use of the two agents in an attempt to reproduce the syn-ergism and enhanced lytic efficacy that had been reported in studies with animals.[55–57] Empirical observations of this type of combi-nation therapy have not suggested a prohibi-tive increase in bleeding complications.[58] Abciximab may be more effective in acute thrombotic situations, while lytic agents may be better suited to treat an established throm-bus that persists after an acute thrombotic episode.

Rotational atherectomy

Recent studies have suggested that following rotational atherectomy, the incidence of periprocedural non-Q MI may be as high as 19–25%.[59] Retrospective studies of other agents (namely Integrilin in the IMPACT II study) sug-gested that GPIIb/IIIa-targeted therapy may be effective in reducing the incidence of abrupt clo-sure, and the composite of death, MI, and urgent intervention.[60] Braden et al[61] conducted a randomized trial of abciximab in patients undergoing rotational atherectomy. They noted that abciximab significantly reduced the peak level of creative kinase (CK) and the frequency of CK elevation above normal. A retrospective recent report by Diez suggested a significant effect of abciximab in reducing the incidence of thrombolysis in myocardial infarction (TIMI) grade O/I flow (but not TIMI grade II flow) following rotational atherectomy.[62] Platelet aggregation in association with rotational atherectomy has been shown to be rotation speed-dependent;[63] Moreover rotation speed-dependent platelet activation can be inhibited by abciximab in vivo.[64] Hence, GPIIb/IIIa-targeted therapy may have a very important role in redu-cing the potential consequences of high-speed rotational atherectomy.

Retreatment

Another difficult question that arises is the issue of retreatment. Since abciximab is a chimeric antibody, it contains some murine-derived sequences, and there is a potential for immunogenic reactions, either as a primary phenomenon, or upon reexposure. Current commercial labeling of ReoPro does not advo-cate retreatment, although there are anecdotal reports of uncomplicated retreatment. Three potential adverse outcomes may arise from retreatment:

(1) Anaphylaxis;
(2) Decreased therapeutic efficacy; and
(3) Enhanced risk of thrombocytopenia.

Thrombocytopenia appears to be the only major complication reported in the literature to date.[65,66] Nevertheless, some asymptomatic patients have developed human antichimeric antibodies (HACA) specific to the murine epi-tope of the Fab fragment.[67] No association has been made, however, regarding efficacy or safety of re-administration in the presence of these antibodies. One recommendation that might be considered if retreatment is deemed to be clinically necessary is to obtain an early (2–4 h) postbolus platelet count, with the hope that if an abrupt drop in platelet count occurs, it can be identified and abciximab discontin-ued promptly, before profound thrombocy-topenia ensues. If profound thrombocytopenia were to develop, it is usually readily reversible, responding to platelet transfusion, unlike heparin-induced thrombocytopenia (HIT). Anecdotal reports, however, have suggested that the thrombocytopenia observed after retreatment with abciximab may be somewhat more aggressive, and may require more than a single platelet transfusion before it fully resolves. The mechanism of abciximab-associated thrombocytopenia may be ligand-induced binding site-mediated (LIBS), and completely different from that of HIT. Since heparin is frequently employed concomitantly with abciximab, it is important to attempt to exclude the presence of HIT. To date there is no documented association between abciximab-associated thrombocytopenia and the development of thrombosis as found with HIT.

Tcheng et al have reported the interim results of the ReoPro Readministration Registry, a phase IV, multicenter prospective registry evaluation the safety and efficacy of the readministration of abciximab for coronary intervention.[68] The investigators also sought to evaluate the implications of HACA positivity and the frequency of new HACA positivity after readministration of abciximab. Clinical data from 500 patients are available. These patients were drawn from an overall cohort of 23 453 total patients undergoing intervention at the 18 participating sites; of these, 9 627 (41%) received abciximab for the intervention. Clinical success in the retreatment group was high (93.6%) and did not differ among HACA-positive and HACA-negative patients; adverse events included myocardial infarction in 3.2% and urgent intervention in 0.8%; there were no deaths. Access site bleeding was noted in 2.2%. The overall incidence of thrombocytopenia (platelet count less than 100 000, with over a 25% decrease) was low (4.4%); 1.4% had a nadir between 50–100 000, 0.8% had a nadir 20–50 000, while 2.2% had a nadir less than 20 000. New HACA positivity developed in 20.2% of patients, which is higher than previous reports on first administration (approx 5–6%). HACA-positive patients also had a higher incidence of thrombocytopenia but there was no difference in the incidence of thrombocytopenia in patients who became HACA positive after the second administration versus those who were already HACA positive at the time

of readministration (7.6% vs. 8.7% respectively; $p = $ NS).

Duration of therapy

The proper duration of therapy with abciximab is still incompletely defined. As mentioned earlier, additional abciximab is necessary beyond the bolus dose to address the mobilized internal pool of GPIIb/IIIa that come to the platelet surface membrane. This was clinically manifested in EPIC, where a 12-h infusion of abciximab was necessary to achieve salutary responses; bolus treatment alone was insufficient. In the ERASER study there was no clinical advantage of longer, 24-h postprocedural infusions, although there may be certain clinical situations where a longer duration of therapy might be desirable, as in acute coronary syndromes. Platelet deposition can take place at the site of endothelial injury for upwards of 100–120 h; therefore the relatively long pharmacodynamic effects of abciximab may prove to be advantageous in circumstances where a longer period of inhibition is necessary. As mentioned previously, the CAPTURE study involved an 18–24-hour infusion of abciximab prior to the interventional procedure, but only 1 h postprocedure therapy and showed no benefit at 6 months. Horrigan et al[69] showed that stabilization of unstable angina patients in EPIC with heparin before angioplasty tended to reduce complications. Whether this can be enhanced with more potent antiplatelet therapy remains to be shown. Nevertheless, a minimum of 12 h therapy following intervention appears necessary.

Cost-effective use

Kereiakes reported the experience of the Ohio Heart Center in which they evaluated 321 consecutive patients with unstable angina undergoing intervention between January and June of 1997.[70] In these patients, 70%

received adjunctive abciximab, and stents were deployed in 60%. Adverse outcomes (death, emerged revascularization, O-wave MI) occurred in only 7 patients, which was 2.2% of the total. Compared with a cohort of 95 patients with unstable angina undergoing intervention in the second quarter of 1995 (deregulatory abciximab was used in 16% and stents deployed in 19%), the average total cost per patient declined by 28% despite the aggressive utilization of expertise and new forms of technology. In the more recent cohort the average preprocedural length of stay was 0.51 days and total hospital length of stay was 1.75 days, compared with 0.96 days and 2.82 days in the earlier, less technology-intense cohort.

Non-interventional applications

Thrombus and thrombosis clearly play a major role in the pathogenesis of acute coronary syndromes, such as unstable angina and acute myocardial infarction. Since an activated platelet membrane is the surface upon which coagulation proceeds, potent antiplatelet therapies may be particularly useful in the treatment of acute coronary syndromes.

Preliminary studies

In the CAPTURE trial of refractory unstable angina patients undergoing intervention GPIIb/IIIa-targeted therapy was associated with fewer repetitive ischemic events, and a reduced total ischemic burden. During the medical management phase, there was a prominent divergence of events even prior to the interventional procedure (Figure 8.10). This raises the issue of whether GPIIb/IIIa-targeted therapy might be employed to avoid the necessity for coronary interventions. Although

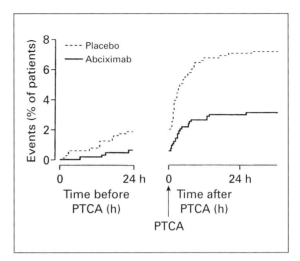

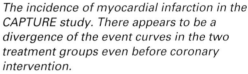

Figure 8.10
The incidence of myocardial infarction in the CAPTURE study. There appears to be a divergence of the event curves in the two treatment groups even before coronary intervention.

there have been large-scale studies with Eptifibatide and Tirofiban (see Chapter 9) in patients with acute coronary syndromes, there are, as yet, only limited data on the use of abciximab in this clinical scenario.

Simoons et al[71] reported the results the randomized pilot study preceding CAPTURE in which 60 patients with refractory unstable angina were randomized to receive either abciximab or placebo. The study population was a selected group of patients with angiographically documented lesions suitable for PTCA, who demonstrated dynamic ST–T segment changes and recurrent pain despite bedrest and medical treatment with intravenous heparin and nitrates. Patients were treated with 18–24 h of study drug before a second angiogram and PTCA. Patients treated with abciximab had fewer episodes of ischemia (9 versus 16 with placebo), fewer major events (1 versus 12 with placebo), improved TIMI flow grade, and significant improvement in quantitatively measured angiographic parameters (compared with placebo-treated patients, who showed no such improvement).

Gold et al noted that in a non-randomized open-label study of the murine m7E3 Fab in patients with unstable angina, anginal pain was abolished during the first few hours after a bolus drug was administered.[72] When the bleeding time fell below 10 min, however, pain recurred in several patients. In the TAMI 8 pilot study,[73] patients with acute myocardial infarction, treated with tissue plasminogen activator (tPA), aspirin, and heparin, were randomized to receive m7E3 F(ab')$_2$ or placebo. Patients who received m7E3 had better coronary artery patency and a trend toward fewer ischemic events. There did not appear to be a significantly increased risk of bleeding above that seen with tPA alone, although the overall event rates were high.

In animal studies the addition of potent GPIIb/IIIa-target therapy to thrombolytic therapy markedly enhances the speed and effectiveness of thrombolytic agents.[55-57] Clinically, when abciximab is administered in acutely thrombotic circumstances in the catheterization laboratory, at least some degree of thrombus dissolution is observed.[74-76] While abciximab is not itself a thrombolytic agent, by blocking the progression of thrombus, it serves to augment the efficacy of endogenous thrombolytic activity. By the same token, the effects of exogenously administered thrombolytic therapy may also be markedly enhanced. Recent trials have studied this strategy as an adjunct to r-tPA for the treatment of acute myocardial infarction.

Gold et al[77] have also reported the efficacy of abciximab therapy alone in achieving recanalization in a canine experimental model of coronary thrombosis, and in a preliminary series of 13 patients with acute myocardial infarction. They reported that flow increased by at least 1 TIMI grade in 11/13 (85%) patients, and achieved TIMI grade 2 or 3 in 7/13 (54%) patients. While subsequent, larger, randomized clinical trials have not confirmed some of the initial optimism, there continues to be much interest in the potential role of abciximab in the immediate management of patients with acute myocardial infarction.

There are also anecdotal reports of circumstances where abciximab has been used alone, without additional interventions, for the treatment of intracoronary thrombus, such as in the setting of abrupt closure or subacute stent thrombosis. Anderson et al[76] have shown that treatment with abciximab abolishes post-PTCA cyclic flow variations in humans.

GRAPE study

The GRAPE (Glycoprotein Receptor Antagonist Patency Evaluation) study was an open-label, non-randomized pilot trial in 60 patients evaluating the effect of abciximab in re-establishing patency in patients undergoing primary PTCA for acute MI.[78] Qualifying acute MI patients received aspirin (160 mg chewed), heparin (5000 U i.v. bolus), and abciximab (250 µg/kg bolus, 10 µg/min infusion) in the emergency room, and were brought to the catheterization laboratory. Angiography (and PTCA, if necessary) were performed, and the abciximab infusion was continued for 12 h after the procedure. At the time of initial angiography (a mean of 45 min after administration of abciximab), of patients achieved TIMI grade III flow, and approximately 40% of infarct-related arteries were patent (TIMI grade II or III flow).

TIMI 14 study

The TIMI 14 study was a prospective, multicenter, randomized, controlled trial of combined therapy with thrombolytic agents and the platelet GPIIb/IIIa antagonist abciximab in patients with acute myocardial infarction (AMI).[79] A total of 888 patients were treated with aspirin and randomized to standard front-loaded tPA (100 mg), streptokinase (500 000, 750 000, 1 250 000, or 1 500 000 U) plus abciximab, low-dose tPA (20, 35, 50, or 65 mg) plus abciximab, or abciximab alone. In the streptokinase groups, lytic therapy was administered as a 30–50-min infusion. In the tPA groups, lytic therapy was administered as either a bolus, a bolus plus a 30-min infusion, or a bolus plus a 60-min infusion. The primary endpoint of the study was the incidence of TIMI grade 3 flow at 90-minute angiography. In TIMI 14 the incidence of TIMI 3 flow at 90 min was 57% in the tPA-alone arm, 32% in the abciximab-alone arm and 41%, 34%, 46%, and 80% ($n = 5$; discontinued because of excessive bleeding and excess mortality) in the respective streptokinase plus abciximab groups. In the tPA plus abciximab groups, the incidence of TIMI 3 flow at 90 min ranged from 38% in the lower dose groups, up to 76% with a 15 mg bolus and a 35 mg infusion over 60 min. This dose was tested in a subsequent dose-confirmation phase in conjunction with either low-dose or very low dose heparin. In this phase, TIMI-3 flow rates with abciximab plus tPA were significantly higher than with tPA alone at both 60 min (72% versus 43%) and 90 min (77% versus 62%). The incidence of major bleeding was 6% with tPA alone; 6% with abciximab alone; 5%, 8%, 14%, and 67% (discontinued arm) in the respective streptokinase groups; and 7% in the 50 mg tPA plus abciximab (low dose heparin) and 1% in the 50 mg tPA plus abciximab (very low dose heparin) groups. Thus, in the TIMI 14 study, abciximab alone was able to achieve TIMI 3 flow rates compa-rable with those for streptokinase therapy alone in previous studies. The combination of reduced-dose thrombolytic therapy and abciximab appeared to augment appreciably the rate and extent of thrombolysis. Reducing the dose of heparin dramatically reduced the bleeding complications.

SPEED trial

The SPEED trial was a dose-escalation study evaluating the combination of r-PA and the platelet GPIIb/IIIa antagonist, abciximab, in patients with acute MI.[80] A total of 305 patients with acute MI were randomized (to treatment with abciximab alone, or one of several different doses of r-PA plus abciximab. All patients received aspirin (150–325 mg) and heparin (60 U/kg bolus (max 4000 U) followed by an 800 U/h infusion). Catheterization and angiography was performed 60–90 minutes after initiation of therapy (median 62–64 min). The incidence of TIMI grade 3 flow at 60–90 min was 28% in the abciximab alone group, 53% in the 5 U r-PA plus abciximab group, 46% in the 7.5 U r-PA plus abciximab group, 44% in the 10 U r-PA plus abciximab group, 48% in the 5 U/2.5 U r-PA group, and 63% in the 5/5 U r-PA group. Corresponding patency rates (TIMI grade 2 or 3 flow) were 48%, 72%, 70%, 80%, 70%, and 83%. Hemorrhagic complications were not significantly increased with combination therapy. A second, as yet unreported, phase of the trial is a dose-confirmation study comparing 5/5 U r-PA plus abciximab with standard r-PA therapy. Thus, in SPEED, combination of low-dose lytic therapy with r-PA and a GPIIb/IIIa antagonist appears to improve patency and TIMI grade 3 flow at 60 min, without an increase in major hemorrhagic complications.

GUSTO IV

The forthcoming large-scale GUSTO IV trial

will look at the use of abciximab in patients with acute MI and unstable angina. The MI arm of the trial will compare abciximab plus a lytic agent (r-PA) versus conventional lytic therapy alone in patients with ST-segment elevation MI. The unstable angina arm of the trial will compare the adjunctive use of abciximab with conventional medical therapy in patients with unstable angina and non-Q wave MI. When added to the data from the prior PURSUIT, PRISM, and PRISM-PLUS trials involving other GPIIb/IIIa antagonists, and also data from the forthcoming TACTICS-TIMI 18 trial, the GUSTO IV study will help to more clearly define the role of adjunctive GPIIb/IIIa therapy in patients across the entire spectrum of acute coronary syndromes.

Treating the window of vulnerability

In aggregate, the data on the clinical use of abciximab strongly support the role of potent antiplatelet therapy in the early phase of injury to the vessel wall. This would be true whether it occurs in the form of spontaneous plaque rupture (as in the acute coronary syndromes), or is iatrogenically induced (as in coronary interventional procedures). In both scenarios, there is a 'window of vulnerability' (Figure 8.11a) during which therapeutic efforts are directed at passivating activated platelets, passivating the vessel wall, and passivating an activated coagulation system. The exact duration of this 'window of vulnerability' is unknown, although it appears to persist for up to 1 week, and even perhaps longer in some cases. In fact, each of the three processes, platelet activation, vessel wall injury, and an activated coagulation system may have relatively (although not completely) independent periods during which passivation takes place.

If therapy is successful in covering the entire 'window of vulnerability', the benefits achieved will be sustained (as shown in the EPIC, EPILOG, and EPISTENT trials). However, if the duration of therapy is inadequate following injury to the vessel wall (as in the EPIC study bolus-alone group and in the CAPTURE trial), there is the potential for a 'catch-up' phenomenon once therapy is discontinued, and the benefits will not be sustained. It is also clear that abciximab, despite its theoretical potential (sustained presence on the platelet, cross-reacting with the vitronectin receptor, and so on) does not significantly affect restenosis or intimal hyperplasia within stents. The benefits are achieved generally early on in the treatment process, rather than occurring late in the post-treatment period.

In this regard, to truly target recurrent events (see Figure 8.11b), two therapeutic strategies appear most promising: reducing the likelihood of plaque rupture (perhaps with lipid-lowering therapy) and reducing the likelihood of thrombus formation if vessel injury takes place (perhaps with chronic antiplatelet therapy). There is every hope that abciximab, as one of the most potent forms of antiplatelet therapy available, will become a very useful tool in the array of clinical implements. There is considerable potential for combining intravenous GPIIb/IIIa antagonists with newer anticoagulant agents, for example low-molecular-weight heparin and the direct thrombin antagonists, as well as with other new chronic forms of antiplatelet therapy, such as aspirin plus ticlopidine or clopidogrel, and even the oral GPIIb/IIIa antagonists.

The primary role that abciximab will play in the numerous permutations and combinations of new (and old) anticoagulant, antiplatelet, and lytic therapies is that of acute therapy. Given its prolonged presence on the platelet and its relatively long pharmacody-

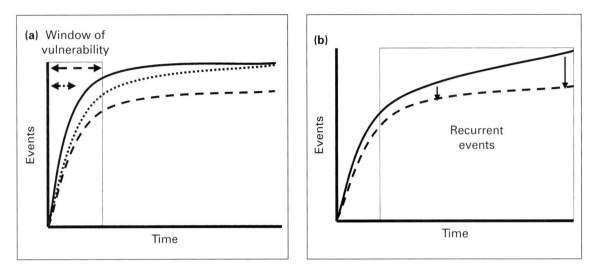

Figure 8.11
(a) *Initial benefit during the 'window of vulnerability'. If the treatment duration adequately covers the vulnerable period, the benefits will be sustained. If it does not, there may be loss of benefit over the subsequent time period.* **(b)** *Recurrent events, outside the 'window of vulnerability' depend on long-term therapeutic mechanisms, such as reducing the likelihood of plaque rupture, and/or reducing the likelihood of thrombus formation.*

namic effects, however, it seems ideally suited to covering as much as possible of the 'window of vulnerability' associated with injury to the vessel wall.

Summary

In this chapter we have summarized the data currently available on the use of abciximab, both in the catheterization laboratory and in other clinical scenarios. The use of this potent platelet inhibitor has evolved substantially over the last 3–4 years, and several very exciting applications are looming on the horizon. The real challenge for the future will come as we begin to interdigitate abciximab into existing treatment algorithms, and combine it with low-molecular-weight heparin, new thienopyridines plus aspirin and, possibly, with oral forms of the GPIIb/IIIa antagonists.

References

1. Coller BS, Peerschke EI, Scudder LE, Sullivan CA. A murine monoclonal antibody that completely blocks the binding of fibrinogen to platelets produces a thrombasthenic-like state in normal platelets and binds to glycoprotein IIb and/or IIIa. *J Clin Invest* 1983;**72**:325–38.

2. Coller BS. A new murine monoclonal antibody reports an activation-dependent change in the conformation and/or microenvironment of the platelet glycoprotein IIb/IIIa complex. *J Clin Invest* 1985;**76**:101–108.

3. Coller BS, Scudder LE. Inhibition of dog platelet function by in vivo infusion of F(ab′)2 fragments of a monoclonal antibody. *Blood* 1985;**66**:1456–9.

4. Jordan RE, Wagner CL, McAleer MF, Spitz MS, Mattis JA. Evaluation of the potency and immunogenicity of 7E3 F(ab′)$_2$ and Fab fragments in monkeys. *Circulation* 1990;**82** (**Suppl. III**):661.

5. Coller BS, Folts JD, Smith SR, Scudder LE, Smith SR. Antithrombotic effect of a monoclonal antibody to the platelet glycoprotein IIb/IIIa receptor in an experimental animal model. *Blood* 1986;**68**:783–6.

6. Coller BS, Folts JD, Smith SR, Scudder LE, Jordan R. Abolition of *in vivo* platelet thrombus formation in primates with monoclonal antibodies to the platelet GPIIb/IIIa receptor. *Circulation* 1989;**80**:1766–73.

7. Mickelson JK, Simpson PJ, Lucchesi BR. Antiplatelet monoclonal F(ab′)$_2$ antibody directed against the platelet GPIIb/IIIa receptor complex prevents coronary artery thrombosis in the canine heart. *J Mol Cell Cardiol* 1989;**21**:393–405.

8. Bates ER, McGillem MJ, Mickelson JK, Pitt B, Mancini GBJ. A monoclonal antibody against the platelet glycoprotein IIb/IIIa receptor complex prevents platelet aggregation and thrombosis in a canine model of coronary angioplasty. *Circulation* 1991;**84**:2463–9.

9. Ellis SG, Tcheng JE, Navetta FI, et al. Safety and antiplatelet effect of murine monoclonal antibody 7E3 Fab directed against platelet glycoprotein IIb/IIIa in patients undergoing elective coronary angioplasty. *Coronary Artery Dis* 1993;**4**:167–75.

10. Gold HK, Gimple LW, Yasuda T, et al. Pharmacodynamic study of F(ab′)$_2$ fragments of murine monoclonal antibody 7E3 directed against human platelet glycoprotein IIb/IIIa in patients with unstable angina pectoris. *J Clin Invest* 1990;**86**:651–9.

11. Kohmura C, Gold HK, Yasuda T, et al. A chimeric murine/human antibody Fab fragment directed against the platelet GPIIb/IIIa receptor enhances and sustains arterial thrombolysis with recombinant tissue-type plasminogen activator in baboons. *Arterio Thromb* 1993;**13**:1837–42.

12. Faulds D, Sorkin EM. Abciximab (c7E3 Fab) Fab): a review of its pharmacology and therapeutic potential in ischemic heart disease. *Drugs* 1994;**48**:583–98.

13. The EPILOG Investigators. Platelet glycoprotein IIb/IIIa receptor blockade and low-dose heparin during percutaneous coronary revascularization. *N Eng J Med* 1997;**336**(24):1689–96.

14. The CAPTURE Investigators. Randomized placebo-controlled trial of abciximab before and during coronary intervention in refractory unstable angina: the CAPTURE study. *Lancet* 1997;**349**:1429–35.

15. Brener SJ, Barr LA, Burchenal JEB, Katz S, George BS, Jones AA et al on behalf of the ReoPro and Primary PTCA Organization and Randomized Trial (RAPPORT) Investigators. Randomized, placebo-controlled trial of platelet glycoprotein IIb/IIIa blockade with primary angioplasty for acute myocardial infarction. *Circulation* 1998; **98**:734–41.

16. Ellis SG, Serruys PW, Popma JJ, et al. Can abciximab prevent neointimal proliferation in Palmaz-Schatz stents? The final ERASER results. *Circulation* 1997;**96** (**Suppl. I**):I-87 (abstract).

17. The EPISTENT Investigators. Randomized

placebo controlled and balloon-angioplasty-controlled trial to assess safety of coronary stenting with use of platelet glycoprotein-IIb/IIIa blockade. *Lancet* 1998;352:87–92.

18. Bhattacharya S, Weisman HF, Morris KG, et al. Chimerization of monoclonal antibody 7E3 preserves the GP IIb/IIIa receptor-blockade and platelet functional inhibition of murine 7E3 (abstract). *Clin Res* 1991;39:196A.

19. Kleiman NS, Raizner AE, Jordan R, et al. Differential inhibition of platelet aggregation induced by adenosine diphosphate or a thrombin receptor-activating peptide in patients treated with a bolus chimeric 7E3 Fab: implications for inhibition of the internal pool of GPIIb/IIIa receptors. *J Am Coll Cardiol* 1995; 26:1665–71.

20. Mascelli MA, Lance ET, Damaraju L, Wagner CL, Weisman HF, Jordan RE. Pharmacodynamic profile of short-term abciximab treatment demonstrates prolonged platelet inhibition with gradual recovery from GPIIb/IIIa receptor-blockade. *Circulation* 1998;97:1680–88.

21. Tam SH, Sassoli PM, Jordan RE, Nakada MT. Abciximab (ReoPro, chimeric 7E3 Fab) demonstrates equivalent affinity and functional blockade of glycoprotein IIb/IIIa and $\alpha_v\beta_3$ integrins. *Circulation* 1998;98:1085–91.

22. Lefkovits J, Topol EJ. Platelet glycoprotein IIb/IIIa receptor antagonists in coronary artery disease. *Eur Heart J* 1996;17:9–18.

23. The EPIC Investigators. Use of a monoclonal antibody directed against the platelet glycoprotein IIb/IIIa receptor in high-risk coronary angioplasty. *N Engl J Med* 1994;330:956–61.

24. Topol EJ, Califf RM, Weisman HF, et al on behalf of the EPIC Investigators. Randomized trial of coronary intervention with antibody against platelet IIb/IIIa integrin for reduction of clinical restenosis results at six months. *Lancet* 1994;343:881–6.

25. Topol EJ, Ferguson JJ, Weisman HF, Tcheng JE, Ellis SG, Kleiman NS, et al for the EPIC Investigator Group. Long-term protection from myocardial ischemic events in a randomized trial of brief integrin beta3 blockade with percutaneous coronary intervention. *J Am Med Assoc* 1997;278:479–84.

26. Lincoff AM, Califf RM, Anderson KM, Weisman HF, Aguirre FV, Kleiman NS, et al for the EPIC Investigators. Evidence for prevention of death and myocardial infarction with platelet membrane glycoprotein IIb/IIIa receptor blockade by abciximab (c7E3 Fab) among patients with unstable angina undergoing percutaneous coronary revascularization. *J Am Coll Cardiol* 1997;30:149–56.

27. Lefkovits J, Ivanhoe RJ, Califf RM, Bergelson BA, Anderson KM, Stoner GL, et al for the EPIC Investigators. Effects of platelet glycoprotein IIb/IIIa receptor blockade by a chimeric monoclonal antibody (abciximab) on acute and 6-month outcomes after percutaneous transluminal coronary angioplasty for acute myocardial infarction. *Am J Cardiol* 1996;77:1045–51.

28. Boehrer JD, Ellis SG, Pieper K, et al. Directional atherectomy versus balloon angioplasty for coronary ostial and nonostial left anterior descending coronary artery lesions: results from a randomized multicenter trial. The CAVEAT-I Investigators. Coronary Angioplasty Versus Excisional Atherectomy Trial. *J Am Coll Cardiol* 1995;25(6):1380–86.

29. Holmes DR Jr, Topol EJ, Califf RM, et al. A multicenter randomized trial of coronary angioplasty versus directional atherectomy for patients with saphenous vein bypass graft lesions. CAVEAT-II Investigators. *Circulation* 1995;91(7):1966–74.

30. Lefkovits J, Blankenship JC, Anderson KM, et al. Increased risk of non-Q wave myocardial infarction after directional atherectomy is platelet dependent: evidence from the EPIC trial. Evaluation of c7E3 Fab for the Prevention of Ischemic Complications. *J Am Coll Cardiol* 1996;28:849–55.

31. Lefkovits J, Stoner GL, Anderson KM, Weisman HF, Topol EJ for the EPIC Investigators. Can conjunctive platelet glycoprotein IIb/IIIa receptor blockade improve outcomes of coronary interventions for restenotic lesions? [Abstract]. *Circulation* 1995;95:1–607.

32. Mak KH, Challapalli R, Eisenberg MJ, Anderson KM, Califf RM, Topol EJ for the EPIC Investigators. Effect of platelet glycoprotein IIb/IIIa receptor inhibition on distal embolization during percutaneous revascularization of aortocoronary saphenous vein grafts. *Am J Cardiol* 1997;80:985–8.

33. Moliterno DJ, Califf RM, Aguirre FV, et al, for the EPIC Investigators: Special considerations for diabetics receiving platelet IIb/IIIa antagonists during coronary interventions: results from the EPIC trial. [Abstract]. *J Am Coll Cardiol* 1995;**25**:155A–156A.

34. Moliterno DJ, Califf RM, Aguirre FV, et al for the EPIC Study Investigators. Effect of platelet glycoprotein IIb/IIIa integrin blockade on activated clotting time during percutaneous transluminal coronary angioplasty or directional atherectomy (the EPIC trial). *Am J Cardiol* 1995;**75**:559–62.

35. Aguirre FV, Ferguson JJ, Blankenship JC, et al for the IMPACT-II Investigators. Association of pre-intervention activated clotting times (ACT) and clinical outcomes following percutaneous coronary revascularization: results from the IMPACT-II trial. [Abstract]. *J Am Coll Cardiol* 1996;**27**(Suppl A):83A.

36. Ammar T, Scudder LE, Coller BS. In vitro effects of the platelet glycoprotein IIb/IIIa receptor antagonist c7E3 Fab on the activated clotting time. *Circulation* 1997;**95**:614–17.

37. Boehrer JD, Kereiakes DJ, Navetta FI, Califf RM, Topol EJ for the EPIC Investigators. Effects of profound platelet inhibition with c7E3 before coronary angioplasty on complications of coronary bypass surgery. *Am J Cardiol* 1994;**74**:1166–70.

38. Mark DB, Talley JD, Topol EJ, et al for the EPIC Investigators. Economic assessment of platelet glycoprotein IIb/IIIa inhibition for the prevention of ischemic complications of high-risk angioplasty. *Circulation* 1996;**94**:629–35.

39. Lincoff AM, Tcheng JE, Califf RM, Bass T, Popma JJ, Teirstein PS, et al for the PROLOG Investigators. Standard versus low-dose weight adjusted heparin in patients treated with the platelet glycoprotein IIb/IIIa receptor antibody fragment abciximab (c7E3 Fab) during percutaneous coronary revascularization. *Am J Cardiol* 1997;**79**:286–91.

40. Kleiman NS, Lincoff AM, Kereiakes DJ, Miller DP, Aguirre FV, Anderson KM, et al for the EPILOG Investigators. Diabetes mellitus, glycoprotein IIb/IIIa blockade, and heparin. Evidence for a complex interaction in a multicenter trial. *Circulation* 1998; **97**:1912–20.

41. Kereiakes DJ, Lincoff AM, Miller DP, Tcheng JE, et al. Abciximab therapy and unplanned coronary stent deployment: favorable effects on stent use, clinical outcomes, and bleeding complications. EPILOG Trial Investigators. *Circulation* 1998;**97**:857–64.

42. Lincoff AM, Tcheng JE, Califf RM, Kereiakes DJ, Kelly TA, Timmis GC, et al for the EPILOG Investigators. Sustained suppression of ischemic complications of coronary intervention by platelet GP IIb/IIIa blockade with abciximab. One-year outcome in the EPILOG trial. *Circulation* 1999;**99**:1951–8.

43. Klootwijk P, Meij S, Melkert R, Lenderink T, Simoons ML. Reduction of recurrent ischemia with abciximab during continuous ECG-ischemia monitoring in patients with unstable angina refractory to standard treatment. *Circulation* 1998;**98**:1358–64.

44. Hamm CW, Heeschen B, Goldmann A, Vahanian A, Adgey J, Miguel CM, et al for the c7E3 Fab Antiplatelet Therapy in Unstable Refractory Angina (CAPTURE) Study Investigators. Benefit of abciximab in patients with refractory unstable angina in relation to serum troponin T levels. *N Engl J Med* 1999;**340**:1623–9.

45. Heeschen C, Hamm CW, Goldmann BU, Wohlrath S, Deu A. Recurrence of symptoms in patients with refractory unstable angina during treatment with abciximab before coronary revascularization results from the CAPTURE trial. *Circulation* 1998;**98**(Suppl.):I-358.

46. Lincoff AM, Tcheng JE, Califf RM, Cabot CF, Booth JE, Godfrey NK, et al. The EPISTENT trial at 6 months: relative and combined effects of abciximab and stenting on reduction of acute ischemic events and late revascularization. [Abstract]. *Circulation* 1998;**19**(Suppl.):I-767.

47. Cura FA, L'Allier PL, Sapp S, Lincoff AM, Ellis SG, Topol EJ, for the EPISTENT Investigators. Comparison of the protection against restenosis afforded by stenting or abciximab. *J Am Coll Cardiol* 1999;**33**:11A (abstract).

48. Lincoff AM, Moliterno DJ, Ellis SG, Debowey D, Cabot CF, Booth JE, et al. 6-month angiographic outcome with abciximab and stents: The EPISTENT angiographic substudy. *Circulation* 1998;**19** (Suppl.):I-768.

49. Neumann F-J, Blasini R, Schmitt C, Alt E,

Dirschinger J, Gawaz M, et al. Effect of glyco-protein IIb/IIIa receptor blockade on recovery of coronary flow and left ventricular function after the placement of coronary-artery stents in acute myocardial infarction. *Circulation* 1998;**98**:2695–701.

50. Brezina K, Murphy M, Stonner T. Care of the patient receiving ReoPro™ following angio-plasty. *J Invasive Cardiol* 1994;**6**(**Suppl A**): 38A–42A.

51. Lincoff AM. Heparin and control bleeding complications during platelet glycoprotein IIb/IIIa receptor antagonist therapy during per-cutaneous coronary revascularization. *J Invasive Cardiol* 1996;**8**(**Suppl. B**):15B–20B.

52. Gammie JS, Zenati M, Kormos RL, Hattler BG, Wei LM, Pellegrini RV, et al. Abciximab and excessive bleeding in patients undergoing emergency cardiac operations. *Ann Thorac Surg* 1998;**65**:465–9.

53. Alvarez JM. Emergency coronary bypass graft-ing for failed percutaneous coronary artery stenting: increased costs and platelet trans-fusion requirements after the use of abciximab. *J Thoracic Cardiovasc Surg* 1998;**115**(**2**): 472–3.

54. Booth JE, Patel VB, Balog C, Sapp S, Templin M, LeNarz L, et al. Is bleeding risk increased in patients undergoing urgent coronary bypass surgery following abciximab? *Circulation* 1998;**19**(**Suppl. 1**):I-845.

55. Coller BS. Platelets and thrombolytic therapy. *N Engl J Med* 1990;**322**:33–42.

56. Gold HK, Coller BS, Yasuda T, et al. Rapid and sustained coronary artery recanalization with combined bolus injection of recombinant tissue-type plasminogen activator and monoclonal antiplatelet GPIIb/IIIa antibody in a canine preparation. *Circulation* 1988; **77**: 670–77.

57. Yasuda T, Gold HK, Fallon JT, et al. Mono-clonal antibody against the platelet glycopro-tein (GP) IIb/IIIa receptor prevents coronary artery reocclusion after reperfusion with recombinant tissue-type plasminogen activator in dogs. *J Clin Invest* 1988; **81**:1284–91.

58. Reddy KJ, Khoshnevis R, Simek S, et al. Reo-Pro as an adjunct to intracoronary throm-bolytic therapy. [Abstract]. *J Invas Cardiol* 1996;**8**:66.

59. Teirstein PS, Warth DC, Haq N, Jenkins NS, McCowan LC, Aubanel-Reidel P, et al. High-speed rotational coronary atherectomy for patients with diffuse coronary artery disease. *J Am Coll Cardiol* 1991;**18**:1694–701.

60. Teirstein PS, Yakubov SJ, Thel MC, Wilder-man N, Kereiakes DJ, Popma JJ, et al. Platelet IIb/IIIa blockade with integrelin: atherectomy patients. [Abstract]. *J Am Coll Cardiol* 1996; **27**:334A.

61. Braden GA, Applegate RJ, Young TM, Love WW, Sane DC. Abciximab decreases both the incidence and magnitude of creatine kinase ele-vation during rotational atherectomy. [Abs-tract]. *J Am Coll Cardiol* 1997;**29**:449A.

62. Diez JG, Fish RD, Croitoru M, Haas CP, Fer-guson JJ. The slow-flow, no-flow phenomena during rotational atherectomy: Does abcix-imab help? *Circulation* 1998;**98**(**Suppl. I**): I-558.

63. Reisman M, Shuman B, Fei R, Dillard D, Nguyen S, Gordon L. Analysis and comparison of platelet aggregation with high-speed rota-tional atherectomy. [Abstract]. *J Am Coll Car-diol* 1997;**27**:186A.

64. Williams MS, Coller BS, Väänänen HJ, Scud-der LE, Sharma SK, Marmur JD. Activation of platelet-rich plasma by rotablation is speed-dependent and can be inhibited by abciximab (c7E3 Fab; ReoPro™). *Circulation* 1998;**98**: 742–8.

65. Berkowitz SD, Harrington RA, Rund MM, Tcheng JE. Acute profound thrombocytopenia after c7E3 Fab (abciximab) therapy. *Circula-tion* 1997;**95**:809–13.

66. Berkowitz SD, Sane DC, Sigmon KN, Shaven-der JH, Harrington RA, Tcheng JE, et al. Occurrence and clinical significance of throm-bocytopenia in a population undergoing high-risk percutaneous coronary revascularization. Evaluation of c7E3 Fab for the Prevention of Ischemic Complications (EPIC) Study Group. *J Am Coll Cardiol* 1998;**32**:311–19.

67. Ferguson JJ, Kereiakes DJ, Adgey AA, et al. Safe use of platelet GPIIb/IIIa inhibitors. *Am Heart J* 1998;**135**:S77–S89.

68. Tcheng JE, Kereiakes DJ, Braden GA, Lincoff AM, Mascelli MA, Langrall MA, et al. Safety of abciximab retreatment: final clinical report of the ReoPro readministration registry (R[3]). [Abstract]. *Circulation* 1998;**19**(**Suppl.**):I-17.

69. Horrigan MCG, Eccleston DS, Wilderman NM, Sigmon KA, Califf RM, Topol EJ, for the Epic Investigators. Heparin pretreatment may confer additional benefit in patients treated with 7E3 and PTCA for unstable coronary syndromes. [Abstract]. *J Am Coll Cardiol* 1995;**25**:420A.

70. Kereiakes, DJ. Preferential benefit of platelet glycoprotein IIb/IIIa receptor blockade: specific considerations by device and disease state. *Am J Cardiol* 1998;**81**(7A):49D–54E.

71. Simoons ML, de Boer MJ, van den Brand MJ, van Miltenburg AJ, Hoorntje JC, Heyndrickx GR, et al. Randomized trial of a GP IIb/IIIa platelet receptor blocker in refractory unstable angina. European Cooperative Study Group. *Circulation* 1994;**89**:596–603.

72. Gold HK, Gimple LW, Yasuda T, Leinbach RC, Werner W, Hold R, et al. Pharmacodynamic study of F(ab')2 fragments of murine monoclonal antibody 7E3 directed against human platelet glycoprotein IIb/IIIa in patients with unstable angina pectoris. *J Clin Invest* 1990;**86**:651–9.

73. Kleiman NS, Ohman EM, Califf RM, George BS, Kereiakes D, Aguirre FV. Profound inhibition of platelet aggregation with monoclonal antibody 7E3 Fab after thrombolytic therapy. Results of the Thrombolysis and Angioplasty in Myocardial Infarction (TAMI) 8 Pilot Study. *J Am Coll Cardiol* 1993;**22**:381–9.

74. Muhlestein JB, Karagounis LA, Treehan S, Anderson JL. 'Rescue' utilization of abciximab for the dissolution of coronary thrombus developing as a complication of coronary angioplasty. *J Am Coll Cardiol* 1997;**30**:1729–34.

75. Anderson HV, Revana M, Rosales O, Brannigan L, Stuart Y, Weisman H, et al. Intravenous administration of monoclonal antibody to the platelet GP IIb/IIIa receptor to treat abrupt closure during coronary angioplasty. *Am J Cardiol* 1992;**69**:1373–6.

76. Anderson HV, Kirkeeide RL, Krishnaswami A, Weigelt LA, Revana M, Weisman HF, et al. Cyclic flow variations after coronary angioplasty in humans: clinical and angiographic characteristics and elimination with 7E3 monoclonal antiplatelet antibody. *J Am Coll Cardiol* 1994;**23**:1031–7.

77. Gold HK, Garabedian HD, Dinsmore E, Guerrero LJ, Cigarroa JE, Palacios IF, et al. Restoration of coronary flow in myocardial infarction by intravenous chimeric 7E3 antibody without exogenous plasminogen activators. Observation in animals and humans. *Circulation* 1997;**95**:1755–9.

78. van den Merkhof LFM, Zijlstra F, Olsson H, Grip L, Veen G, Bär FWHM, et al. Abciximab in the treatment of acute myocardial infarction eligible for primary percutaneous transluminal coronary angioplasty. Results of the Glycoprotein Receptor Antagonist Patency Evaluation (GRAPE) Pilot Study. *J Am Coll Cardiol* 1999;**33**:1528–32.

79. Antman EM, Giugliano RP, Gibson CM, McCabe CH, Coussement P, Kleiman NS, et al for the TIMI 14 Investigators. Abciximab facilitates the rate and extent of thrombolysis. Results of the thrombolysis in myocardial infarction (TIMI) 14 trial. *Circulation* 1999;**99**:2720–32.

80. Ohman EM, Lincoff AM, Bode C, Bachinsky WB, Ardissino D, Matteo I, et al. Enhanced early reperfusion at 60 minutes with low-dose retaplase combined with full dose abciximab in acute myocardial infarction: preliminary results from GUSTO-4 pilot (SPEED) dose ranging trial. *Circulation* 1998;**98**: I-504 (abstract).

9

Peptide and non-peptide inhibitors of platelet glycoprotein IIb/IIIa

Robert A Harrington and John Alexander

Atherosclerosis, vascular injury, and coronary thrombosis

Formation and progression of atherosclerotic plaque involves a complex interaction of lipids, inflammation, thrombosis, and mechanical shear forces.[1] The pathologic underpinnings of acute coronary syndromes (ACS), including unstable angina and acute myocardial infarction, and the acute complications of percutaneous coronary intervention both result from the rupture, fissuring, or erosion of an atherosclerotic plaque, with subsequent intracoronary thrombosis formation (Figure 9.1).[2] In the setting of an ACS, plaque injury is spontaneous and unpredictable; however, in coronary intervention, vascular injury is induced by the coronary interventionist in an attempt to expand the obstructed coronary lumen. Following either spontaneous or planned plaque injury, acute thrombosis of a coronary vessel leads to subtotal or total vascular occlusion with interruption of normal blood flow, causing myocardial ischemia and, if persistent, necrosis.

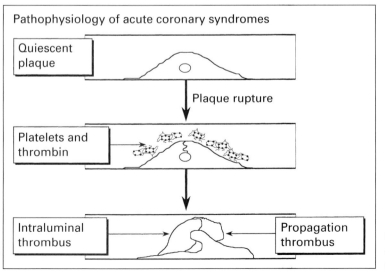

Figure 9.1
Pathophysiology of acute coronary syndromes.

145

The initial hemostatic response to such vascular injury is platelet deposition over the injured endothelium. Activation of platelets by any of a number of agonists, including adenosine diphosphate (ADP), epinephrine (adrelatine), collagen, thrombin, or shear stress, leads to ongoing platelet activation and aggregation. The resulting core of platelet-rich thrombus provides the necessary phospholipid surface on which assembly of the prothrombinase complex occurs, precipitating the conversion of prothrombin to thrombin, which then catalyses the conversion of fibrinogen to fibrin.[3] In addition to its role in the formation of fibrin, thrombin, as the central enzyme of the coagulation cascade, activates factors V, VIII, and XIII, activates platelets, and controls its own regulation through its effects on thrombomodulin and protein C.[4]

Rationale for antithrombotic therapies in the acute ischemic coronary syndromes

Given the central role of thrombosis in the pathophysiologic mechanism of unstable angina and acute myocardial infarction, the use of antithrombotic agents in the treatment of patients who present with acute ischemia seems reasonable. Oral antiplatelet therapy with aspirin provides impressive clinical benefits to patients presenting with a spectrum of vascular diseases, and reduces the risk of death, myocardial infarction, and stroke by approximately one-third (Figure 9.2).[5,6] Recently, the antiplatelet agent clopidogrel, which inhibits ADP-induced activation of platelets, was shown to be marginally superior to aspirin alone in reducing the risk from the composite of vascular death, myocardial infarction, and stroke in patients with an array of atherosclerotic vascular disease.[7]

Despite the wide use of antiplatelet therapy, primarily with aspirin, in patients with atherosclerotic disease, there remains significant morbidity and mortality associated with acute ischemia; thus, there is a clinical need for alternative antiplatelet therapies. Aspirin, ticlopidine, and clopidogrel are all relatively weak antiplatelet agents. Additionally, there is a group of patients, perhaps as high as 15–30% of patients treated with aspirin, who are non-responders or 'resistant' to the antiplatelet effects of aspirin and who appear to be at increased risk for subsequent vascular events.[8–10]

For these reasons, recent research has focused on the development of new, more potent antiplatelet therapies as a means of combating the problem. Platelet aggregation occurs via fibrinogen binding to the cellular receptor, glycoprotein (GP) IIb/IIIa, on adjacent platelets. This receptor belongs to a family of integrins that are involved in the processes of cellular adhesion. On circulating and quiescent platelets, the GPIIb/IIIa receptor is incapable of binding other circulating molecules like fibrinogen or von Willebrand factor (i.e. it is ligand-unresponsive). After activation, however, the platelet GPIIb/IIIa receptor undergoes a conformational change that permits the binding of adhesion molecules, primarily fibrinogen, and facilitates platelet aggregation. Interfering with the ability of platelet GPIIb/IIIa receptors to bind fibrinogen thus inhibits the 'final common pathway' of platelet aggregation and provides an attractive target for a cardiovascular therapeutic agent.

Platelet GPIIb/IIIa inhibition

Coller et al[11] reported on the first experience with a murine monoclonal antibody that

Category of trial	No. of trials with data	MI, stroke, or vascular death		Stratified statistics		Odds ratio and confidence interval (antiplatelet: control)	% Odds reduction (8D)
		Antiplatelet	Adjusted controls	O-E	Variance		
Prior MI	11	1991/9877 (13.6%)	1693/9914 (17.1%)	−158.3	561.6		25% (4)
Acute MI	9	992/9388 (10.6%)	1348/9385 (14.4%)	−177.9	510.3		29% (4)
Prior stroke/TIA	18	1076/5837 (18.4%)	1301/5870 (22.2%)	−98.5	388.5		22% (4)
Other high-risk patients	104	784/11 434 (6.9%)	1058/11 542 (9.2%)	−134.0	352.5		32% (4)
ALL HIGH-RISK patients (four main categories)	142	4183/36 536 (11.4%)	5400/36 711 (14.7%)	−568.8	1810.9		27% (2)
ALL LOW-RISK patients (primary prevention)	3	652/14 608 (4.46%)	708/14 694 (4.85%)	−28.5	273.5		10% (6)
ALL TRIALS (high- or low-risk)	145	4836/51 144 (9.5%)	6108/51 315 (11.9%)	−597.3	2084.4		25% (2)

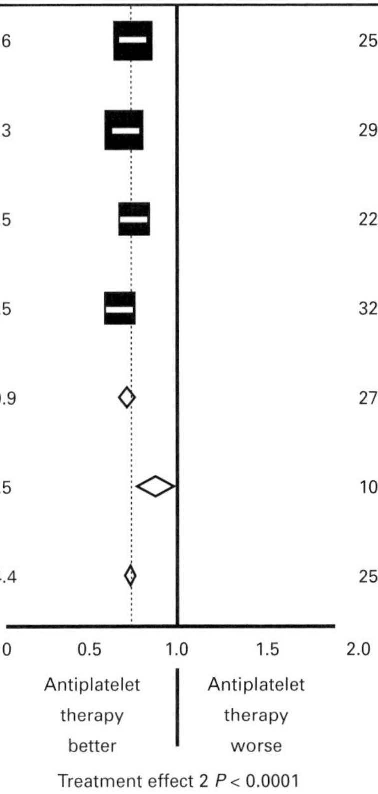

0   0.5   1.0   1.5   2.0

Antiplatelet therapy better — Antiplatelet therapy worse

Treatment effect 2 $P < 0.0001$

Figure 9.2
Proportional effects of antiplatelet therapy (145 trials) on vascular events (myocardial infarction, stroke, or vascular death) in four main high-risk categories of trial and in low-risk categories (primary prevention). (Stratified ratio of odds of an event in treatment groups to that in control groups is plotted for each group of trials (black square) along with its 99% confidence interval (horizontal line). Overviews of results for certain subtotals (and 95% confidence intervals) are represented by diamonds. Odds reductions observed in particular groups of trials are given to right of solid vertical line.) TIA, transient ischemic attack; MI, myocardial infarction.

almost completely inhibited the ability of platelets to aggregate. Refinement of this initial work led to the development of the chimeric monoclonal antibody fragment, abciximab.[12] In a series of trials, studying a variety of patient populations and interventional strategies, abciximab was then shown to be effective in reducing the acute ischemic complications in a broad spectrum of patients undergoing percutaneous coronary intervention.[13-17] Abciximab is discussed extensively in Chapter 8.

In addition to abciximab, several other intravenous GPIIb/IIIa inhibitors have been developed. These are commonly referred to as 'small-molecule inhibitors', to contrast them with the monoclonal antibody GPIIb/IIIa inhibitor, abciximab. In extensive clinical trial work, including over 33 000 randomized patients, the intravenous GPIIb/IIIa inhibitors have been demonstrated to reduce acute ischemic complications in patients undergoing percutaneous coronary intervention and in patients presenting with non-ST-segment elevation ACS.[18] The remainder of this chapter will focus on the intravenous small molecule inhibitors of the GPIIb/IIIa receptor. Specific clinical indications are discussed separately in Chapters 12–17.

Small-molecule GPIIb/IIIa inhibitors

Around the same time that Coller[11] was working on a monoclonal antibody approach to GPIIb/IIIa antagonism, other investigators were attempting to interfere with the GPIIb/IIIa receptor through small molecule inhibitors. These agents, both peptides and nonpeptide mimetics, are small-molecule inhibitors that were developed using the knowledge that fibrinogen binding to the receptor occurs via RGD amino acid sequences (arginine-glycine-aspartic acid).[19] Key differences between the small-molecule inhibitors and the monoclonal antibody GPIIb/IIIa antagonist can be seen in Table 9.1. Three intravenous small-molecule inhibitors are currently under clinical development, eptifibatide, tirofiban, and lamifiban. Eptifibatide and tirofiban have been approved for clinical

Properties	Monoclonal antibody fragment	Small-molecule inhibitors
Chemical nature	Antibody	Peptides and peptidomimetics
Size	Large (approximately 48 kD)	Small (<1 kD)
Onset of platelet aggregation inhibition	Rapid	Rapid
Plasma half-life	Very short (<10 min)	Moderate (1–2 h)
Reversibility of platelet aggregation inhibition	Slow	Rapid
Binds non-GPIIb/IIIa integrins	Yes	No (GPIIb/IIIa specific)
Antigenicity	Yes (human anti-chimeric antibodies)	No

GP, glycoprotein.

Table 9.1
Similarities and differences among clinically available GPIIb/IIIa.

GPIIb/IIIa Antagonists	Approved indications	Major clinical trials
Eptifibatide (Integrilin™)	PCI Non ST-segment elevation ACS	IMPACT II[20] ($n = 4010$): Elective and high-risk PCI PURSUIT[21,25] ($n=10,948$): Non ST-segment elevation ACS
Tirofiban (Aggrastat™)	Non ST-segment elevation ACS	RESTORE[22] ($n = 2141$): High-risk PCI PRISM[23,25] ($n = 3232$): Non ST-segment elevation ACS PRISM-PLUS[24,25] ($n = 1915$): Non-ST-segment elevation ACS
Lamifiban	Phase III trials	PARAGON A[25] ($n = 2282$): Non ST-segment elevation ACS PARAGON B ($n = 4000$ planned): Non ST-segment elevation ACS (ongoing trial)

PCI, percutaneous coronary intervention; ACS, acute coronary syndromes.

Table 9.2
Small-molecule GPIIb/IIIa Inhibitors: approved indications and supporting clinical trials.

use in the USA, while lamifiban is in Phase III clinical trials. Table 9.2 lists the agents and summarizes the approved indications and randomized trials of more than 1000 patients.[20–25]

Abciximab binds non-specifically to the GPIIb/IIIa receptor in an irreversible manner and consequently, even after the infusion is terminated, platelet function is maximally (>80% inhibition of platelet aggregation) inhibited for many hours and measurably altered for days to weeks. In addition, because of its non-specificity, abciximab may have other effects on platelet function, the importance of which is not currently understood. In contrast, the small-molecule inhibitors are highly specific competitive antagonists of the GPIIb/IIIa receptor. Thus, after terminating an infusion of one of the short-acting small-mole-

cule inhibitors, platelet function (as measured by inhibition of platelet aggregation) rapidly returns to normal as the competitive antagonist is cleared from the circulation. It is unknown whether such differentiating characteristics as the non-specificity and prolonged duration of the antiplatelet effect translate into differing degrees of clinical benefit. In a recent systematic overview of all randomized clinical trials, including more than 1000 patients and performed with the four major intravenous GPIIb/IIIa antagonists, regardless of agent, the point estimate for clinical benefit consistently favors the platelet inhibitor to a similar degree.[18] In the absence of direct head-to-head trials comparing abciximab and the small-molecule inhibitors, speculation about differential clinical effects is premature.

Small-molecule antagonists: clinical development

Percutaneous coronary intervention and the ACS were chosen as the rational areas in which to develop eptifibatide, tirofiban, and lamifiban, given the pivotal role that the platelet plays in the pathophysiology of plaque rupture (whether induced or spontaneous) and subsequent arterial thrombosis. Perceived advantages to the small-molecule inhibitors, compared with the monoclonal antibody inhibitor, included their rapid reversibility, their specificity for GPIIb/IIIa and not other cellular integrins, and their likely lack of immunogenicity. Rapid reversibility appeared to be an especially attractive safety feature in an era of balloon angioplasty, without coronary stenting, when more than 5% of patients would require emergency bypass surgery to salvage a failed percutaneous procedure. In addition, rapid recovery of platelet function was felt to be necessary if these agents were to be used as empirical therapy for patients presenting with ACS. At the time of patient presentation, the clinician must make a treatment decision without knowing the patient's coronary anatomy and, consequently, before knowing whether the patient would require surgical intervention.

Eptifibatide

Eptifibatide (Integrilin™, COR Therapeutics, South San Francisco) is the prototypical peptide inhibitor of platelet GPIIb/IIIa. It is a cyclic heptapeptide modeled on the structure of barbourin, a specific inhibitor of GPIIb/IIIa found in the venom of the Southeastern pygmy rattlesnake. Replacing lysine for arginine results in a KGD sequence that provides eptifibatide with high affinity and specificity for the GPIIb/IIIa receptor.[26] Eptifibatide is cleared predominantly through renal mechanisms and has a circulating plasma half-life of approximately 150 min. Inhibition of platelet aggregation, in response to a variety of agonists, is dose-dependent and predictable based on plasma concentrations.[27,28] Preclinical experience with animal models of arterial thrombus showed eptifibatide to be a potent agent at inhibiting platelet-dependent arterial thrombosis.[29] Studies in normal human volunteers demonstrated that eptifibatide had a rapid onset of action and was readily reversible with a calculated plasma half-life in normals of approximately 1 h.[29]

Eptifibatide development: percutaneous coronary intervention

Although the first Phase II trial with eptifibatide was in patients with unstable angina,[30] percutaneous coronary intervention was the area chosen for the first full development trial with this new agent. The acute ischemic complications of these procedures include death, myocardial infarction, and the need for repeat urgent procedures. These complications were believed to be, at least in part, platelet-mediated events, as demonstrated by the benefits conferred by aspirin in lowering the risk of these complications.[5] This chapter will review the highlights of the completed trials with all three small molecule inhibitors of GPIIb/IIIa. Details of the benefits of GPIIb/IIIa inhibition in patients undergoing percutaneous coronary intervention can be found in Chapter ?.

Two small, Phase II, dose-finding trials were completed with eptifibatide before a large Phase III project in coronary intervention: IMPACT (Integrilin to Manage Platelet Aggregation and Prevent Coronary Thrombosis)[27] and IMPACT Hi-Lo.[28] The IMPACT trial enrolled 150 patients undergoing elective angioplasty; the patients were randomized to treatment with eptifibatide (90 µg/kg bolus with 1.0 µg/kg-min infusion for either 4 h or 12 h) or placebo. All patients received both heparin and aspirin. Clinical efficacy and safety results in this small number of patients appeared promising. Platelet function studies, performed on a subset of 31 patients, revealed that eptifibatide provided rapid and readily reversible inhibition of ex-vivo ADP-induced platelet aggregation but with a wider degree of variability than had been seen in the normal volunteer studies.

The IMPACT Hi-Lo trial[28] was performed to better delineate doses of eptifibatide that reliably inhibited platelet aggregation to the degree seen in the recently completed and reported abciximab trial in coronary angioplasty (approximately 80% inhibition of platelet aggregation with 20 µM ADP).[14] IMPACT Hi-Lo was a small trial of 73 patients undergoing coronary intervention who were randomized to receive placebo or eptifibatide in addition to aspirin and heparin. Pharmacodynamic and pharmacokinetic data were used to identify a bolus dose of eptifibatide that provided rapid and intense (more than 80%) inhibition of platelet aggregation (135 µg/kg) and two dosing strategies for the subsequent infusion. In light of the excessive bleeding noted in the EPIC trial using abciximab, it was hypothesized that a strategy that provided potent antiplatelet action at the actual time of the procedure but that was followed by a gradual lessening of the intensity might be effective at reducing ischemic complications while improving the safety profile of GPIIb/IIIa inhibition. In the IMPACT Hi-Lo study, the 0.75 µg/kg-min infusion provided sustained levels of platelet inhibition for the duration of the infusion while the 0.50 µg/kg-min infusion allowed some recovery of platelet function over the 18–24-h infusion period. As

hoped, there was no increase in serious bleeding observed in the patients treated with eptifibatide.

Using the dosing information from the Phase II trials, the IMPACT II study was designed to test the hypothesis that a bolus plus an 18–24-h infusion of eptifibatide given with aspirin and heparin would be superior to aspirin and heparin alone in reducing the ischemic complications of percutaneous coronary intervention.[20] The trial, conducted in the USA, randomized 4010 patients who were undergoing either elective or high-risk coronary intervention to treatment with one of two doses of eptifibatide (135 µg/kg bolus followed by an infusion of either 0.5 µg/kg/min or 0.75 µg/kg/min) or placebo. The primary endpoint was the 30-day composite of death, myocardial infarction, urgent revascularization, or stent placement for abrupt closure. Treatment with the eptifibatide 135 µg/kg bolus, 0.5 µg/kg/min infusion modestly reduced the risk of the composite endpoint compared with placebo (9.1% versus 11.6%, $p = 0.035$). A smaller benefit was seen with the higher dose of eptifibatide (135 µg/kg bolus, 0.75 µg/kg/min infusion) (9.9% versus 11.6%, $p = 0.18$). These beneficial effects were realized without an increase in major bleeding. The beneficial effects occurred early during eptifibatide infusion and were maintained to the primary endpoint determination at 30 days and, subsequently, to 6 months.

While there was clear evidence that treatment with eptifibatide exerted a beneficial effect for patients undergoing coronary intervention, the magnitude of the benefit (both absolute and relative) was less than the original study projections. Subsequent work by Phillips and others[31] revealed that, because the early dose-finding work with eptifibatide had been performed using sodium citrate as the anticoagulant in the collection tubes, the antiplatelet effects of eptifibatide had been overestimated ex vivo. This is because the ability of eptifibatide to interact with the receptor is a calcium-dependent process that is not accurately determined in the presence of citrate, which chelates and lowers the calcium concentration, providing an overestimation of the platelet inhibitory effect ex vivo. Phillips et al[31] suggested that the doses of eptifibatide used in the IMPACT II trial actually provided between 30% and 50% inhibition of platelet aggregation and might explain the less than expected magnitude of benefit. Collection of plasma samples into PPACK, an anticoagulant that does not chelate calcium, seems to provide a more accurate measure of the platelet inhibitory effect of eptifibatide.

Subsequent subgroup analyses[32] of patients undergoing percutaneous coronary intervention in the large PURSUIT trial of patients presenting with ACS without persistent ST-segment elevation (see ACS section later) support the notion that a higher dose of eptifibatide may increase the magnitude of benefit during coronary intervention. Further dose-finding work is ongoing with eptifibatide to examine higher doses that provide a greater degree of platelet inhibition and to determine if such doses correlate with improved clinical outcomes.[33]

Eptifibatide development: ACS without persistent ST-segment elevation

Antithrombotic therapy with aspirin (antiplatelet) and heparin (anticoagulant) has been the mainstay of therapy for patients presenting with ACS without persistent ST-segment elevation.[34] Despite these and other standard therapies, including beta-blockers, nitrates, ACE inhibitors, lipid-lowering agents, and coronary revascularization, the morbidity and mortality in this group of patients remains high. Owing to the key role of the platelet in the thrombotic process responsible for the ACS, the addition of more potent GPIIb/IIIa inhibitors to the standard antithrombotic armamentarium seemed a logical step.

Eptifibatide was the first platelet GPIIb/IIIa inhibitor to be used for the treatment of patients with non-ST-elevation ACS. Schulman et al[35] studied 227 patients with unstable angina in a dose-finding pilot study of eptifibatide plus heparin versus heparin plus aspirin. The doses of eptifibatide were substantially lower than were used in the percutaneous intervention studies: a bolus of either 45 µg/kg or 90 µg/kg followed by infusions of either 0.5 µg/kg/min or 1.0 µg/kg/min. The primary endpoint was recurrent ischemia in the first 24 h of therapy as measured by Holter monitoring. Despite using doses of eptifibatide that would subsequently be shown to be inadequate for substantial platelet inhibition, there was a measurable and significant effect of eptifibatide on reducing Holter-recorded myocardial ischemia. Patients receiving the highest dose of eptifibatide plus heparin had fewer and less severe episodes of ischemia than patients receiving aspirin plus heparin.

The largest trial performed to date using a platelet GPIIb/IIIa inhibitor in any clinical setting is the PURSUIT (Platelet Glycoprotein IIb/IIIa in Unstable Angina: Receptor Suppression Using Integrilin Therapy) trial.[21] Patients were eligible for enrollment who had at presentation typical symptoms of ischemic chest pain within 24 h and evidence of either ischemia (ST deviation but not persistent ST-segment elevation) or myocardial necrosis (positive CK-MB isoenzymes). Patients were randomized to one of two doses of eptifibatide (180 µg/kg bolus followed by a 2.0 µg/kg/min or 1.3 µg/kg/min infusion) or placebo. In keeping with the large, simple trial philosophy, all other treatment decisions, including use of heparin, aspirin, and invasive cardiac procedures, were left to the discretion of the treating physicians. The primary endpoint was the composite of 30-day death or myocardial infarction. The PURSUIT trial enrolled 10 948 patients in 28 countries. As had been prespecified in the protocol, the lower dose was discontinued after approximately 3200 patients had been enrolled and the safety of the higher dose was confirmed. The primary comparison was between the eptifibatide 180 µg/kg and 2.0 µg/kg/min dose ($n = 4722$) and placebo ($n = 4739$). There was a statistically significant 1.5% absolute reduction in the composite endpoint among patients receiving eptifibatide compared with those receiving placebo (15.7% versus 14.2%, $p = 0.04$). Not unexpectedly in this large, international mega-trial, the estimate of the effect varied among the geographic regions involved. The estimate of the effect was greatest (more than 3.0% absolute reduction) among patients enrolled in North America (predominantly the USA), where the rates of invasive cardiac procedures (including cardiac catheterization, percutaneous intervention, and coronary surgery) were substantially higher than in the rest of the world. Patients benefited from treatment with eptifibatide regardless of treatment strategy (revascularization or medical), although the magnitude of the benefit was greater among those patients treated with coronary revascularization. After adjusting for the patient differences between the treatment strategies, there was a consistent and similar benefit to treatment with eptifibatide.[36] Importantly, a reduction in death or myocardial infarction was observed even before coronary intervention, supporting the strategy of using eptifibatide upon presentation, before cardiac catheterization and coronary intervention, if

needed. Bleeding occurred more frequently among patients treated with eptifibatide than with placebo, primarily at arterial access sites. Rates of thrombocytopenia were similar between the groups.

Eptifibatide development: ACS with persistent ST-Segment elevation

Although antiplatelet therapy in the form of aspirin adds substantial benefit to fibrinolysis for patients presenting with acute myocardial infarction with persistent ST-segment elevation,[37] limited data support the use of more potent platelet GPIIb/IIIa antagonists concurrently with fibrinolysis. Only four completed trials have reported on the effects of this strategy[38–41] and all have been small-dose exploration trials. Eptifibatide has been evaluated as an adjunct to full-dose fibrinolysis in two trials.[39,41]

In the IMPACT-AMI trial, 180 patients with ST-segment elevation myocardial infarction were randomized to receive escalating doses of eptifibatide or placebo in addition to receiving the standard dose of alteplase, heparin, and aspirin. Reperfusion was accelerated with the use of eptifibatide as determined by TIMI flow at 90 min and by resolution of ST-segment elevation on continuous ST monitoring. At 90 min, there was TIMI grade 3 flow in 66% of eptifibatide-treated patients versus 39% of placebo patients ($p = 0.006$). There was also an excess of access-site bleeding among the eptifibatide-treated patients. Clinical outcomes were similar between the treatment groups, but the small sample size limits the significance of the observation.

Eptifibatide has also been evaluated in a small trial ($n = 181$) as an adjunct to streptokinase for the treatment of acute myocardial infarction.[42] Patients presenting with

ST-segment elevation were eligible for randomization to escalating doses of eptifibatide or placebo. All patients received 1.5 million units of streptokinase and underwent 90-min angiography for determination of TIMI flow. TIMI grade 3 flow was increased among patients receiving eptifibatide compared with placebo, but non-central nervous system bleeding and transfusion requirements were also increased to a degree that led to termination of the trial.

While it appears from these small, dose-finding studies that eptifibatide combined with standard fibrinolytic regimens improves angiographic outcomes, there are insufficient clinical outcome data to conclude that this combination strategy is actually effective and safe. In particular, emerging data suggest that reduced doses of the fibrinolytic agent in combination with the antiplatelet agent might preserve the observed reperfusion benefit, improve clinical outcomes (mortality), and have an acceptable, perhaps even improved, safety profile. Phase II dose-finding work is continuing in the INTRO-AMI (Integrilin and Reduced dose of Thrombolytics in Acute Myocardial Infarction) trial. Although the combination of GPIIb/IIIa inhibitors and fibrinolytic therapy appears promising, large-scale trials with adequate statistical power are needed before these strategies are adopted into clinical practice.

Tirofiban

Tirofiban is the prototypical non-peptide, small-molecule inhibitor of platelet GPIIb/IIIa. This tyrosine derivative is an active antagonist against the RGD binding site of the GPIIb/IIIa receptor.[43] Cleared predominantly via renal mechanisms, tirofiban has a plasma half-life of approximately 2 h.[44] In a small dose-finding study of patients undergoing percutaneous coronary intervention, Kereiakes et al[45] reported that tirofiban provided dose-dependent inhibition of ex-vivo ADP-mediated platelet aggregation. The highest doses of tirofiban (bolus of 10 µg/kg/min followed by an infusion of either 0.10 µg/kg/min or 0.15 µg/kg/min) provided greater than 90% ADP-induced aggregation inhibition when measured at 5 min after the bolus and greater than 80% (0.10 dose) 90% (0.15 dose) inhibition at the end of the 16–24-h infusion. There was rapid reversibility of the platelet inhibitory effect, with less than 50% inhibition remaining, even at the highest tirofiban doses 4 h after the termination of the infusion. Of note, inhibition of platelet aggregation with tirofiban was measured using 5 µM ADP as an agonist, while both abciximab and eptifibatide studies used 20 µM ADP as the stimulus to platelet aggregation. More inter-patient variability occurs at doses of ADP below 10 µM. Therefore, testing at the 5 µM ADP level may lead to an overestimation of the antiplatelet effect in large populations.[46]

Tirofiban development: percutaneous coronary intervention

Like eptifibatide, tirofiban was first studied as an adjunct to heparin and aspirin in the setting of percutaneous coronary intervention. The Randomized Efficacy Study of Tirofiban for Outcomes and Restenosis (RESTORE)[22] limited enrollment to a group of patients who were felt to be at high risk for the ischemic complications of percutaneous intervention, as in the EPIC trial,[14] which was the first trial using abciximab. In the RESTORE trial, patients were eligible for randomization to either tirofiban (10 µg/kg bolus followed by 0.15 µg/kg/min infusion for 36 h) or placebo if they were within 72 h of presenting with an

ACS. The primary endpoint was the 30-day composite of death, myocardial infarction, repeat intervention (percutaneous or surgical), or stent placement for threatened or actual abrupt closure. Although 2212 patients were randomized into the trial, only the 2141 patients who actually received study drug were considered in the primary safety and efficacy analyses. At 2 days there was a 3.3% absolute reduction in the composite endpoint ($p = 0.005$), which did not meet statistical significance at the primary endpoint measurement at 30 days (12.2% placebo versus 10.3% tirofiban, $p = 0.16$). As had been seen in the other trials of GPIIb/IIIa blockade in the setting of percutaneous intervention, the early effect was at its maximum during the time of study drug infusion but there was no loss (rebound) in the absolute benefit for at least the first 30 days. Bleeding was similar between the two groups and in general, was quite low.

Tirofiban is not currently approved for use during routine coronary intervention. Subset analyses of patients undergoing percutaneous coronary intervention as part of the PRISM-PLUS trial[24] (see later) revealed a consistent effect of tirofiban in reducing the composite of death, myocardial infarction, and refractory ischemia at 7 days. Further work is required to determine the optimal dosing strategy and to demonstrate definitive clinical benefits in the broad group of patients presenting for percutaneous coronary intervention.

Tirofiban development: ACS without persistent ST-segment elevation

Like eptifibatide, tirofiban has more recently (in the Spring 1998) been approved for use in the treatment of patients presenting with ACS without persistent ST-segment elevation. Two trials support the claim that tirofiban is benefi-cial in this group of patients: the Platelet Receptor Inhibition in Ischemic Syndrome Management (PRISM) and the Platelet Receptor Inhibition in Ischemic Syndrome Management in Patients Limited by Unstable Signs and Symptoms (PRISM-PLUS) trials (see Table 9.2).[23,24]

Unlike the PURSUIT investigators who chose to study eptifibatide using the large, simple trial model, the PRISM and PRISM-PLUS investigators chose to use two separate and smaller trials with more controlled treatment characteristics to answer individual questions about the utility of tirofiban in specific clinical settings. The primary endpoints of these trials were early, reflecting their limited size. Despite the differences in trial design and methodology, taken together the PURSUIT, PRISM, and PRISM-PLUS trials studied more than 16 000 randomized patients and confirmed the benefits of small-molecule inhibitors of GPIIb/IIIa in the treatment of patients with non-ST-segment elevation ACS.[46]

The PRISM trial was designed to test the hypothesis that medical stabilization with tirofiban plus aspirin, but without heparin, would improve 48-h clinical outcomes compared with aspirin plus heparin in low- to moderate-risk patients with ACS. In this study, 3232 patients were randomized to tirofiban (0.6 µg/kg bolus followed by an infusion of 0.15 µg/kg-min) or heparin for 48 h, during which time cardiac catheterization and revascularization were discouraged. Heparin therapy was blinded and the level of anticoagulation was controlled by an investigator not involved with the patient's care. The primary endpoint was the composite at 48 h of death, myocardial infarction, or refractory ischemia.

At the primary endpoint measurement at 48 h, fewer composite events had occurred in the tirofiban group than in the placebo group (3.8% versus 5.6%, $p = 0.01$). The beneficial effects of tirofiban were mainly a reduction of refractory ischemia (3.5% versus 5.3%, $p = 0.01$). At 30 days, the effect trended in the direction favoring tirofiban but was no longer significant (15.9% versus 17.1%, $p = 0.34$). Major bleeding was very low, as would be expected in a trial that discouraged invasive procedures, and similar in both treatment groups (0.4% versus 0.4%). Thrombocytopenia occurred infrequently but more often among patients treated with tirofiban than with placebo (1.1% versus 0.4%, $p = 0.04$).

The PRISM-PLUS[24] trial was designed to complement the PRISM trial. Enrollment was expanded to include a more high-risk group of patients and tirofiban was studied with and without heparin, compared with placebo and heparin. Tirofiban doses differed depending on whether heparin was given (0.6 µg/kg bolus + 0.15 µg/kg/min infusion without heparin versus 0.4 µg/kg bolus + 0.1 µg/kg/min infusion with heparin). Cardiac catheterization was still discouraged for the first 48 h but was then specifically encouraged for all patients with coronary intervention to be performed if anatomically appropriate. The primary endpoint was the composite of death, myocardial infarction, and refractory ischemia at 7 days. Since the prespecified analysis plan was to compare each of the tirofiban strategies to placebo, the nominal level of statistical significance for the trial was set at a p-value of 0.025.

In the PRISM-PLUS study, 1915 patients were randomized. The tirofiban without heparin arm was discontinued prematurely after enrollment of 345 patients when an independent Data and Safety Monitoring Board noted an increase in 7-day mortality in this group compared with placebo (4.6% versus 1.1%, $p = 0.012$). The trial continued to its completion with enrollment into the two remaining treatment groups. Tirofiban with heparin significantly reduced the 7-day pri-

mary composite endpoint compared with placebo with heparin (12.9% versus 17.9%, $p = 0.004$). The composite of death and myocardial infarction was also reduced at 7 days (4.9% versus 8.3%, $p = 0.006$), but no longer maintained the prespecified level of statistical significance at 30 days (8.7% versus 11.9%, $p = 0.03$). Almost 90% of patients underwent cardiac catheterization during the index hospitalization, with 30.5% having percutaneous intervention. As seen with eptifibatide in the PURSUIT trial, GPIIb/IIIa blockade with tirofiban appeared especially beneficial among those patients having percutaneous revascularization. The rates of major bleeding and thrombocytopenia were low and increased non-significantly in patients who received tirofiban compared with placebo.

In these percutaneous intervention and ACS trials, tirofiban appears to improve clinical outcomes consistently; however, several questions remain unanswered. Since the initial dose-finding work with tirofiban was performed with 5 µM ADP and because the dose of tirofiban differed in each of the trials, the optimal dose of tirofiban for clinical use remains unclear. In addition, the discontinuation of the tirofiban without heparin arm in the PRISM-PLUS study is confusing. This treatment arm used the same dose that was found to be better than placebo in the PRISM trial. It is unknown whether the higher mortality seen in the tirofiban-alone arm of PRISM-PLUS was caused by chance (a significant mortality difference was not apparent at other time points) or whether the higher mortality reflected a problem when higher-risk patients were deprived of concomitant antithrombin therapy; this question needs further study. Finally, further work will be required to evaluate tirofiban as an adjunct to fibrinolysis for acute ST-segment elevation myocardial infarction.

Lamifiban

Lamifiban is a non-peptide inhibitor of GPIIb/IIIa that, like the other small molecule antagonists, is excreted renally. It has been studied in several small ACS trials in patients with and without ST-segment elevation. To date no large, definitive trial has been completed and consequently, lamifiban is not yet available for clinical use.

Theroux et al[47] first studied lamifiban in a Phase II dose-finding trial, the Canadian Lamifiban Study. Patients with unstable angina (86%) or myocardial infarction without ST-segment elevation (14%) were randomized in a parallel fashion to one of four lamifiban doses or placebo ($n = 123$):

(1) bolus 150 µg plus 1.0 µg/min infusion ($n = 40$);
(2) bolus 300 µg plus 2.0 µg/min ($n = 41$);
(3) bolus 600 µg plus 4.0 µg/min ($n = 120$); or
(4) bolus 750 µg plus 5.0 µg/min ($n = 41$).

Heparin was given at the investigator's discretion to approximately 28% of the patients. Inhibition of platelet aggregation was measured in response to 10 µM ADP and 100 µM thrombin receptor agonist peptide. Lamifiban provided a dose-dependent inhibition of aggregation with 100% ADP-induced aggregation inhibition measured at the two highest doses at steady state. Major bleeding was more frequent with lamifiban versus placebo (2.9% versus 0.8%). At 30 days, among patients receiving the two highest lamifiban doses, there was a reduction in the composite of death and myocardial infarction compared with placebo (2.5% versus 8.1%, $p = 0.03$). Based on the encouraging results of this Phase II trial, a larger dose-exploration study was performed.

The Platelet IIb/IIIa Antagonism for the Reduction of Acute coronary syndrome events in a Global Organization Network (PARAGON) trial[48] employed a modified three-by-two factorial design to evaluate two doses of lamifiban (300 µg bolus + 1.0 µg/min infusion or 750 µg bolus + 5.0 µg/min infusion) with and without heparin, against placebo with heparin in patients presenting with an ACS without persistent ST-segment elevation. All patients received aspirin. The primary endpoint was the 30-day composite of death and myocardial infarction. This was the first trial with a platelet GPIIb/IIIa antagonist to randomize heparin therapy in addition to the platelet inhibitor. Although a modest trial in size ($n = 2282$), the investigators sought to gain some insight into whether heparin provided additional benefit in patients being treated with potent platelet inhibition.

In PARAGON A, there was no difference in the composite endpoint between any lamifiban dose and placebo at 30 days; however, by 6 months there was continued divergence of the event curves so that a significant reduction in the composite endpoint was observed in the low-dose lamifiban group compared with placebo (13.7% versus 18.1%, $p = 0.02$). The 6-month composite endpoint occurred in 16.4% of patients receiving high-dose lamifiban. Bleeding was highest among those patients receiving high-dose lamifiban, particularly when combined with heparin.

Lamifiban has also been evaluated in the setting of acute myocardial infarction with ST-segment elevation. In the Platelet Aggregation Receptor Antagonist Dose Investigation and reperfusion Gain in Myocardial infarction (PARADIGM) trial, 353 patients presenting within 12 h of an acute ST-segment elevation myocardial infarction were enrolled in a dose-escalation study of standard-dose fibrinolysis (either t-PA or streptokinase) with lamifiban.[40] The choice of thrombolytic agent was left to the discretion of the investigator. In an open-label fashion, a dose of lamifiban was identified that provided greater than 85% ADP-induced inhibition of platelet aggregation; patients were then randomized to receive this dose of lamifiban or placebo, along with the fibrinolytic agent. Those receiving t-PA also received heparin, while those treated with streptokinase did not.

In the PARADIGM study, the highest dose of lamifiban (400 μg bolus +2.0 μg-min infusion for 48 h) resulted in a 91% median (interquartile range, 84–95%) inhibition of aggregation at steady-state measurement. There was also an improvement in myocardial reperfusion as measured by continuous ST-segment monitoring with less time to ST-segment resolution and less time to ST-segment steady state. Both these variables were shown in previous trials to correlate with an improvement in 30-day clinical outcomes.[49] There was an increased risk of bleeding among patients treated with lamifiban compared with placebo, although there were too few patients to make reliable observations about the risk of intracranial hemorrhage associated with the combination strategy.

Unresolved issues

A systematic overview of the trials with the small molecule GPIIb/IIIa antagonists supports the hypothesis that this class of agent benefits patients presenting with ACS without persistent ST-segment elevation (Figure 9.3).[18] The benefits of the small-molecule inhibitors also appear to extend to coronary intervention, although only eptifibatide is approved for use in this indication. More work is required on the potential role of these agents in patients with ACS with persistent ST-segment elevation.

While these agents clearly represent a major therapeutic advance for the treatment of patients with acute ischemic heart disease, many questions remain regarding their use. Firstly, there are similarities and differences among the three small-molecule inhibitors. Whether these differences are clinically important is unknown; this question will only be answered using head-to-head comparator trials. Without such trials, speculation about meaningful differences is inappropriate, given the major differences in clinical trial design even within a common indication. Similarly, the question of whether the small-molecule inhibitors and the monoclonal antibody antagonist are clinically different is unknown; determining the answer likewise requires head-to-head trials.

Secondly, the optimal dosing strategy for each of these agents remains unknown. Future trials will need to consider using point-of-care platelet aggregation testing[50] to define better the level of inhibition achieved in individual patients. Studies also need to be performed to determine more acurately the level of platelet inhibition that is associated with maximum benefit.[46] PARAGON B, an ongoing study with lamifiban in patients with ACS without persistent ST-segment elevation is testing whether a dosing strategy that takes into consideration individual patient characteristics such as age, gender, weight, and renal function, can lead to more optimal drug concentrations and to improved patient outcomes.

Finally, in addition to these GPIIb/IIIa inhibitors, there exist fibrinolytics and novel antithrombins, including low-molecular-weight heparins and direct thrombin inhibitors that are approved for use or being studied for use in patients with acute ischemic heart disease. The combination of potent antiplatelet therapies with novel antithrombins and fibrinolytics needs further investigation. The small

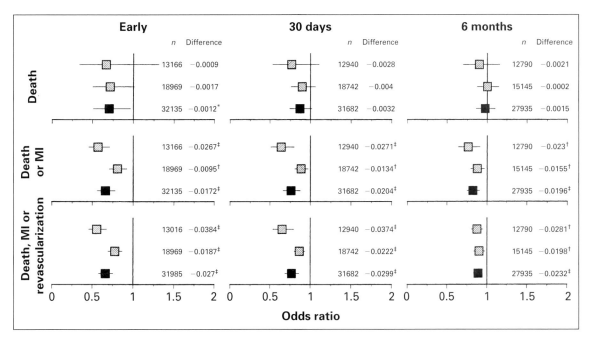

Figure 9.3
Odds ratios (OR) and 95% confidence intervals (CI) for risk of death, death or myocardial infarction (MI), and death, MI, or revascularization (Revasc) 48 to 96 h, 30 days, and 6 months after randomization to a glycoprotein IIb/IIIa inhibitor (versus placebo). ORs are given for combined percutaneous intervention trials (▨), combined non-ST-segment elevation acute coronary syndromes trials (▧), and all collected trials (■). n, sample size; Difference, risk difference. *p < 0.05; †p < 0.01; ‡p < 0.001.

dose-finding studies using GPIIb/IIIa antagonists and full-dose fibrinolytic therapy appear promising. Several trials are underway with lower doses of the fibrinolytic agents that, in combination with GPIIb/IIIa inhibitors, improve angiographically determined myocardial perfusion. Much larger trials, enrolling tens of thousands of patients, are needed to show the safety and efficacy of this approach.

References

1. Tolleson TR, Harrington RA. Thrombosis in acute coronary syndromes and coronary interventions. In: Lincoff AM, Topol EJ (eds) *GPIIb/IIIa Inhibitors in Cardiology*. (Humana Press, Totowa, NJ, 1998).

2. Fuster V, Chesebro JH. Mechanisms of unstable angina. *N Engl J Med* 1986;**315**:1023–5.

3. Alexander JH, Harrington RA: Antiplatelet and antithrombin therapies in the acute coronary syndromes. *Curr Opin Cardiol* 1997; **12**:427–37.

4. Harrington RA, Macik BG. Monitoring the coagulation system after thrombolytic therapy. In: Califf RM, Mark DB, Wagner GS (eds) *Acute Coronary Care*, 2nd edn. (Mosby, St. Louis, 1995) 469–80.

5. Antiplatelet Trialists' Collaboration. Collaborative overview of randomized trials of antiplatelet therapy—I: Prevention of death, myocardial infarction, and stroke by prolonged antiplatelet therapy in various categories of patients. *Br Med J* 1994;**308**:81–106.

6. Jack DB. One hundred years of aspirin. *Lancet* 1997;**350**:437–39.

7. CAPRIE Steering Committee. A randomized, blinded, trial of clopidogrel versus aspirin in patients at risk of ischaemic events (CAPRIE). *Lancet* 1996;**348**:1329–39.

8. Helgason CM, Bolin KM, Winkler SR, Mangat A, Tortorice KL, Brace LD. Development of aspirin resistance in persons with previous ischemic stroke. *Stroke* 1994;**25**:2331–6.

9. Farrell TP, Hayes KA, Tracey PB, Sobel BE, Schneider DJ. Unexpected, discordant effects of aspirin on platelet activity. *J Am Coll Cardiol* 1998;**31**:352A[Abstract].

10. Buchanan MR, Brister SJ. Individual variation in the effects of ASA on platelet function: implications for the use of ASA clinically. *Can J Cardiol* 1998;**11**:221–7.

11. Coller BS, Peerschke EI, Scudder LE, Sullivan CA. A murine monoclonal antibody that completely blocks the binding of fibrinogen to platelets produces a thrombasthenic-like state in normal platelets and binds to glycoproteins IIb and/or IIIa. *J Clin Invest* 1983;**72**:325–38.

12. Coller BS, Folts JD, Smith SR, Scudder LE, Jordan R. Abolition of in vivo platelet thrombus formation in primates with monoclonal antibodies to the platelet GPIIb/IIIa receptor. Correlation with bleeding time, platelet aggregation, and blockade of GPIIb/IIIa receptors. *Circulation* 1989;**80**:1766–74.

13. Simoons ML, de Boer MJ, van den Brand MJBM, et al. Randomized trial of a GPIIb/IIIa platelet receptor blocker in refractory unstable angina. *Circulation* 1994;**89**:596–603.

14. EPIC Investigators. Use of a monoclonal antibody directed against the platelet glycoprotein IIb/IIIa receptor in high-risk coronary angioplasty. *N Engl J Med* 1994;**330**:956–61.

15. The EPILOG Investigators. Platelet glycoprotein IIb/IIIa receptor blockade and low-dose heparin during percutaneous coronary revascularization. *N Engl J Med* 1997;**336**:1689–96.

16. The CAPTURE Investigators. Randomised placebo-controlled trial of abciximab before and during coronary intervention in refractory unstable angina: the CAPTURE study. *Lancet* 1997;**349**:1429–35.

17. Brener SJ, Barr LA, Burchenal J, et al. A randomized, placebo-controlled trial of abciximab with primary angioplasty for acute MI. The RAPPORT trial. *Circulation* 1997;**96**:I-473 [Abstract].

18. Kong DF, Califf RM, Miller DP, et al. Clinical outcomes of therapeutic agents that block the platelet glycoprotein IIb/IIIa integrin in ischemic heart disease. *Circulation* 1998;**98**: 2829–35.

19. Kleiman NS, Lincoff AM, Ohman EM, Harrington RA. Glycoprotein IIb/IIIa inhibitors in acute coronary syndromes: pathophysiologic foundation and clinical findings. *Am Heart J* 1998;**136**:S32–S42.

20. Anonymous. Randomized placebo-controlled trial of effect of eptifibatide on complications of percutaneous coronary intervention:

IMPACT-II. Integrilin to Minimise Platelet Aggregation and Coronary Thrombosis—II. *Lancet* 1997;**349**:1422–8.

21. The PURSUIT Trial Investigators. Inhibition of platelet glycoprotein IIb/IIIa with eptifibatide in patients with acute coronary syndromes. *N Engl J Med* 1998;**339**:436–43.

22. The RESTORE Investigators. Effects of platelet glycoprotein IIb/IIIa blockade with tirofiban on adverse cardiac events in patients with unstable angina or acute myocardial infarction undergoing coronary angioplasty. *Circulation* 1997;**96**: 1445–53.

23. The Platelet Receptor Inhibition in Ischemic Syndrome Management (PRISM) Study Investigators. A comparison of aspirin plus tirofiban with aspirin plus heparin for unstable angina. *N Engl J Med* 1998;**338**:1498–505.

24. The Platelet Receptor Inhibition in Ischemic Syndrome Management in Patients Limited by Unstable Signs and Symptoms (PRISM-PLUS) Study Investigators. Inhibition of the platelet glycoprotein IIb/IIIa receptor with tirofiban in unstable angina and non-Q-wave myocardial infarction. *N Engl J Med* 1998;**338**:1488–97.

25. Alexander JH, Harrington RA. Recent antiplatelet drug trials in the acute coronary syndromes: clinical interpretation of PRISM, PRISM-PLUS, PARAGON A and PURSUIT. *Drugs* 1998;**56**:[In press].

26. Scarborough RM, Naughton MA, Teng W, et al. Design of potent and specific integrin antagonists. Peptide antagonists with high specificity for glycoprotein IIb-IIIa. *J Biol Chem* 1993;**268**:1066–73.

27. Tcheng JE, Harrington RA, Kottke-Marchant K, et al. Multicenter, randomized, double-blind, placebo-controlled trial of the platelet integrin glycoprotein IIb/IIIa blocker integrelin in elective coronary intervention. *Circulation* 1995;**91**:2151–7.

28. Harrington RA, Kleiman NS, Kottke-Marchant K, et al. Immediate and reversible platelet inhibition after intravenous administration of a peptide glycoprotein IIb/IIIa inhibitor during percutaneous coronary intervention. *Am J Cardiol* 1995;**76**:1222–7.

29. Tardiff BE, Miller JM, Harrington RA, Tcheng JE, Califf RM. Integrilin: synthetic peptides against the platelet glycoprotein IIb/IIIa receptor. In: Sasahara AA, Loscalzo J (eds) *New Therapeutic Agents in Thrombosis and Thrombolysis.* (Marcel Dekker, New York, 1997) 333–54.

30. Schulman SP, Goldschmidt-Clermont PJ, Navetta FI, et al. Integrelin in unstable angina: a double-blind randomized trial. *Circulation* 1993;**88**(Suppl. I):I-608[Abstract].

31. Phillips DR, Teng W, Arfsten A, et al. Effect of Ca^{2+} on GPIIb-IIIa interactions with integrilin: enhanced GPIIb-IIIa binding and inhibition of platelet aggregation by reductions in the concentration of ionized calcium in plasma anticoagulated with citrate. *Circulation* 1997;**96**: 1488–94.

32. Kleiman NS. Primary and secondary safety endpoints from IMPACT II. Integrilin to Minimize Platelet Aggregation and Coronary Thrombosis. *Am J Cardiol* 1997;**80**(4A): 29B–33B.

33. Tcheng JE. PRIDE Study Preliminary Results. *19th Congress of the European Society of Cardiology*, Stockholm, Sweden. 1997.

34. Braunwald E, Mark DB, Jones RH, et al. Unstable Angina: Diagnosis and Management. *Clinical Practice Guideline Number 10.* (Agency for Health Care Policy and Research and the National Heart, Lung, and Blood Institute, Public Health Service, US Department of Health and Human Services, Rockville, MD, 1994).

35. Schulman SP, Goldschmidt-Clermont PJ, Topol EJ, et al. Effects of integrelin, a platelet glycoprotein IIB/IIIa receptor antagonist, in unstable angina. A randomized multicenter trial. *Circulation* 1996;**94**:2083–9.

36. Kleiman NS, Lincoff AM, Miller DP, et al. Abciximab (c7E3) reduces death and myocardial infarction but not target vessel revascularization in diabetics undergoing percutaneous transluminal coronary angioplasty: the EPILOG experience. *Eur Heart J* 1997; **18**(Suppl.):13[Abstract].

37. ISIS-1 (First International Study of Infarct Survival) Collaborative Group. Randomised trial of intravenous atenolol among 16 027 cases of suspected acute myocardial infarction: ISIS-1. *Lancet* 1986;**2**:57–66.

38. Kleiman NS, Ohman EM, Keriakes DJ, et al. Profound platelet inactivation with 7E3 shortly

after thrombolytic therapy for acute myocardial infarction: Preliminary results of the TAMI 8 trial. *Circulation* 1991;**84**:II-522[Abstract].

39. Ohman EM, Kleiman NS, Gacioch G, et al. Combined accelerated tissue-plasminogen activator and platelet glycoprotein IIb/IIIa integrin receptor blockade with Integrilin in acute myocardial infarction: results of a randomized, placebo-controlled, dose-ranging trial. *Circulation* 1997;**95**:846–54.

40. The PARADIGM Investigators. Combining thrombolysis with the platelet glycoprotein IIb/IIIa inhibitor lamifiban: results of the Platelet Aggregation Receptor Antagonist Dose Investigation and reperfusion Gain in Myocardial infarction (PARADIGM) trial. *J Am Coll Cardiol* 1998; [In press].

41. Simoons ML, Wijns W, Balakumaran K, et al. The effect of intracoronary thrombolysis with streptokinase on myocardial thallium distribution and left ventricular function assessed by blood-pool scintigraphy. *Eur Heart J* 1982;**3**: 433–40.

42. Ronner E, van Kesteren HAM, Zijnen P, et al. Combined therapy with streptokinase and Integrilin. *J Am Coll Cardiol* 1998;**31**(**Suppl. A**):191A[Abstract].

43. Peerlinck K, De Lepeleire I, Goldberg M, et al. MK-383 (L-700,462), a selective non-peptide platelet glycoprotein IIb/IIIa antagonist, is active in man. *Circulation* 1993; **88**:1512–17.

44. Deckelbaum LI, Sax FL, Grossman W. Tirofiban, a non-peptide inhibitor of the platelet glycoprotein IIb/IIIa receptor. In: Sasahara AA, Loscalzo J (eds) *New Therapeutic Agents in Thrombosis and Thrombolysis*. (Marcel Dekker, New York, 1997).

45. Kereiakes DJ, Kleiman NS, Ambrose J, et al. Randomized double-blind, placebo-controlled dose-ranging study of tirofiban (MK-383) platelet IIb/IIIa blockade in high-risk patients undergoing coronary angioplasty. *J Am Coll Cardiol* 1996;**27**:536–42.

46. Harrington RA, Kleiman NS, Granger CB, Ohman EM, Berkowitz SD. Relation between inhibition of platelet aggregation and clinical outcomes. *Am Heart J* 1998;**136**:S43–S50.

47. Theroux P, Kouz S, Roy L, et al. Platelet membrane receptor glycoprotein IIb/IIIa antagonism in unstable angina—the Canadian lamifiban study. *Circulation* 1996;**94**:899–905.

48. Anonymous. International, randomized, controlled trial of lamifiban (a platelet glycoprotein IIb/IIIa inhibitor), heparin, or both in unstable angina. The PARAGON Investigators. Platelet IIb/IIa Antagonism for the Reduction of Acute coronary syndrome events in a Global Organization Network. *Circulation* 1998;**97**:2386–95.

49. Krucoff MW, Green CL, Trollinger KM, et al. ST-segment recovery parameters predictive of outcome in AMI: variability with infarct artery location and implications for therapeutic targets. *J Am Coll Cardiol* 1997;**29**(**Suppl.A**): 412A[Abstract].

50. Berkowitz SD, Frelinger AL, Hillman RS. Progress in point-of-care laboratory testing for assessing platelet function. *Am Heart J* 1998;**136**:S51–S65.

10

Oral platelet glycoprotein IIb/IIIa blockers

Christopher P Cannon

Introduction

Every year more than four million patients are admitted to hospitals worldwide with the diagnosis of unstable angina or acute myocardial infarction (MI).[1,2] The initiating event of unstable coronary syndromes is atherosclerotic plaque rupture followed by local thrombosis.[3] Antithrombotic therapy, currently aspirin and heparin, is the mainstay of therapy, and numerous trials have documented a dramatic 25–50% benefit on death and/or MI with aspirin in acute coronary syndromes.[4]

The importance of *antiplatelet* therapy comes from the broad experience with aspirin, which has dramatic effects in reducing both mortality and non-fatal events in patients across the spectrum of acute coronary syndromes.[4–11] In addition, the newer class of antiplatelet agents, the thienopyridines (ticlopidine and clopidogrel), which inhibit platelet function are stronger antiplatelet agents than aspirin, have been shown to be beneficial in reducing clinical events compared with aspirin alone in coronary stenting,[12–14] and in symptomatic patients with atherosclerosis.[4,15–17] This wealth of data has focused attention on the platelet, as a target for more potent therapies, notably the inhibitors of the platelet glycoprotein (GP) IIb/IIIa, which mediates platelet aggregation.

Glycoprotein IIb/IIIa blockers

GPIIb/IIIa blockers are a new, potent class of platelet inhibitors. GPIIb/IIIa receptor antagonists block the binding of fibrinogen to specific membrane GPIIb/IIIa integrin receptors, thus preventing platelet aggregation induced by various platelet agonists.[18,19] Platelet GPIIb/IIIa is a member of the integrin receptor superfamily of complexes that mediate cell–protein and cell–cell interactions.[18] GPIIb/IIIa is a calcium-dependent heterodimer, composed of two different subunits (a_{IIb} and b_3), both of which span the platelet membrane. The GPIIIa subunit contains a four-amino acid sequence, which is crucial for binding of fibrinogen and other ligands.[18] The first three amino acids are arginine-glycine-aspartic acid (RGD) while the fourth amino acid may vary. Low-molecular-weight peptide and non-peptide GPIIb/IIIa inhibitors have been developed to bind to the RGD sequence of the receptor, thereby interfering with the binding of fibrinogen to GPIIb/IIIa.

Mechanisms of action of ASA, ticlopidine, and GPIIb/IIIa inhibitors

The mechanisms of action of the current antiplatelet agents and GPIIb/IIIa inhibitors are quite distict. Aspirin permanently acetylates cyclo-oxygenase, thereby blocking the synthesis of thromboxane A_2 (TXA_2) by the platelet.[20] By decreasing the amount of TXA_2 released, which would act to stimulate other platelets, there is a decrease in overall platelet aggregation. This inhibition of cyclo-oxygenase is permanent, thus the antiplatelet effects last for the lifetime of the platelets, that is, between 7 and 10 days.

The thienopyridine class of agents (ticlopidine and clopidogrel) are believed to act by blocking the ADP receptor.[17,21,22] They may also inhibit intracellular processing of activation of the ADP pathway but have no effect on the numerous other stimulants to platelet aggregation, such as thrombin and collagen.[22] Their onset of antiplatelet effect is delayed, with peak inhibition occuring 2–4 days after the start of therapy, although clopidogrel has more rapid onset.

In contrast, GPIIb/IIIa inhibitors bind to the GPIIb/IIIa receptor and thereby block the final common pathway of platelet aggregation. By binding to the receptor, they prevent the binding of fibrinogen to the platelet and thereby prevent formation (or progression) of a platelet plug. Thus, no matter what stimuli to platelet activation exist, the platelet is inhibited by the GPIIb/IIIa inhibitor—making it a great deal more able to inhibit platelet aggregation than aspirin (or ticlopidine). When testing platelet aggregation in the laboratory, aspirin inhibits ADP-induced platelet aggregation by approximately 10%, ticlopidine and clopidogrel by approximately 30–40%,[23] and the doses of the GPIIb/IIIa inhibitors being tested clinically inhibit platelet aggregation by approximately 80–90%.[24] Several potential mechanisms exist to explain how GPIIb/IIIa inhibition may improve clot resolution and clinical outcome in patients with acute coronary syndromes. Firstly, by blocking platelet aggregation in the platelet-rich arterial thrombus, propagation of the thrombus is prevented;

GPIIb/IIIa inhibitors may also *disaggregate* a recently-formed platelet plug. Second, by preventing accumulation of a large number of platelets at the lesion, it decreases the amount of platelet phospholipid membrane, a cofactor for thrombin generation and of the clotting cascade. Thirdly, a thrombus rich in platelets may resist thrombolysis (either thrombolytic therapy or endogenous thrombolysis) owing in part to the increased presence of plasminogen activator inhibitor (PAI-1), a potent natural inhibitor of fibrinolysis that exists in high concentrations in platelets.

Potential risks of GPIIb/IIIa inhibition

Bleeding

The major concerns with any antithrombotic agents are bleeding, and for platelet inhibitors, thrombocytopenia. As with any antithrombotic agent, the potential for increased bleeding exists. Although the initial EPIC study showed increased bleeding using abciximab plus heparin during angioplasty compared with heparin alone,[25] a strong interaction with the dose of heparin was observed, such that in the EPILOG trial, the rate of major bleeding was identical in heparin control patients and in those receiving abciximab and low-dose heparin.[26] Similarly, the rate of major bleeding has generally not been found to increase significantly in other trials using intravenous[27,28] or oral GPIIb/IIIa inhibitors.[29] Thus, the use of lower doses of heparin and careful monitoring of the level of anticoagulation will avoid bleeding complications in patients receiving GPIIb/IIIa inhibitors. With regard to monitoring the degree of platelet inhibition, trials to date have used fixed dosing; however, investigation is currently underway to determine when and where monitoring of platelet function may be clinically useful.[30]

Thrombocytopenia

Thrombocytopenia is the other important side-effect of GPIIb/IIIa inhibition. Platelet counts falling below 100 000 occur in approximately 1–2% of patients treated with GPIIb/IIIa inhibitors, while platelet counts falling to below 50 000 occurs in less than 0.5% of patients.[26,28,31] In the initial trials, thrombocytopenia generally occurred on either the first day after beginning therapy, or after approximately 2 weeks' of therapy. The mechanism by which it occurs is not defined completely, but appears to involve immune mechanisms. Fortunately, it is nearly always reversible, with platelet counts returning to normal after a few days.

Types of GPIIb/IIIa inhibitors

There are three broad categories of GPIIb/IIIa inhibitors:

(1) The Fab fragment of a monoclonal antibody to the GPIIb/IIIa receptor, abciximab (ReoPro™) (see Chapter 8);

(2) The intravenous peptide and non-peptide small-molecule inhibitors, such as eptifibatide (Integrilin™) and tirofiban (Aggrastat™) (see Chapter 4);

(3) The oral GPIIb/IIIa inhibitors, such as xemilofiban, orbofiban, sibrafiban, roxifiban and many others.

Abciximab

Abciximab, the monoclonal antibody, binds very tightly to the GPIIb/IIIa receptor.[32] Thus, the antiplatelet effect lasts much longer than the infusion period—a potential benefit on improving efficacy. Conversely, if bleeding occurred, stopping the drug will not reverse the antiplatelet effect immediately; transfusion of platelets however, will allow the antibodies to redistribute among all the platelets, thereby reducing the level of platelet inhibition. Abciximab also binds to other integrins on the platelet receptor, such as the vitronectin receptor[18] but the clinical significance of this cross-reactivity is not yet established.

Peptide and non-peptide small-molecule, inhibitors

The peptide and peptidomimetic inhibitors (e.g. tirofiban and eptifibatide) are competitive inhibitors of the GPIIb/IIIa receptor.[33,34] Thus, the level of platelet inhibition is directly related to the drug level in the blood. Since both inhibitors have short half-lives, when the drug infusion is stopped,[33,34] the antiplatelet activity reverses after a few hours, which is potentially beneficial to avoid bleeding complications. Conversely, for prolonged antiplatelet effect, the drug needs to be given intravenously for a longer period of time. The inhibitors developed to date have been targeted specifically to the GPIIb/IIIa receptor and not to cross-react with other integrins.

Oral GPIIb/IIIa inhibitors

The third group of GPIIb/IIIa inhibitors are the oral agents. These agents are also competitive inhibitors, and are usually pro-drugs, which are absorbed and then converted to active compounds in the blood.[29,35,36] The oral agents all have longer half-lives than the intravenous compounds and, as such, they can be given once, twice or three times daily (depending on the half-life) in order to achieve relatively steady levels of GPIIb/IIIa inhibition. With oral dosing, long-term therapy (i.e. over 1 year) is possible. However, the long half-life also means that, if bleeding occurs, the drug must be removed from the circulation in order to reduce the antiplatelet effect. Currently this can be accomplished acutely using hemodialysis or charcoal hemoperfusion. The development of specific antidotes would be an attractive alternative method for removing the drug quickly from the circulation.

Initial clinical trials with intravenous GPIIb/IIIa inhibitors

Numerous trials have shown that intravenous GPIIb/IIIa inhibitors are beneficial in acute settings (see Chapters 8 and 9).[25–28,31,37–40] In studies of intravenous GPIIb/IIIa antagonists in coronary angioplasty and unstable angina, there have been significant reductions in recurrent ischemic events. For example, in the PRISM-PLUS trial, patients with unstable angina or non-Q-wave MI treated with aspirin, heparin, and a 2–4-day infusion of tirofiban had a 32% reduction in death, MI, or refractory ischemia at 7 days compared with placebo (12.9% versus 17.9%, $p = 0.004$), and a 30% risk reduction in death or MI at 30 days ($p = 0.03$).[31] A significant improvement in death or MI was also observed in the larger PURSUIT trial with a 3-day infusion of eptifibatide.[38] A logical extension of the potent form of therapy is to develop strategies for more sustained or chronic GPIIb/IIIa inhibitor with long-term treatment. Thus, the hypothesis for current trials is that oral GPIIb/IIIa inhibitors will provide a novel form of therapy to prevent early and late recurrent thrombotic complications in patients with acute coronary syndromes or those undergoing percutaneous coronary intervention (PCI).

Rationale for long-term GPIIb/IIIa inhibition

The rationale for long-term platelet inhibition comes from both biological and clinical observations. From the biological standpoint, as already discussed, platelet function tests show that platelets remain activated long after a patient is stabilized clinically. Active thrombus has been observed by coronary angioscopy even 1 month following acute coronary syndromes,[41] indicating the long period of time that is needed for complete antithrombotic treatment of a culprit lesion. Similarly, in the TIMI 12 trial of an oral GPIIb/IIIa inhibitor in patients stabilized after an acute coronary syndrome, we observed high levels of activated platelets in patients at the start of the study but also 1 month later (Table 10.1) despite oral GPIIb/IIIa treatment.[43] Thus, there is an active, prothrombotic 'milieu' in patients following acute coronary syndromes, which could potentially benefit from more aggressive antithrombotic therapy than just aspirin.

From the clinical standpoint, one observation supporting a potential role for long-term GPIIb/IIIa inhibition is that greater benefit appears to be achieved with longer duration of GPIIb/IIIa inhibition. When contrasting the statistically significant results obtained with abciximab use during angioplasty[25,26,39,40] with the loss of early benefit in angioplasty trials seen after the shorter infusions (24–36 h) of tirofiban and eptifibatide,[27,28] abciximab had a very long duration of action on the platelet, with antiplatelet activity detected up to 1–2 weeks after administration.[44] This suggests that the prolonged antiplatelet effect of abciximab may be responsible for some of its sustained beneficial effect.

Further support for this hypothesis comes from the RESTORE and PRISM-PLUS trials. In the RESTORE trial, tirofiban was adminis-

Agonist	Baseline (%)	Day 7(%)	Day 28 (%)
Spont.	28 ± 19	*17 ± 13	**20 ± 14
0 µM ADP	36 ± 17	*24 ± 17	*25 ± 15
1 µM ADP	48 ± 19	**44 ± 20	***40 ± 17
5 µM ADP	65 ± 19	68 ± 18	64 ± 18

* $p < 0.001$; ** $p < 0.05$; *** $p = 0.005$.
Data from Ault et al.[42]

Table 10.1
P Selectin results from the TIMI 12 study.

tered for 36 h, and a 26% reduction in MI and no difference in death at 30 days was observed. In the PRISM-PLUS trial, in which patients received 48–72 h therapy with tirofiban, those undergoing PTCA had a 45% reduction in death or MI at 30 days.[27,31] These comparisons are not randomized but are consistent with the hypothesis that a longer duration of GPIIb/IIIa inhibition is more beneficial than a shorter duration of platelet inhibition.

The second clinical observation is that the benefit of intravenous GPIIb/IIIa inhibitors is achieved *only during the infusion*. Owing to the potent platelet inhibition, the benefits are maintained but no *added* benefit is observed after the infusions are stopped. For example, in the PURSUIT trial in unstable angina and non-Q-wave MI, eptifibatide reduced death or MI by an absolute 1.7% at 72 h; the reduction was similar (1.5%) at 30 days.[38] Similarly, in PRISM-PLUS, tirofiban plus heparin reduced death or MI by 3.4% at 7 days, and by 3.2% at 30 days.[31] It is hypothesized that chronic dosing with oral GPIIb/IIIa antagonists will demonstrate ongoing benefit throughout the period of treatment and thereby amplify the benefits seen to date with the intravenous GPIIb/IIIa inhibitors.

Potential role for long-term oral GPIIb/IIIa inhibition

Oral GPIIb/IIIa receptor antagonists offer the potential for long-term treatment with many possible clinical applications (Table 10.2). Potential applications include:

(1) The early phase of acute coronary syndromes;
(2) Secondary prevention of events after stabilization from an acute coronary syndrome; and
(3) Both acute treatment and secondary prevention.

By extension, oral GPIIb/IIIa inhibitors could also potentially inhibit the development of athero(thrombo)sclerosis, which is sometimes augmented by microthrombotic events within the plaque. In addition, these agents may be useful for percutaneous coronary intervention, and also in stroke, for both early treatment and secondary prevention.

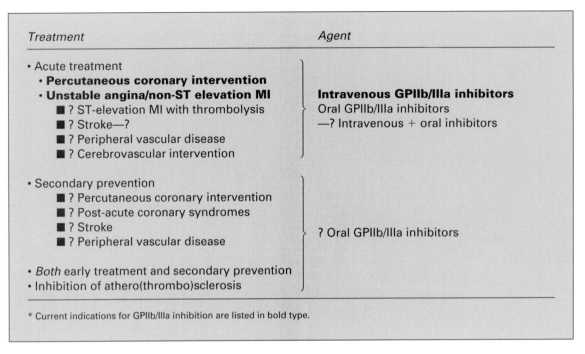

Treatment	Agent

• Acute treatment
  • **Percutaneous coronary intervention**
  • **Unstable angina/non-ST elevation MI**
    ■ ? ST-elevation MI with thrombolysis
    ■ ? Stroke—?
    ■ ? Peripheral vascular disease
    ■ ? Cerebrovascular intervention
	Intravenous GPIIb/IIIa inhibitors
	Oral GPIIb/IIIa inhibitors
	—? Intravenous + oral inhibitors

• Secondary prevention
    ■ ? Percutaneous coronary intervention
    ■ ? Post-acute coronary syndromes
    ■ ? Stroke
    ■ ? Peripheral vascular disease
 	
• *Both* early treatment and secondary prevention
• Inhibition of athero(thrombo)sclerosis
	? Oral GPIIb/IIIa inhibitors

* Current indications for GPIIb/IIIa inhibition are listed in bold type.

Table 10.2
Current and future indications for GPIIb/IIIa inhibition.*

Initial clinical experience
Pharmacokinetics and pharmacodynamics

Several orally active platelet GPIIb/IIIa inhibitors have been studied in clinical trials (Table 10.3). These agents are usually in a pro-drug form and require hepatic conversion to an active moiety. Absolute bioavailability is generally low as shown in Table 10.3. Currently available data suggest these agents produce inhibition of *ex vivo* platelet aggregation in response to various agonists (e.g. ADP, collagen, thrombin receptor activating peptide (TRAP)) that correlates closely with plasma level of active metabolite. In addition, the dose/concentration-response is maintained without evidence for tolerance or tachyphylaxis over time. Differences in drug half-life may result in drug accumulation and more pronounced platelet inhibition during chronic therapy depending on the dose-interval employed. The pharmacokinetic and pharmacodynamic response to most oral GPIIb/IIIa inhibitors can be illustrated by comparing and contrasting the responses of short-acting (xemilofiban, half-life 4.1 h) and longer-acting (sibrafiban and orbofiban; half-lives approximately 10–11 h) agents on roxifiban (18–24 hours).

Oral agent	Pharmaceutical company	Trials	Phase	Study population	Drug half-life (h)	Absolute bio-availability
Xemilofiban	GD Searle	ORBIT EXCITE	II III	Coronary intervention	4.1	13%
Sibrafiban	Roche Genentech	TIMI 12 Symphony	II III	Post-acute coronary syndrome	11	NA
Orbofiban	GD Searle	SOAR OPUS-TIMI 16	II III	Acute coronary syndrome	10	13%
Lotrafiban	SmithKline-Beecham	APLAUD BRAVO	II III	Acute coronary syndrome TIA, post-ischemic stroke	4–8	NA
Klerval	RPR	TIMI 15	II (discontinued)	Acute coronary syndrome	4–5	NA
Lefradifiban	Boehringer Ingelheim	FROST	II	Acute coronary syndrome		NA
Roxifiban	DuPont	ROCKET	II	Acute coronary syndrome	18–24	NA

Table 10.3
Clinical trials of oral GPIIb/IIIa inhibitors.

Xemilofiban

The first clinical trials of oral GPIIb/IIIa inhibition were with xemilofiban.[23,35,45] As shown in Figure 10.1, platelet inhibition was achieved in a dose-dependent fashion with this oral GPIIb/IIIa inhibitor. It had a relatively short half-life and thus is given three times daily. The drug was well tolerated by patients in this study.

The Oral Glycoprotein IIb/IIIa Receptor Blockade to Inhibit Thrombosis (ORBIT) trial was a randomized dose-ranging trial of xemilofiban in patients undergoing percuta-neous intervention.[46] Peak inhibition of platelet aggregation was similar following the same dose of xemilofiban administered on Days 14 and 28 of the trial. The time to peak blood level following the same dose of xemilofiban was reduced from 4 h following the first dose of drug to 2 h with steady-state dosing during chronic therapy.[46]

The incidence and severity of bleeding events with 2 and 4 weeks of therapy by pharmacologic treatment regimen in the ORBIT trial is shown in Table 10.4. Most bleeding events were observed during the first 2 weeks

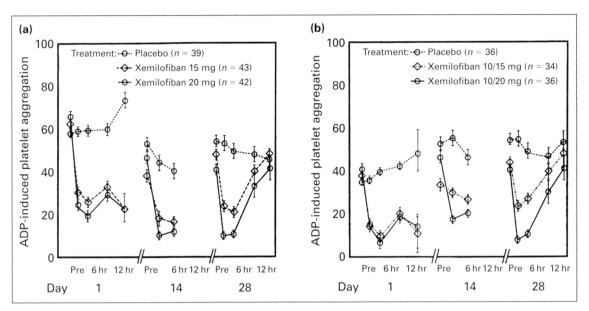

Figure 10.1
Platelet inhibition achieved by xemilofiban: **(a)** *without antecedent abciximab therapy;* **(b)** *with antecedent abciximab therapy. Data expressed as mean ± SEM (Reproduced with permission from Kereiakes et al[46]).*

	Placebo		Xemilofiban (10/15 mg)*		Xemilofiban (10/20 mg)*	
	Abciximab	No Abciximab	Abciximab	No Abciximab	Abciximab	No Abciximab
Event at 2 weeks (%)						
Insignificant	12	19	18	26	23	32
Mild	0	5	11	10	4	11
Moderate	6	0	2	1	0	2
Severe	0	0	0	2	2	0
Event at 4 weeks (%)						
Insignificant	17	24	23	32	34	38
Mild	4	6	13	11	6	13
Moderate	6	0	2	1	0	2
Severe	0	0	0	2	2	0

* Xemilofiban dosing regimen as outlined in Figures 10.1 and 10.2.

Table 10.4
Bleeding events in ORBIT trial (Data from ref. 46).

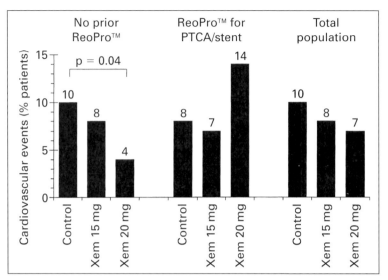

Figure 10.2
Cardiac events at 90 days in the ORBIT trial.[46]

of therapy on a three times per daily dosing regimen. Further bleeding events were uncommon during the final 2 weeks of treatment on a twice-daily dosing regimen and the requirement for blood transfusion was infrequent.

An intriguing difference in cardiac events was observed in the ORBIT trial. In the xemilofiban 20 mg group, there was a trend toward benefit at 90 days in the composite clinical endpoint. Curiously, there was an *increase* in cardiac events during the first weeks of therapy but a late decrease in events, among patients who had not received abciximab for their index PCI (Figure 10.2). Among those who received abciximab, there was actually an increase in cardiac events; however, since the number of patients in the trial was modest (just over 500), it is the larger Phase III trials that will establish the effects of oral GPIIb/IIIa inhibitors on cardiac events (see below).

The TIMI 12 trial

The Thrombolysis in Myocardial Infarction (TIMI) 12 trial was a Phase II, double-blind, dose-ranging trial designed to evaluate the pharmacokinetics (PK), pharmacodymamics (PD), safety and tolerability of sibrafiban in 329 patients post-acute coronary syndromes.[29] In the PK/PD cohort of the TIMI 12 study 106 patients were randomized to receive one of seven dosing regimens of sibrafiban, ranging from 5 mg daily to 10 mg twice daily for 28 days. In the safety cohort, 223 patients were randomized to one of four dose regimens of sibrafiban (ranging from 5 mg twice daily to 15 mg once daily) or aspirin for 28 days.

High levels of platelet inhibition were achieved: mean peak values ranged from 47% to 97% inhibition of 20 μM ADP-induced platelet aggregation on Day 28 across the

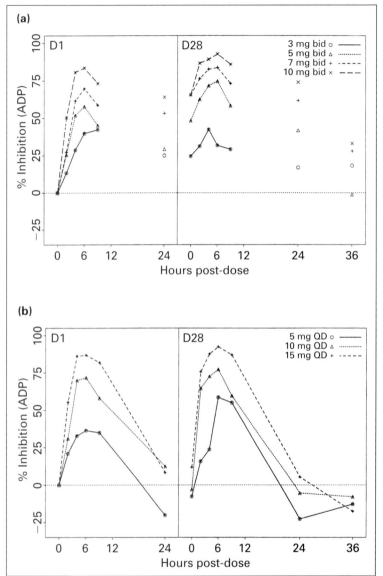

Figure 10.3
*Inhibition of ex vivo platelet aggregation in the TIMI trial[29] in response to 20 μM ADP on Day 1 (D1) and Day 28 (D28): **(a)** Twice daily (bid) dosing regimens; and **(b)** during daily (QD) dosing regimens (Reproduced with permission from Cannon et al[29]).*

seven doses (Figure 10.3). Twice daily dosing provided more sustained platelet inhibition (mean inhibition 36–86% on Day 28), while platelet inhibition returned to baseline levels by 24 h with once daily dosing.[29] Major

hemorrhage was rare (1.5%) in patients treated with sibrafiban or aspirin (1.9%). Protocol-defined 'minor' bleeding, usually mucocutaneous, occurred in 0–32% of patients in the various sibrafiban groups,

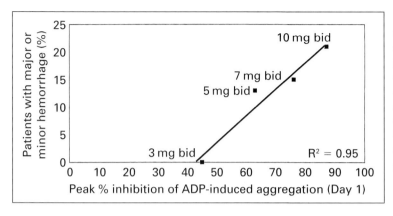

Figure 10.4
Relationship between major or minor hemorrhage (% of patients) and peak inhibition (%) of ADP (20 μM) induced platelet aggregation on Day 1. Mean levels of platelet inhibition achieved by twice daily (bid) study drug administration are shown.[29] (Reproduced with permission from Cannon et al[29]).

compared with none of the aspirin-treated patients. In a multivariate model, minor bleeding was related to total daily dose ($p = 0.002$), once- versus twice-daily dosing ($p < 0.0001$), renal function ($p < 0.0001$), and presentation with unstable angina ($p < 0.01$).[29] Thus, the oral GPIIb/IIIa antagonist sibrafiban achieved effective, chronic platelet inhibition with a clear dose-response but at the expense of a relatively high incidence of minor bleeding. The mucocutaneous bleeds appeared to be related to plasma drug concentrations, the degree of platelet inhibition (Figure 10.4) and other patient factors (e.g. weight, renal function). One lesson learned is that dosing of sibrafiban (or other oral agents) based on such clinical factors, might help improve the safety profile of the drug with regard to minor bleeding.

'Peak-to-trough ratios'

In the TIMI 12 study, the rate of minor bleeding was approximately double with once-daily dosing compared with a similar total daily dose of twice daily dosing (e.g. 15 mg once daily versus 7 mg twice daily). This may indicate that the higher peak drug concentrations and degree of platelet inhibition (sometimes 100%) may be related to the bleeding episodes observed. The timing of the bleeding appeared to occur approximately 6 h after study drug ingestion, which correlates with the peak blood level. Thus, these data suggest that using dosing regimens that avoid high peaks may decrease the risk of bleeding.

Variability

Given the inter-patient variability observed in drug level and degree of platelet inhibition, another potential dosing strategy for any GPIIb/IIIa antagonist is to monitor the degree of platelet inhibition or drug level achieved in individual patients and adjust the dose to a target level, as is currently performed with anticoagulant therapy. By avoiding higher levels of platelet inhibition, this strategy may reduce bleeding complications. Potentially, this could be accomplished with a bedside assay for platelet inhibition.[30] An alternative strategy for adjusting the dose of an oral GPIIb/IIIa inhibitor is to begin using a fixed dose initially but to lower the dose if the patient experienced minor bleeding. Such strategies may improve the overall safety profile of these potent platelet antagonists.

Future questions to be answered

Many questions remain about the use of GPIIb/IIIa inhibitors, particularly those relating to the numerous pharmacokinetic and pharmacodynamic issues with oral agents (Table 10.5). One key question is whether there are differences between the various drugs. There are some compounds with very tight prolonged binding to the receptor (e.g. roxifiban) which may translate into greater antithrombotic effects. Two other questions are the degree of variability in the drug level (and the degree of platelet inhibition) and the incidence of excessive bleeding. In the TIMI 12 trial, a considerable degree of variability in both drug level and the degree of platelet inhibition was observed using oral agents,[24] although it should be noted that intravenous GPIIb/IIIa inhibitors also demonstrate some variability. The peak (and trough) levels of platelet inhibition also appear to be related to clinical effects, such as bleeding. In the TIMI 12 study, at the doses that caused high peaks in the level of inhibition, the rate of bleeding

---

Receptor interactions
(a) Selectivity for αIIb/B3
    Cross-reactivity with αv/B3 (vitronectin) receptor
    Leukocyte Mac-1 αM/B2 interactions
(b) Competitive binding to receptor – 'tightness' of binding
(c) Ligand-induced binding sites (LIBS)
(d) Internalization of drug in platelet granules

Variability in drug level: pharmacokinetic considerations
(a) Absorption, bioavailability (absolute %, consistency, food effect)
(b) Metabolism (active drug versus pro-drug; active metabolite)
(c) Volume of distribution; internalization in platelets
(d) Half-life; peak–trough ratio, dosing regimen
(e) Route of excretion

Platelet inhibition
(a) Relationship of drug level to platelet inhibition (steepness of curve, tightness of correlation)
(b) Synergism with aspirin

Adverse effects
(a) Thrombocytopenia (early versus late, mild versus profound)
(b) Bleeding
    Related to degree of inhibition
    Relationship of high peaks = added risk
(c) Immunogenicity
(d) Other unexpected adverse effects

Table 10.5
Issues to consider when assessing GPIIb/IIIa antagonists.

was higher than in those with lower 'peak–trough' ratios. In addition, the absolute degree of inhibition achieved appeared to correlate with the amount of minor bleeding, raising the important issue of what level of platelet inhibition will be tolerable for long-term treatment.

Degree of platelet inhibition

Previous animal and clinical studies have suggested that the maximum benefit of GPIIb/IIIa inhibition occurs when the degree of platelet inhibition is greater than 80%.[25,26] Currently, it is not clear whether lower levels of platelet inhibition would also be beneficial. The IMPACT II study showed a strong trend toward the reduction of recurrent ischemic events after coronary angioplasty at a dose of eptifibatide that achieved only 50–60% inhibition.[28] Thus, it remains to be determined whether 80% platelet inhibition is a 'threshold level' to achieve clinical benefit with GPIIb/IIIa inhibitors or whether there is a graded benefit across a range of platelet inhibition.

Degree of platelet inhibition and bleeding

As observed in the TIMI 12 study, increasing the degree of platelet inhibition may produce a higher incidence of minor bleeding events.[29] This suggests that a lower degree of platelet inhibition may be better tolerated during chronic, oral therapy. Nevertheless, major hemorrhage appears to be rare in the initial experience with oral GPIIb/IIIa inhibitors, even at high levels of platelet inhibition. Therefore, one possible dosing strategy for GPIIb/IIIa inhibitors may be to tailor the dose to the risk of recurrent ischemic events, thus optimizing the degree of platelet inhibition and minimizing the risk of minor bleeding. For example, patients might be given a higher dose during the early phase of their acute coronary syndrome, when they are at highest risk of recurrent ischemic events. The dose could then be lowered during the chronic phase, when the risk of recurrent ischemic events is lower, thereby decreasing the risk of bleeding.

Need for aspirin

An important aspect of oral GPIIb/IIIa inhibition is concomitant therapy with aspirin. There are several factors suggesting the benefit of the combination of aspirin and an oral GPIIb/IIIa inhibitor. Firstly, synergism has been demonstrated for inhibition of platelet aggregation in response to collagen, with a greater degree of platelet inhibition with the combination of aspirin plus the GPIIb/IIIa inhibitor.[46] Secondly, the action of aspirin is to decrease the synthesis of thromboxane A_2 by the platelet, which decreases platelet *activation*, a step proximal to platelet aggregation. Thus, aspirin and GPIIb/IIIa inhibitors inhibit different steps in the formation of a platelet thrombus. In addition, reduction in thromboxane A_2 reduces local coronary vasospasm, which helps to reduce the ischemia. Additional factors favoring the combination are the efficacy for primary and secondary prevention of ischemic events of aspirin,[4] its relatively good safety profile, and its low cost. Finally, aspirin would provide antiplatelet effects during the troughs in GPIIb/IIIa blockade that may occur between doses. The potential adverse effect of concomitant aspirin is increased risk of bleeding, particularly gastrointestinal bleeding. In addition, it has been argued that the effects of GPIIb/IIIa inhibitor are an order of magnitude stronger than those of aspirin – and thus adding aspirin is redundant to the antiplatelet effects of the GPIIb/IIIa inhibitor.

The first Phase III trial of an oral II/IIIa inhibitor in patients with acute coronary syndromes was the OPUS-TIMI 16 trial, the preliminary results of which were presented at the American College of Cardiology in March 1999. This trial involved 10 302 patients randomized at 888 hospitals in 28 countries worldwide. The inclusion criteria were: onset within the last 72 hours of an acute coronary syndrome defined as rest ischemic pain lasting at least 5 min associated with either ECG changes, positive cardiac enzymes, or a prior history of vascular disease. Major exclusion criteria included renal insufficiency (creatinine >1.6 mg/dl or an estimated creatinine clearance of <40 cc/min, increased bleeding risk, or need for warfarin.

Eligible patients were treated with 150–162 mg of ASA, and were randomized, in double-blind fashion, to one of two dosing strategies of orbofiban given twice daily, or placebo. In one dose orbofiban was given 50 mg twice daily throughout the trial (50/50 group), in the other, the 50 mg twice daily dose was given for the first 30 days (the highest risk period), and then the dose was reduced to 30 mg twice daily (50/30 group). Other medical and interventional therapy was at the discretion of the treating physician. Patients are seen at 14 and 30 days and every 3 months. The primary endpoint was a composite of death, MI, recurrent ischemia leading to rehospitalization or urgent revascularization, or stroke. The planned sample size was to be 12 000 patients, but the trial was stopped prematurely after an unexpected finding of increased mortality at 30 days was observed in one of the orbofiban groups.

The preliminary findings on interim data showed: composite endpoint rates at 30 days were 10.7% in the placebo group vs. 9.5% in the two orbofiban groups ($p = 0.05$). Mortality at 30 days was 1.4% in the placebo group vs. 2.3% in the 50/30 group and 1.6% in the 50/50 group. Through follow-up, 300-day event rates were: 20.5, 20.2 and 19.5% respectively ($p = $ NS). The safety profile was acceptable, with the rate of major hemorrhage and thrombocytopenia within the expected range for this class of drugs. Subsequent exploratory analyses found greater benefit in patients who underwent percutaneous coronary intervention while on study drug and those who were stable on admission (Killip class I).

Data from the EXCITE trial of the agent xemilofiban in patients undergoing percutaneous coronary intervention were also presented, with similar results. No significant benefit was observed at 6 months.

Many lessons were learned from OPUS-TIMI 16, the first large trial of oral IIb/IIIa inhibition in acute coronary syndromes, which will be helpful in planning future trials of other IIb/IIIa inhibitors. First, it appears that it will be beneficial to optimize the dosing strategy used with the oral agents, potentially to mimic the stable antiplatelet effect achieved by the intravenous drugs. This would mean trying to reduce the inter- and intra-patient variability, potentially adjusting the dose by weight and/or renal function, as has been done in the SYMPHONY trials. One might also use plasma drug level and/or bedside platelet function test to adjust the dose. Second, out data suggest that one could target stabilized patients. In addition, several new and planned trials will be testing different drugs (e.g. with tight IIb/IIIa receptor binding), hence the field is moving forward.

Conclusions

Oral GPIIb/IIIa inhibitors may represent a major advance in the treatment of acute coronary syndromes, percutaneous coronary interventions, and stroke. They may also play a role not only in early treatment but also secondary prevention. In early treatment, they may either be a substitute for, or a follow-up to, intravenous compounds. To date, data are available only on the pharmacokinetic and pharmacodynamic effects of these agents. Numerous questions remain, such as what level of platelet inhibition is optimal, how efficacy and safety can best be balanced, whether other adjunctive agents are needed, and whether monitoring of platelet function will assist in the use of these agents. Ongoing large-scale clinical trials will assess many of these issues and the clinical effects of this promising class of agents.

References

1. Braunwald E, Mark DB, Jones RH, Cheitlin MD, Fuster V, McCauley KM, et al. *Unstable Angina: Diagnosis and Management. Clinical Practice Guideline Number 10.* (Rockville, MD: Agency for Health Care Policy and Research and the National Heart, Lung, and Blood Institute, Public Health Service, U.S. Department of Health and Human Services, 1994).

2. Ryan TJ, Anderson JL, Antman EM, Braniff BA, Brooks NH, Califf RM, et al. ACC/AHA guidelines for the management of patients with acute myocardial infarction: a report of the American College of Cardiology/American Heart Association Task Force on Practice Guidelines (Committee on Management of Acute Myocardial Infarction). *J Am Coll Cardiol* 1996;**28**:1328–428.

3. Fuster V, Badimon L, Badimon JJ, Chesebro JH. The pathophysiology of coronary artery disease and the acute coronary syndromes. *N Engl J Med* 1992;**326**:242–50, 310–18.

4. Antiplatelet Trialist' Collaboration. Collaborative overview of randomized trials of antiplatelet therapy—I: prevention of death, myocardial infarction and stroke by prolongued antiplatelet therapy in various categories of patients. *Br Med J* 1994;**308**:81–106.

5. Steering Committee of the Physicians' Health Study Research Group. Final report on the aspirin component of the ongoing Physicians' Health Study. *N Engl J Med* 1989;**321**:129–35.

6. Ridker PM, Manson JE, Gaziano JM, Buring JE, Hennekens CH. Low-dose aspirin therapy for chronic stable angina. A randomized, placebo-controlled clinical trial. *Ann Intern Med* 1991;**114**:835–9.

7. Lewis HD, Davis JW, Archibald DG, Steinke WE, Smitherman TC, Doherty JE, et al. Protective effects of aspirin against acute myocardial infarction and death in men with unstable angina. *N Engl J Med* 1983;**309**:396–403.

8. Cairns JA, Gent M, Singer J, Finnie KJ, Froggatt GM, Holder DA, et al. Aspirin, sulfinpyrazone, or both in unstable angina. *N Engl J Med* 1985;**313**:1369–75.

9. Theroux P, Ouimet H, McCans J, Latour J-G, Joly G, Levy G, et al. Aspirin, heparin or both to treat unstable angina. *N Engl J Med* 1988;**319**:1105–11.

10. The RISC Group. Risk of myocardial infarction and death during treatment with low-dose aspirin and intravenous heparin in men with unstable coronary artery disease. *Lancet* 1990;**336**:827–30.

11. ISIS-2 (Second International Study of Infarct Survival) Collaborative Group. Randomized trial of intravenous streptokinase, oral aspirin, both, or neither among 17,187 cases of suspected acute myocardial infarction: ISIS-2. *Lancet* 1988;**2**:349–60.

12. Schömig A, Neumann F-J, Kastrati A, Schühlen H, Blasini R, Hadamitzky M, et al. A randomized comparison of antiplatelet and anticoagulant therapy after the placement of coronary-artery stents. *N Engl J Med* 1996;**334**:1084–9.

13. Bertrand M, Legrand V, Boland J, Fleck E, Bonnier J, Emmanuelson H, et al. Full anticoagulation versus ticlopidine plus aspirin after stent implantation: a randomized multicenter European study: the FANTASTIC trial. *Circulation* 1996;**94**(Suppl. I):I-685.

14. Leon MB, Baim DS, Gordon P, Giambartolomei A, Williams DO, Diver DD, et al. Clinical and angiographic results from the STent Anticoagulation Regimens Study. *Circulation* 1996;**94**(Suppl. I):I-685.

15. Balsano F, Rizzon P, Violi F, Scrutinio D, Cimminiello C, Aguglia F, et al for the Studio della Ticlopidina nell'Agnina Instabile Group. Antiplatelet treatment with ticlopidine in unstable angina: a controlled multicenter clinical trial. *Circulation* 1990;**82**:17–26.

16. CAPRIE Steering Committee. A randomized, blinded, trial of clopidogrel versus aspirin in

patients at risk of ischaemic events (CAPRIE). *Lancet* 1996;**348**:1329–39.

17. Sharis PJ, Cannon CP, Loscalzo J. The antiplatelet effects of ticlopidine and clopidogrel. *Ann Intern Med* 1998;**129**:394–405.

18. Lefkovits J, Plow EF, Topol EJ. Platelet glycoprotein IIb/IIIa receptors in cardiovascular medicine. *N Engl J Med* 1995;**332**:1553–9.

19. Cannon CP. Platelet glycoprotein IIb/IIIa receptor inhibitors in the management of acute coronary syndromes and coronary intervention. In: Braunwald E (ed.) *Heart Disease, Clinical Updates.* (Philadelphia, WB Saunders), [In press].

20. Patrono C. Aspirin as an antiplatelet drug. *N Engl J Med* 1994;**330**:1287–94.

21. Verstraete M, Zoldhelyi P. Novel antiplatelet drugs in development. *Drugs* 1995;**49**:856–84.

22. Schafer AI. Antiplatelet therapy. *Am J Med* 1996;**101**:199–209.

23. Kereiakes DJ, Kleiman NS, Ferguson JJ, Runyon JP, Broderick TM, Higby NA, et al. Sustained platelet glycoprotein IIb/IIIa blockade with oral xemilofiban in 170 patient following coronary stent deployment. *Circulation* 1997;**96**:1117–21.

24. Coller BS, Scudder LR. Inhibition of dog platelet function by in vivo infusion of $F(ab')_2$ fragments of a monoclonal antibody to the platelet glycoprotein IIb/IIIa receptor. *Blood* 1985;**66**:1456–9.

25. The EPIC Investigators. Use of a monoclonal antibody directed against the platelet glycoprotein IIb/IIIa receptor in high-risk angioplasty. *N Engl J Med* 1994;**330**:956–61.

26. The EPILOG Investigators. Platelet glycoprotein IIb/IIIa receptor blockade and low-dose heparin during percutaneous coronary revascularization. *N Engl J Med* 1997;**336**:1689–96.

27. The RESTORE Investigators. The effects of platelet glycoprotein IIb/IIIa blockade with tirofiban on adverse cardiac events in patients with unstable angina or acute myocardial infarction undergoing coronary angioplasty. *Circulation* 1997;**96**:1445–53.

28. The IMPACT-II Investigators. Randomized placebo-controlled trial of effect of eptifibatide on complications of percutaneous coronary intervention: IMPACT-II. *Lancet* 1997;**349**:1422–8.

29. Cannon CP, McCabe CH, Borzak S, Henry TD, Tischler MD, Mueller HS, et al for the TIMI 12 Investigators. A randomized trial of an oral platelet glycoprotein IIb/IIIa antagonist, sibrafiban, in patients after an acute coronary syndrome: results of the TIMI 12 trial. *Circulation* 1998;**97**:340–49.

30. Coller BS, Land D, Scudder LE. Rapid and simple platelet function assay to assess glycoprotein IIb/IIIa receptor blockade. *Circulation* 1997;**95**:860–67.

31. The Platelet Receptor Inhibition for Ischemic Syndrome Management in Patients Limited by Unstable Signs and Symptoms (PRISM-PLUS) Trial Investigators. Inhibition of the platelet glycoprotein IIb/IIIa receptor with tirofiban in unstable angina and non-Q-wave myocardial infarction. *N Engl J Med* 1998;**338**: 1488–97.

32. Coller BS, Folts JD, Scutter LE, Smith SR. Antithrombotic effect of a monoclonal antibody to the platelet glycoprotein IIb/IIIa receptor in an experimental model. *Blood* 1986;**68**:783–6.

33. Kereiakes DJ, Kleiman NS, Ambrose J, Cohen M, Rodriguez S, Palabrica T, et al. Randomized, double-blind, placebo-controlled dose-ranging study of tirofiban (MK-383) platelet IIb/III blockade in high risk patients undergoing coronary angioplasty. *J Am Coll Cardiol* 1996;**27**:536–642.

34. Tcheng JE, Harrington RA, Kottke-Marchant K, Kleiman NS, Ellis SG, Kereiakes DJ, et al. Multicenter, randomized, double-blind, placebo-controlled trial of the platelet integrin glycoprotein IIb/IIIa blocker integrelin in elective coronary intervention. *Circulation* 1995; **91**:2151–7.

35. Kereiakes DJ, Runyon JP, Kleiman NS, Higby NA, Anderson LC, Hantsbarger G, et al. Differential dose-response to oral xemilofiban after antecedant intravenous abciximab. Administration for complex coronary intervention. *Circulation* 1996;**94**:906–10.

36. Ferguson JJ, Deedwania PD, Kereiakes DJ, Fitzgerald D, Anders RJ, Burns DM, et al. Sustained platelet GPIIb/IIIa blockade with oral orbofiban: interim pharmacodynamic results of the SOAR study. *J Am Coll Cardiol* 1998;**31** (**Suppl.A**):185A.

37. The Platelet Receptor Inhibition For Ischemic

Syndrome Management (PRISM) Study Investigators. A comparison of aspirin plus tirofiban with aspirin plus heparin for unstable angina. *N Engl J Med* 1998;**338**:1498–505.

38. The PURSUIT Trial Investigators. Inhibition of platelet glycoprotein IIb/IIIa with eptifibatide in patient with acute coronary syndromes. *N Engl J Med* 1998;**339**:436–43.

39. The CAPTURE Investigators. Randomized placebo-controlled trial of abciximab before and during coronary intervention in refractory unstable angina: the CAPTURE study. *Lancet* 1997;**349**:1429–35.

40. The EPISTENT Investigators. Randomized placebo-controlled and balloon-angioplasty-controlled trial to assess the safety of coronary stenting with use of platelet glycoprotein-IIb/IIIa blockade. *Lancet* 1998;**352**:87–92.

41. Van Belle E, Lablanche J-M, Bauters C, Renaud N, McFadden EP, Bertrand ME. Coronary angioscopic findings in the infarct-related vessel within 1 month of acute myocardial infarction. Natural history and the effect of thrombolysis. *Circulation* 1998;**97**:26–33.

42. Ault et al. *J Am Cordiol*. In Press.

43. Cannon CP, Ault K, Mitchell J, McCabe CH, Braunwald E. P-selectin in patients post acute coronary syndromes treated with sibrafiban, an oral IIb/IIIa antagonist: Results from TIMI 12. *Circulation* 1997;**96**(Suppl. I):I-169.

44. Mascelli MA, Lance ET, Dararaju L, Wagner CL, Weisman HF, Jordan RE. Pharmacodynamic profile of short-term abciximab treatment demonstrates prolonged platelet inhibition with gradual recovery from GPIIb/IIIa receptor blockade. *Circulation* 1998;**97**:1680–88.

45. Simpfendorfer C, Kottke-Marchant K, Topol EJ. First experience with chronic platelet GPIIb/IIIa receptor blockade: a pilot study of xemlofiban, an orally active antagonist in unstable angina patients eligible for PTCA. *J Am Coll Cardiol* 1996;**27**(Suppl. A):242A.

46. Kereiakes DJ, Kleiman NS, Ferguson JJ, Masud ARZ, Broderick TM, Abbottsmith CW, et al for the Oral Glycoprotein IIn/IIa Receptor Blockade to Inhibit Thrombosis (ORBIT) Trial Investigators. Pharmacodynamic efficacy, clinical safety, and outcomes after prolonged platelet glycoprotein IIb/IIIa receptor blockade with oral xemilofiban: results of a multicenter, placebo-controlled, randomized trial. *Circulation* 1998;**98**:1268–78.

47. Willerson JT, McNatt JM, Clubb FJ, Jr., Nicholson N, Herman MP, Ferguson JJ, III, et al. Xemilofiban, an oral GPIIb/IIIa receptor antagonist is enhanced by aspirin in inhibiting neoimtimal proliferation following percutaneous coronary angioplasty. *Circulation* 1997;**96** (Suppl. I):I-168.

11

Miscellaneous antiplatelet agents: A physiologically based overview of platelet antagonist therapy

Richard C Becker

Introduction

The development of pharmacologic agents that offer platelet antagonist capabilities is a direct extension of our understanding of normal physiology and the laws that govern cellular events in the circulatory system. Under normal conditions, platelets circulate freely within the vasculature in a non-stimulated state and, as a result, little meaningful interaction takes place with other platelets, leukocytes or the vessel wall. It has become increasingly evident, however, that many of the recognized risk factors for atherosclerosis, and certainly atherosclerosis itself, have a profound impact on platelets, in essence, 'priming' them for future cell–cell and cell–vessel wall encounters. In the presence of advanced endothelial cell dysfunction, disruption or atheromatous plaque rupture, a complex chain of events is rapidly initiated, leading to platelet-rich thrombus formation. The responsible biochemical and cellular processes can be divided conceptually into five general categories:

(1) Platelet adhesion;
(2) Activation;
(3) Secretion;
(4) Aggregation; and
(5) Support of coagulation.

Platelet adhesion

Platelets quickly and efficiently recognize abnormalities within the vascular system and adhere by means of adhesive proteins that interact with specific platelet membrane glycoproteins (receptors). To date, nine of the predominant and physiological important platelet membrane glycoproteins have been characterized.[1-4] The most common nomenclature for identification is based on polyacrylamide gel separation (Table 11.1, Figure 11.1). Most platelet membrane receptors consist of non-covalent complexes of individual glycoproteins or heterodimers (integrins) derived from α and β subunits. Platelets express at least two β subunits (β_1 and β_2) and five α subunits, which in varying combinations, identify distinct surface receptors.[5]

The initial events in adhesion are contact and binding, accomplished predominately by an interaction between the platelet glycoprotein Ib-IX complex and vonWillebrand factor.[6] Other ligand–receptor interactions typically play a supportive role.

Platelet activation

Platelet activation can be triggered by a wide variety of biochemical and mechanical stimuli (in addition to platelet adhesion). Many of the biochemical agonists are produced or released by platelets themselves after vessel wall adhesion,

Receptor	Ligand	Integrin components	Biologic function
GPIa/IIa	Collagen	$\alpha_2\beta_1$	Adhesion
GPIb/IX	von Willebrand factor	—	Adhesion
GPIc/IIa	Fibronectin	$\alpha_5\beta_1$	Adhesion
GPIIb/IIIa	Collagen	$\alpha_{IIb}\beta_3$	Aggregation
	Fibrinogen		(secondary role in
	Fibronectin		adhesion under
	Vitronectin		high shear stress)
	von Willebrand factor		
GPIV	Thrombospondin	—	Adhesion
(GPIIb)	Collagen		
Vitronectin	Vitronectin	$\alpha_v\beta_3$	Adhesion
VLA 6	Laminin	$\alpha_6\beta_1$	Adhesion

* GP, glycoproteins.

Table 11.1
Platelet surface membrane glycoproteins.*

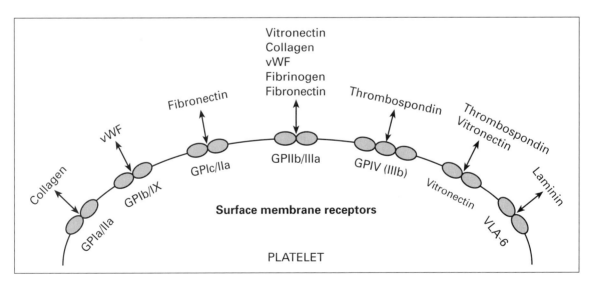

Figure 11.1
Diagram showing platelet surface membrane interactions. Properties inherent to platelets, including adhesion, activation, and aggregation are governed by membrane glycoproteins (receptors) that recognize one or more proteins (ligands). GP, glycoprotein; VFW, vonWillebrand factor.

initiating a positive feedback loop that amplifies the response to a given stimulus. The list of biochemical agonists is extensive, numbering 100 or more. The most physiologically relevant agonists are outlined in Table 11.2.

Platelet agonists bind surface glycoprotein receptors and stimulate signal transmission across the membrane via a messenger protein that, in turn, triggers one of two intracellular pathways. The phosphoinositide pathway is initiated by activation of phospholipase C. Phosphatidylinositol 4-5-biphosphate (PIP_2) is cleaved to form two secondary messengers, inositol 1,4,5 triphosphate (IP_3) and diacylglycerol.[7] IP_3 stimulates calcium mobilization from the dense tubular system. Increased cellular Ca^{2+} concentrations are required for activation of other intracellular enzymes responsible for physiologic platelet responses.[8] Diacylglycerol activates protein C, causing protein phosphorylation, granule secretion and fibrinogen receptor expression.

The second pathway (phosphatidylcholine) that can be initiated following platelet activation involves phospholipase A_2, which liberates arachidonate from cell membranes. Arachidonate is subsequently converted to thromboxane A_2 (TXA_2) by the platelet's cyclo-oxygenase enzyme system. TXA_2 is a potent platelet agonist in its own right, thus providing yet another positive-feedback mechanism that promotes the thrombotic mechanism (Figure 11.2). The platelet response to activation is summarized as follows:

(1) Conformational change of GPIIb/IIIa (ligand receptive);
(2) Pseudopod formation and platelet shape change;
(3) Surface expression of α-granule proteins (e.g. thrombospondin, fibrinogen);
(4) Surface expression of granule membrane protein (P-selectin, GMP-140, CD62);
(5) Development of coagulant activity through inside-out movement of membrane phospholipids;

Agonist	Source	Receptor(s)
Thrombin	Enzymatic end-product of coagulation cascade	High-affinity (GPIbα) receptor
ADP	Platelet dense body erythrocytes	ADP/aggregin
Collagen	Subendothelial matrix	GPIa/IIa
		GPIIb/IIIa
		GPIV
Serotonin	Platelet dense body	5HT$_2$ receptor
Thromboxane A_2	Platelet membrane	PGH$_2$/TXA$_2$ receptor
Platelet activating factor (PAF)	—	PAF receptor

* PAF, platelet activating factor; prostaglandin H_2; TXA_2, thromboxane A_2; GP, glycoprotein; ADP, adenosine diphosphate.

Table 11.2
Predominant biochemical agonists for platelet activation.*

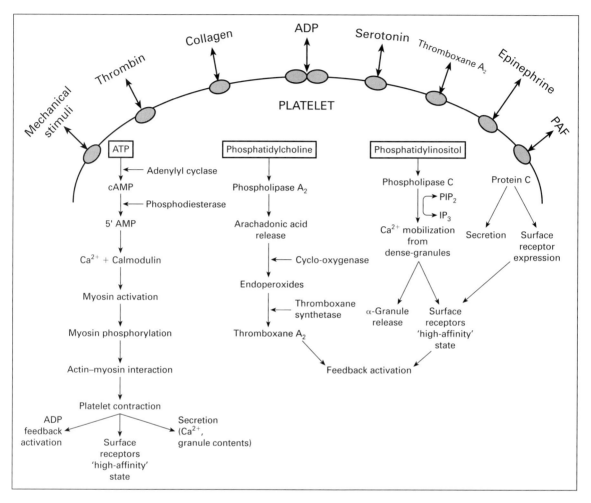

Figure 11.2
Platelet activation. This important process is triggered by a variety of biochemical and mechanical stimuli that provoke a series of internal events following their initial binding to specific surface receptors. The phosphoinositide and phosphotidylcholine pathways ultimately cause the release of calcium and physiologic agonists that stimulate further activation and potentiate aggregation through surface receptor expression. ADP, adenosine diphosphate; PAF, platelet activating factor; PIP$_2$, phosphatidylinositol 4-5-biphosphate; IP$_3$, inositol 1,4,5 triphosphate.

(6) Expression of coagulation proteins (e.g. factor V);

(7) Secretion of α and dense-granule contents;

(8) Increased cystosolic Ca^{2+};

(9) Activation of phospholipase C;

(10) Mobilization of Ca^{2+};

(11) Activation of phospholipase A$_2$; and

(12) Activation of protein kinase C.

Platelet agonists can be classified as strong or weak. Strong agonists, for example, thrombin affect both phosphoinositide hydrolysis and arachidonate metabolism (via phospholipase C and phospholipase A_2). Accordingly, their ability to promote platelet activation and aggregation persists despite inhibition of one of the two pathways. Indeed, it has been shown that even low concentrations of thrombin (≤ 0.1 U/ml) can produce platelet aggregation in the face of inhibition of platelet TXA_2 production.[9] Weak agonists (collagen and adenosine diphosphate, for example) lack the ability to trigger phosphoinositide hydrolysis and are more dependent on TXA_2 formation for their effects. Studies dating back several decades revealed that inhibition of TXA_2 formation could reduce collagen-induced platelet aggregation.[10]

Platelet secretion

Platelet activation prompts the secretion of contents from within three different types of platelet storage granules: lysosomes, α-granules, and dense bodies. The exact mechanism of granule secretion is largely undetermined but it is felt to involve an energy-dependent contractile process, resulting in extrusion of granule contents. Fusion of α-granules with each other and with deep invaginations of the plasma membrane (the open canalicular system) followed by an 'emptying' of contents to the exterior has since been demonstrated.[11,12] It is unclear if other platelet granules use a similar mechanism to release their contents.

Platelet aggregation

Platelet aggregation is considered the physiologic goal of platelet activation because it is through platelet aggregation that primary hemostasis can occur. As already reviewed, a variety of agonists can stimulate platelets via interaction with specific membrane receptors, followed by production of secondary messengers, which in turn promote a series of intracellular events. One of the most important platelet responses triggered is a confirmational change in the glycoprotein (GP)IIb/IIIa membrane receptor that facilitates an interaction between fibrinogen and its receptor and thus forming multiple cross-links between adjacent platelets. This reaction represents the 'final common pathway' for platelet activation and is a vital process in the formation of platelet-rich thrombi. Accordingly, investigators have focused their attention on this fundamental event in attempting to develop new platelet antagonists for clinical use.

Platelet support of coagulation

The phospholipid membrane of activated platelets and of platelet aggregates forms an ideal template for coagulation processes that facilitate thrombus growth (a second-wave phenomenon). The prothrombinase complex, responsible for the conversion of prothrombin to thrombin, consists of factor V_a (provided by activated platelets), factor X_a, phospholipid and calcium. Thrombin, in turn, converts fibrinogen to fibrin that is responsible for stabilization of the platelet-rich thrombus (Figure 11.3). It is very important to recognize that, although platelets are the predominant source of phospholipid in both physiologic hemostasis and pathologic thrombosis, prothrombinase assembly can occur on dysfunctional vascular endothelial cells and factor X_a can be generated through tissue factor that is present in high concentrations within atheromatous plaques and on the surface of activated monocytes.[13,14]

Platelet and vessel wall physiology and pharmacologic interventions

An understanding of platelet behavior provides the cornerstone of pharmacologic

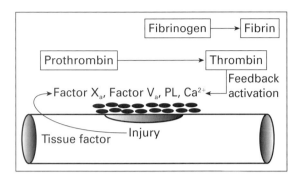

Figure 11.3
Platelet aggregates at a site of vessel wall injury. These serve as a template for assembly and activation of the prothrombinase complex (factor X_a, factor V_a, phospholipid (PL) and calcium), which rapidly converts prothrombin to thrombin. Thrombin, a pivotal enzyme, converts fibrinogen to fibrin and also stimulates autocatalytic activation of factors V, VIII (tenase complex) and X. The prothrombinase complex also can be assembled on dysfunctional vascular endothelial cells and atheromatous plaques where tissue factor serves as a potent stimulus.

approaches to the treatment of patients with disorders characterized by enhanced platelet adhesion, activation, aggregation and/or support of coagulation (prothrombinase assembly and activity).

A summary of agents affecting platelet and vessel wall physiology are summarized in the following list.

(1) *Agents that inhibit platelet adhesion*

- von Willebrand factor monoclonal antibodies
- Aurintricarboxylic acid
- GPIIb/IIIa receptor antagonists (high shear stress)

(2) *Agents that inhibit platelet activation*

- Prostacyclin
- Prostaglandin E_1
- Prostanoid analogs (iloprost, beraprost, cicaprost, ciprostene)
- Thromboxane/endoperoxide receptor antagonists
- Platelet activating factor antagonists

(3) *Agents that inhibit platelet aggregation*

- P_{2T} purinoceptor antagonists
- Nitric oxide/nitric oxide donors
- Apyrase
- GPIIb/IIIa receptor antagonists
- Aspirin
- Non-steroidal anti-inflammatory agents (NSAIDs)
- Dipyridamole
- Ticlopidine
- Clopidogrel
- Dextran
- Omega-3 fatty acids
- Cilostazol
- Ketanserin
- Ridogrel
- Angiotensin converting-enzyme inhibitors
- Vitamin E

(4) *Agents that inhibit platelet secretion*

- Calcium-channel antagonists

(5) *Agents that inhibit prothrombinase assembly on platelet surface*

- Low-molecular-weight heparins
- GPIIb/IIIa antagonists

Platelet antagonists
Agents that inhibit platelet adhesion

The adhesion of platelets to a site of vessel wall injury is mediated by vonWillebrand factor that binds to the platelet GPIb/IX complex receptor (and the GPIIb/IIIa receptor under high shear stress conditions). Monoclonal antibodies to vonWillebrand factor have been developed and tested in animal models,[15] as has aurintricarboxylic acid,[16] which is a triphenylmethyl compound that inhibits von-Willebrand factor binding. To date, investigation in humans has not taken place, perhaps because of concerns regarding the potential risk for hemorrhagic complications.

Although the GPIIb/IIIa receptor antagonists are best known for their ability to inhibit platelet aggregation (discussed in detail in Chapters 8, 9 and 10), under high shear stress conditions von-Willebrand factor can also bind the GPIIb/IIIa receptor, facilitating adhesion. As a result, GPIIb/IIIa antagonists may have an impact on both platelet adhesion and aggregation.

Agents that inhibit platelet activation

As previously discussed, platelet activation is followed by a series of intracellular events that culminate in the release of calcium and substances that augment platelet aggregation and support of the coagulation cascade. Thus, pharmacologic agents that inhibit initial surface receptor-mediated activation also impair platelet aggregation.

Prostaglandin E and prostacyclin

Several natural prostanoids (PGE_1 and PGI_2) can inhibit platelet activation and aggregation by elevating cyclic AMP (cAMP) levels. Although the mechanism is complex, the primary mode of inhibition is through the activation of adenylate cyclase (with a subsequent rise in cAMP concentrations), that in turn, prevents calcium mobilization. The clinical application of PGE_1 and PGI_2 has been limited by their effect on vascular tone, producing

substantial systemic hypotension,[17–19] and by extensive first-pass metabolism in the lungs (70% of the active compound is rapidly cleared).[20,21]

The prostanoid analogs (e.g. iloprost, beraprost, cicaprost, ciprostene) are more stable compounds than PGE_1 and PGI_2; however, their development has focused primarily on potential use in patients with primary pulmonary hypertension.[22]

Thromboxane/endoperoxide receptor antagonists

This class of compounds is designed to prevent platelet activation in response to thromboxane A_2 and other endoperoxides. There is a limited experience with the thromboxane receptor antagonists sulotraban and SQ30741, in patients with myocardial infarction treated with streptokinase[23] and tPA,[24] respectively. Ridogrel, a thromboxane synthetase antagonist, that also has antagonistic effects on the thromboxane receptor, was shown to reduce recurrent ischemia compared with aspirin when used adjunctively with thrombolytic therapy;[25] however, further investigation on a large scale has not yet taken place.

Agents that inhibit platelet aggregation

Serotonin receptor antagonists

Ketanserin, a serotonin receptor antagonist, has been studied in animal models of coronary thrombosis and thrombolysis where it has been shown, when administered concomitantly with a thromboxane A_2 receptor antagonist, to improve reperfusion and decrease reocclusion following tPA administration.[26]

Aspirin and platelet antagonists (see also Chapter 6)

Aspirin acetylates platelet cyclo-oxygenase and impairs prostaglandin metabolism and thromboxane A$_2$ synthesis, is discussed in detail within Chapter 6. The potent class of platelet antagonists that prevent the binding of fibrinogen to its GPIIb/IIIa receptor (GPIIb/IIa receptor antagonists) on the platelet surface is discussed in Chapter 9.

Thromboxane synthetase inhibitors

Thromboxane synthetase antagonists, including dazoxiben and pirmagrel, suppress platelet thromboxane synthesis and platelet aggregation.[41,42] Clinical development has been hampered by the aggregating potential of endoperoxide intermediates and by the incomplete inhibition of thromboxane synthesis by currently available compounds.

Dextran

Dextran is a polysaccharide preparation that ranges in molecular weight from 65–80 kD. It prolongs the bleeding time, probably by interfering with surface membrane receptor function and fibrinogen binding.[43] Dextran also reduces plasma viscosity.

Omega-3 fatty acids

Omega-3 fatty acids decrease platelet membrane arachidonic acid concentration, reducing thromboxane A$_2$ synthesis. The competition of N-3 polyunsaturated fatty acids for cyclo-oxygenase also reduces platelet aggregating capacity by facilitating the synthesis of biologically inactive prostanoids.[44,45]

Nitric oxide

Nitric oxide (NO) is a naturally occurring molecule derived from the amino acid L-arginine. It is a product of normal vascular endothelial cells and plays a critical role in maintaining both vasoreactivity and thromboresistance.

NO prevents platelet adhesion and also inhibits agonist-dependent G-protein-mediated phospholipase C activation with subsequent calcium release. Accordingly, NO prevents P-selectin expression and calcium-dependent conformation change in platelet surface GPIIb/IIIa. It has also been shown to potentiate platelet disaggregation by preventing the stabilization of fibrinogen–GPIIb/IIIa interactions.[46] Beyond having potent platelet inhibitory effects, NO also inhibits neutrophil aggregation in vitro and prevents leukocyte adhesion to vascular endothelium.

Although the endothelial cell is a major source of NO, it is not the sole source. Platelets themselves, and their precursor megakaryocytes, possess NO synthase activity.[47] Vascular endothelial cells produce NO at a basal rate that can be augmented in response to physiologic stimuli including platelet release products, thrombin, shear stress and changes in oxygen tension.

Organic nitrates and other nitrosovasodilators serve as an exogenous source of NO. Both nitroglycerin and nitroprusside have platelet inhibitory effects and promote platelet disaggregation in vitro.[48] The mechanism by which organic nitrates release NO remains controversial but it seems most likely that the former are converted to bioactive NO by a surface enzyme system.[49] In a double-blind randomized, placebo controlled trial, hypercholesterolemic patients were assigned to L-arginine hydrochloride (8.4 g/day orally or placebo) for 2 weeks. Platelet aggregation in response to collagen (5 µg/ml), was increased at baseline in patients with a marked reduction following treatment. The effect lasted for 2 weeks after completion of the treatment phase.[50] L-Arginine has been shown to reduce human monocyte adhesion to endothelial cells and may also decrease the expression of several cellular adhesion molecules.[51]

In addition to their direct effects, organic nitrates undergo denitrification with formulation of S-nitrosothiol (RSNO) intermediates. These species inhibit platelet aggregation through cyclic GMP (cGMP).[52] A poly-nitrosated RSNO, S-nitroso-BSA, administered locally following femoral artery injury in a rabbit model, prevented neointimal proliferation and platelet adhesion.[53] N-acetyl-L-cysteine enhanced the platelet inhibitory effects of nitroglycerin[54] and S-nitroso-N-acetyl-L-cysteine decreased platelet function by reducing the expression of ligand receptive GPIIb/IIIa.[55] In patients with acute coronary syndromes S-nitrosoglutathione reduced platelet activation and GPIIb/IIIa expression.[56]

RSNO$_s$ have been used in animal models to prevent leukocyte-mediated tissue damage and reperfusion injury. In a rat splanchnic artery model of ischemia, the NO donor, S-nitroso-N-acetyl-D,L penicillamine caused reduced leukocyte-endothelial cell interactions.[57] S-Nitrosated tissue plasminogen activator reduced myocardial necrosis and preserved endothelial function in a feline model of ischemia and reperfusion.[58]

NONOates

Complexes of nitric oxide with nucleophiles, known as NONOates, are capable of spontaneously generating NO and, as a result, may offer therapeutic benefit in the treatment of NO deficiency states. The biologic potency, as well as duration of action, can be modified by altering the carrier nucleophile. For example, DEA (diethylamine)/NO possesses a shorter half-life than SPER (spermine)/NO (2.1 min versus 39 min, respectively) resulting in an earlier peak activity (5 min versus 15 min) and a shorter duration of action. In contrast to the acid stability of RSNOs, NONOates are alkali stable and decompose rapidly at low pH.[59]

DEA/NO and SPER/NO have been shown to have potent antiplatelet properties. Platelet aggregation measured in whole blood or platelet-rich plasma (PRP) following the addition of collagen was reduced by DEA/NO in a dose-dependent manner. The effect was similar to aspirin in whole blood. In vivo both agents demonstrated antiplatelet activity that correlated with the rate of release of NO in solution.[60]

A rapid NO donor, PROLI/NO, formed by the reaction of nitric acid with L-proline in methanolic sodium methoxide, dissociates to proline (1 mole) and NO (2 moles) with a half-life of 1.8 s at a PH 7.4 (37°C) and possesses both antiplatelet and vasodilatory properties. When infused into an unheparinized polyester vascular graft (baboon model) platelet deposition was reduced significantly.[61]

Recently, the NONOate group has been incorporated into polymeric matrices that can be applied onto therapeutic surfaces such as vascular grafts. Platelet function in vivo has been evaluated in a baboon artery-to-vein shunt coated with a polymer containing the NONOate functional group. When compared with uncoated grafts, the NO treated grafts were found to be less thrombogenic.[62]

Molsidomine and SIN-1

A novel class of nitrosovasodilators, the sydnonimines, that include molsidomine and its active metabolite SIN-1, has been evaluated clinically as effective NO donors. SIN-1 reacts with molecular oxygen resulting in the spontaneous release of NO through a process that involves a 1-electron abstraction.[63]

It has been suggested that administration of molsidomine and SIN-1 may decrease mortality associated with acute myocardial infarction by up to 35%. To confirm this observation, the ESPRIM (European Study of Prevention of Infarct with Molsidomine) trial randomized 4017 patients with acute myocardial infarction to receive either SIN-1 (1 mg/h intravenously for 48 h) followed by molsidomine (16 mg orally for 12 days) or placebo.

Although there was no difference in all-cause mortality between groups at either 35 days or 13 months; the study was considered inconclusive, based on the inclusion of predominantly low-risk patients.[64]

An oral extended release preparation of molsidomine was evaluated in a small randomized trial of 50 patients with known ischemic heart disease and chronic stable angina to determine its effect on both symptoms and overall exercise capacity. Patients received either study drug or placebo and underwent exercise testing at baseline, 2, 4, 6, 8 and 10 h. Exercise duration and performance were enhanced and ST-segment depression, a marker of ischemia, was reduced up to 10 h following administration of molsidomine. Further, anginal attacks and sublingual nitrate use were reduced in the treatment group.[65]

Molsidome and SIN-1, as NO donors, inhibit vascular smooth muscle cell proliferation. Therefore, it has been suggested that these agents may reduce the occurrence of restenosis following percutaneous coronary interventions. The ACCORD (Angioplastic Coronaire Corvasal Diltiazem) study evaluated 700 stable patients scheduled for coronary angioplasty and randomized them to receive either SIN-1 or diltiazem. Therapy was administered prior to coronary intervention and continued for 6 months afterward. Patients receiving SIN-1 demonstrated a greater luminal diameter pre- and post-angioplasty, as well as at 6-month angiographic follow-up. Although restenosis rates were significantly reduced in the SIN-1 group, this effect did not translate into a difference in combined clinical events, including death and non-fatal MI.[66]

Pirsidomine

Pirsidomine, N-*p*-anisoyl-3-(*cis*-2,6-dimethyl-piperidino) sydnonimine, possesses hemody-namic properties similar to molsidomine, but has a longer duration of action. In animals subjected to coronary arterial occlusion pirisidomine administration reduced the occurrence of ventricular ectopy and delayed the time to onset of ventricular fibrillation. Leukocytes recovered from animals treated with pirsidomine, generated less superoxide as determined by lumino-enhanced chemiluminescence than those not treated.[67]

New NO donors

Several novel NO donors are currently under development. The compound FK 409, (±)(E)-4-ethyl-3[(Z)-hydroxyimino]-5-nitro-3-gexene-1-yl]-3-pyridinecarboxamide, similarly releases NO but at a slower rate. When compared with FR 144420 in an isolated rat aortic preparation, FK 409 demonstrated greater vasorelaxant potency and hemodynamic effects, although its duration of action was shorter than that seen with FR 144420.[68]

IFT 296

The nitrate ester IFT 296, [3-(2-nitro-oxyethyl)-3-4-dihydro-2H-1,3-benzoxazin-4-one] has demonstrated anti-ischemic effects in an isolated rabbit heart model subjected to global ischemia.[69]

SPM-5185

The compound SPM-5185, (N-nitratopivaloyl]-S-(N′-acetylalanyl)-cysteine ethylester, is an effective NO donor. SPM-5185 was compared to nitroglycerin in an ex vivo preparation of human saphenous vein grafts and internal mammary arteries obtained at the time of bypass grafting. SPM-5185 produced comparable relaxation in both arteries and veins, was less prone to the development of tolerance, and effectively produced vasorelaxation in vessels that developed tolerance to nitroglycerin.[70]

Agents that inhibit platelet-dependent prothrombinase assembly and activity

Anticoagulants

The platelet surface serves as a pivotal site for assembly of the procoagulant intrinsic 'tenase' complex, that leads to factor X activation, and prothrombinase. Thus, platelet activation can be viewed as a thrombin-generating system that contributes to a rapid increase in local concentrations of thrombin, as well as a persistent site of thrombin generation.

In a recent series of experiments, platelet activation in response to ADP was greatest in blood anticoagulated with unfractionated heparin compared with hirudin, recombinant tick anticoagulant peptide or enoxaparin (a low-molecular-weight heparin preparation).[71] The effect may have been driven by the negative charge of unfractionated heparin and its tendency to bind thrombospondin, a platelet α-granule adhesive protein, and platelet factor

4, increasing platelet activation in response to biochemical mediators.[72,73] Although the physiologic implications of this observation are yet to be determined, they suggest that platelet activation may be facilitated by unfractionated heparin and attenuated by factor Xa and/or direct thrombin antagonists.

The ability of low-molecular-weight heparin to inhibit platelet-dependent prothrombinase assembly and activity was investigated by Spencer and colleagues.[74] Samples were obtained from patients with a presenting diagnosis of unstable angina or non-ST segment elevation MI who had received enoxaparin (Lovenox®). Using samples obtained 1 h after enoxaparin administration (peak concentration), platelet-dependent prothrombinase activity (thrombin generation represented by prothrombin fragment 1.2) was reduced by approximately 25% compared with baseline (pre-treatment) (Figure 11.4). A similar reduction in prothrombinase activity was observed using samples obtained 24–48 h after the

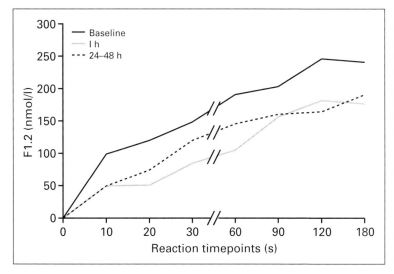

Figure 11.4
Prothrombinase inactivation. This was achieved using the low-molecular-weight heparin preparation, enoxaparin, among patients with unstable angina and non-ST segment elevation MI. Inactivation, as determined by prothrombin fragment 1.2 (F1.2) generation, was greatest with higher plasma concentrations (1 h after a 30 mg intravenous bolus) but was also observed at steady-state concentration (24–48 h on a maintenance dose of 1.0–mg/kg sc twice daily).

initiation of treatment (steady-state enoxaparin concentrations). In a separate series of experiments, samples from patients receiving enoxaparin reduced tissue factor-mediated prothrombinase assembly (and subsequent thrombin generation) (Figure 11.5).

The findings of Spencer and colleagues suggest that enoxaparin is able to inactivate platelet prothrombinase as well as inhibit tissue factor-mediated prothrombinase assembly. Both properties, which may have important implications for the treatment of patients with acute coronary syndromes, could be explained by the ability of enoxaparin to inactivate platelet bound factor X_a. It follows that more potent and specific X_a inhibitors may offer considerable promise in the management of arterial thrombotic disorders.

Platelet antagonists

If platelets contribute substantially to thrombin generation in vivo, it is possible that platelet antagonists themselves can decrease thrombin generation. Decreased platelet deposition, activation and aggregation would reduce the template for thrombin generation and fibrin formation, yielding a less stable thrombus.

Inhibitors of GPIIb/IIIa have received considerable attention, not only as potent platelet antagonists but also as anticoagulants. Initial support for the latter was derived from a large-scale clinical trial (EPIC) in which patients treated with abciximab (ReoPro®) and heparin had longer activated clotting times (ACT) than those receiving heparin alone at the time of coronary interventions.[74] Work in our laboratory supports the ability of other GPIIb/IIIa antagonists to inhibit thrombin generation as well. In vitro experiments with the selective, non-peptide tirofiban identified a dose-dependent inhibition of tissue factor mediated thrombin generation (Figure 11.6). Although the mechanism for the anticoagulant effects is

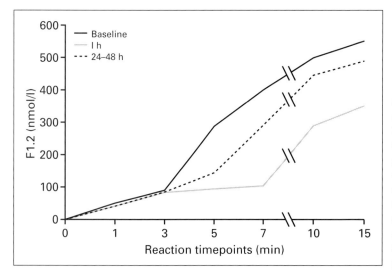

Figure 11.5
Inhibition of prothrombin formation and activity. Plasma samples were obtained from patients with unstable angina or non-ST-segment elevation MI receiving enoxaparin inhibited both prothrombinase formation and activity. Inhibition was greatest 1 hour after a 30 mg intravenous bolus. F1.2, prothrombin fragment F1.2.

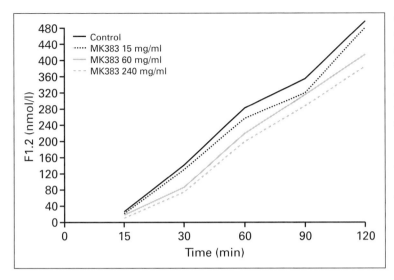

Figure 11.6

Inhibition of tirofiban (MK383) on platelet coagulant activity in the presence of fibrinogen (3 mg/ml) The platelet GPIIb/IIIa surface receptor antagonist tirofiban, in addition to its ability to prevent platelet aggregation, inhibits thrombin generation (F1.2) in a dose-dependent manner. Plasma systems with washed platelets, thrombin, $CaCl_2$, factor V_a, factor X_a, and fibrinogen.

unknown, it is possible that GPIIb/IIIa blockade impairs microparticle formation and prothrombinase assembly. Studies to define the antithrombotic potential of GPIIb/IIIa antagonists in greater detail are ongoing.

New developments in platelet inhibition

An ability to target specific receptors and intracellular signaling events that lead to pathologic thrombosis, offers considerable potential in clinical medicine.

The platelet inhibiting potential of ticlopidine and its derivative, clopidogrel, are well recognized and are discussed in detail in Chapter 7. In order to understand and appreciate the newest class of platelet inhibitors, purine receptor antagonists, some initial discussion of the ADP receptor is required.

The platelet ADP receptor (see also Chapter 7)

Adenosine diphosphate (ADP) was the first nucleotide to be indentified in blood that could account for changes in platelet behavior upon exposure to a foreign surface. In fact, ADP extracted from erythrocyte membranes was shown to increase the ability of platelets to stick to glass.[27,28] Since that time, a wide variety of pharmacologic responses to nucleotides have been identified and a comprehensive classification of nucleotide receptors has been developed.[29–32]

The receptors, classified by their preference for a variety of nucleotide analogs as agonists are referred to as P_2 purinoceptors. This distinguishes them from receptors that recognize adenosine, which are known as P_1 purinoceptors. The P_2 purinoceptor includes three separate categories P_{2X}, P_{2Y} and P_{2T}, based on structural criteria and the order of cloning.

The P_2 receptor has two hydrophobic domains. To date, no specific competitive antagonists have been identified that distinguish between the P_{2X} and P_{2Y} receptors. The P_{2Y} receptor has seven hydrophobic domains and resembles the rhodopsin family of receptors that interact with G-proteins to activate phospholipases, or to stimulate (or inhibit) adenyl cyclase. Both ADP and ATP are agonists for the P_{2X} and P_{2Y} purinoceptors. In contrast, the P_{2T} receptor is activated by ADP, while it is inhibited (by competitive antagonism) by ATP. These unique properties have led to the development of ATP analogs with high potency and specificity for the P_{2T} receptor (discussed later).

Binding

The binding of [^{14}C] ADP to the platelet surface is achieved through a specific receptor site (molecular weight 61 kDa) with approximately 100 000 copies per cell (affinity constant $K = 6.5 \times 10^6$ M^{-1}).[33] Competition for binding at the ADP receptor is as follows: ATP = ADP > AMP >> adenosine.

Mechanisms of action

A variety of platelet responses have been reported following ADP binding to its receptor. These include rapid calcium influx, mobilization of intracellular calcium stores, shape change, inhibition of adenylyl cyclase, stimulation of IP$_3$ formation, expression of GPIIb/IIIa, phospholipase A$_2$ stimulation, release of dense-granule contents and release of α-granule contents (Figure 11.7).

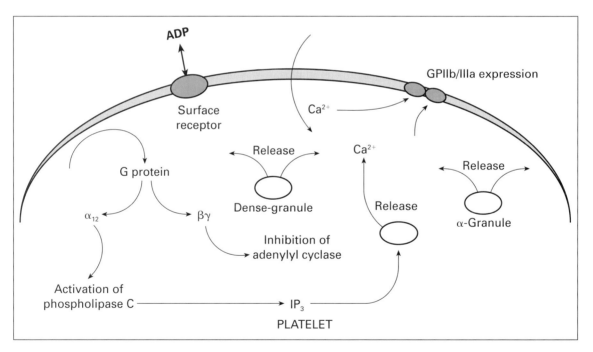

Figure 11.7
Adenosine diphosphate (ADP) binding to the platelet surface. This can happen via one or more membrane receptors. Following receptor stimulation, interval signaling takes place followed by dissociation of heterotrimeric G; protein to α$_{12}$ and β$_y$ subunits that activate phospholipase C and inhibit adenylyl cyclase, respectively. Ultimately, the release of agonists from both dense and alpha granules takes place and surface expression of GPIIb/IIIa is provoked.

ADP receptors on other cells

ADP receptors exist on cells other than platelets and this may have physiologic importance. ADP promotes the binding of fibrinogen to monocytes[34] and stimulates calcium mobilization in megakaryocytes. ADP receptors have also been identified on glioma cells, hepatocytes, and capillary endothelial cells.[35]

P_{2T} purinoceptor antagonists

Adenosine triphosphate (ATP) is a competitive P_{2T} purinoceptor antagonist that can inhibit ADP-mediated platelet aggregation. However, since ATP functions as an agonist at other P_2 receptor sites, efforts are underway to develop selective P_{2T} receptor antagonists that can be used clinically in situations where platelet activation, aggregation, and platelet-rich thromboses are prevalent (e.g. in acute coronary syndromes).

A novel ATP analog, FPL66096 (2-propyl-thio-D-$B_1$4-difluoromethylene ATP) produces a dose-dependent inhibition of ADP-mediated platelet aggregation with a high degree of selectivity for the P_{2T} purinoceptor.[36] The dichloro-derivative molecule, FPL67085 is a potent ADP-mediated platelet antagonist as well, and has been shown to prevent cyclic flow variations in a Folts model.[37] Its antithrombotic effects were similar to those of GPIIb/IIIa antagonists but at much less prolongation in the bleeding time (Figure 11.8).[38]

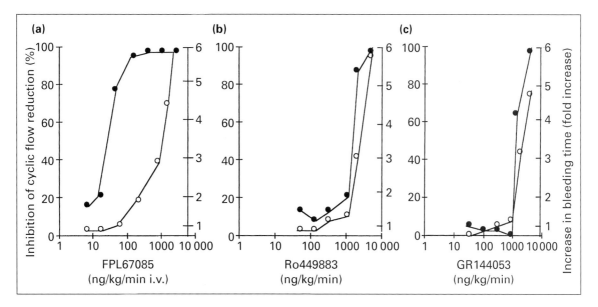

Figure 11.8
*Comparison of the antithrombotic effect of (**a**) the P_{2T} purinoceptor antagonist FPL67085 and two GPIIb/IIIc receptor antagonists (**b**) RO449883 and (**c**) GR144053, in a canine model of coronary thrombosis (●, % inhibition of cyclic flow reduction), (○, bleeding time increase). From Humphries RG, 1995; with permission.*[38]

When compared with ticlopidine and aspirin in an anesthetized rat model[39] FPL 67085 was found to be a more effective inhibitor of ADP-mediated platelet aggregation.

A second novel ATP analog, AR-C69931 MX (2-methylthio-ethyl-2-3,3,3-trifluoropropyl (adenylic acid) is a potent inhibitor of ADP-induced aggregation in human washed platelets (in vitro). It has also been shown to prevent arterial thrombosis in a canine model with minimal prolongation of the bleeding time. The latter observation has also been confirmed in studies of healthy human volunteers in whom platelet aggregation in response to ADP was eventually abolished at doses that prolonged the bleeding time by approximately 2-fold (Figure 11.9). ADP-mediated ex vivo aggregation returned to normal within 20 min of terminating the infusion.[40] The metabolism of AR-C69931 MX is predominately via the hepatic route with less than 10% being excreted through the kidneys.

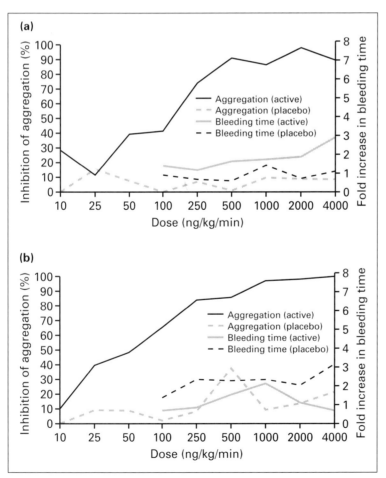

Figure 11.9
*Platelet inhibition and bleeding time prolongation with increasing concentrations of the P_{2T} purinoceptor antagonist: **(a)** ARC 69931 MX, in healthy female subjects; **(b)** ARC69931 MX, in healthy male subjects. Humphries RG, Personal communication.[40]*

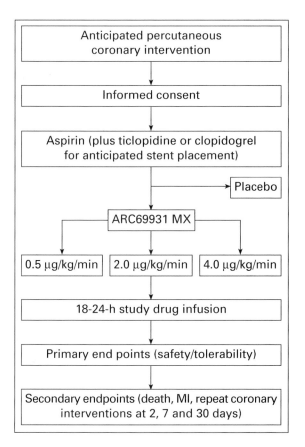

Figure 11.10
Proposed study design for a Phase II clinical trial of ARC69931 MX in patients with coronary artery disease undergoing percutaneous coronary interventions.

Clinical experience

The specific P_{2T} receptor antagonist, AR C69931 MX, has been given to patients with unstable angina and non-ST segment elevation MI in phase II clinical trials. A double-blind, placebo-controlled multicenter dose ranging study of approximately 450 patients is being conducted in the USA to assess the safety and tolerability of intravenous AR C69931 MX (doses: 0.5 µg/kg/min, 2.0 µg/kg/min, 4.0 µg/kg/min) given for 18–24 h in patients undergoing percutaneous coronary interventions (Figure 11.10). Preliminary safety results are favorable and have stimulated further investigation.

Summary

A comprehensive and expanding knowledge of platelet cellular anatomy and physiology, coupled with an understanding of pathobiologic events that govern coronary arterial thrombosis in patients with acute ischemic syndromes has paved the way for pharmacologic advances in antithrombotic therapy. Although much investigation is needed, antagonists of the platelet ADP receptor and nitric oxide derivatives, either alone or administered conjunctively with a GPIIb/IIIa inhibitor, appear particularly attractive for development, and, if deemed worthy, clinical use.

References

1. George JN. Studies on platelet plasma membranes: IV—quantitative analysis of platelet membrane glycoproteins by (^{125}I)-diazotized diiodosulfanilic acid labeling and SDS-polyacrylamide gel electrophoresis. *J Lab Clin Med* 1978;**92**:430.

2. Nurden AT, Caen JP. Membrane glycoproteins and human platelet function. *Br J Haematol* 1978;**38**:155.

3. Phillips DR, Agin PP. Platelet membrane defects in Glanzmann's thromboasthenia. Evidence for decreased amounts of two major glycoproteins. *J Clin Invest* 1997;**60**:535.

4. Phillips DR, Agin PP. Platelet plasma membrane glycoproteins. Evidence for the presence of nonequivalent disulfide bonds using nonreduced-reduced two-dimensional gel electrophoresis. *J Biol Chem* 1997;**252**:2121.

5. Plow EF, Ginsberg MH. The molecular basis of platelet function. In Hoffman R, Benz EJ, Shaltil SJ, Furie B, Cohen HJ (eds) *Hematology. Basic Principles and Practice* (Churchill Livingstone, New York, 1991) 1165.

6. Fauvel F, Grant ME, Legrand YJ, Souchon H, Tobelem G, Jackson DS, Caen JP. Interaction of blood platelets with a microfibrillar extract from adult bovine aorta: requirement for von Willebrand factor. *Proc Natl Acad Sci USA* 1983;**80**:551.

7. Berridge MJ. Inositol triosephosphate and diacylglycerol: Two interacting second messengers. *Ann Rev Biochem* 1987;**56**:159.

8. Rink TJ, Sage SO. Calcium signaling in human platelets. *Ann Rev Physiol* 1990;**52**:431.

9. Packham MA. Platelet reactions in thrombosis. In: Gottlieb AI, Langille BL, Federoff S (eds), *Atherosclerosis. Cellular and Molecular Interactions in the Artery Wall* (New York, Plenum Press, 1991) 209.

10. Kinlough-Rathbone RL, Packham MA, Reimers HJ, Casenave JP, Mustard JF. Mechanisms of platelet shape change, aggregation, and release induced by collagen, thrombin, or A23, 187. *J Lab Clin Med* 1997;**90**:707.

11. Stenberg PE, Shuman MA, Levine SP, Bainton DF. Redistribution of alpha-granules and their contents in thrombin-stimulated platelets. *J Cell Biol* 1984;**98**:748.

12. Ginsberg MH, Taylor L, Painter RG. The mechanism of thrombin-induced platelet factor 4 secretion. *Blood* 1980;**55**:661.

13. Van't Veer C, Hackeng TM, Delahaye C, Sixma JJ, Booma BN. Activated factor X and thrombin formation triggered by tissue factor on endothelial cell matrix in a flow model. *Blood* 1994;**84**:1132–9.

14. Gupta M, Doellgast GJ, Cheng T, Lewis JC. Expression and localization of tissue factor-based procoagulant activity in pigeon monocyte derived macrophages. *Thromb Haemost* 1993;**70**:963–9.

15. Badimon L, Badimon JJ, Chesebro JH, Fuster V. Inhibition of thrombus formation: blockage of adhesive glycoprotein mechanisms versus blockage of the cyclo-oxygenase pathway. *J Am Coll Cardiol* 1988;**11** (**Suppl A**):30A [Abstract].

16. Strony J, Phillips M, Brands D, et al. Aurintricarboxylic acid in a canine model of coronary artery thrombosis. *Circulation* 1990;**81**:1106–14.

17. Emmons PR, Hamptom JR, Harrison MJG, et al. Effect of prostaglandin E_1 on platelet behavior in vitro and in vivo. *Br Med J* 1967;**2**:468–72.

18. Terres W, Beythien C, Kupper W, Bleifeld W. Effects of aspirin and prostaglandin E_1 on in vitro thrombolysis with urokinase. *Circulation* 1989;**79**:1309–14.

19. Weksler BB. Prostaglandins and vascular-function. *Circulation* 1984;**70** (**Suppl. III**):63–71.

20. Sharma B, Wyeth RP, Gimenez HJ, Franciosa JA. Intracoronary prostaglandin E_1 plus streptokinase in acute myocardial infarction. *Am J Cardiol* 1986;**58**:1161.

21. Kleiman NS, Tracy RP, Schaaf LJ, Harris S, Hill RD, Puleo P, Roberts R. Prostaglandin E_1 does not accelerate rTPA-induced thrombolysis

in acute myocardial infarction. *Am Heart J* 1994;**127**:738.

22. Okano Y, Yoshioka T, Shimouchi A, Satoh T, Kuneida T. Orally active prostacyclin analoguie in primary pulmonary hypertension. *Lancet* 1997;**349**:1365–8.

23. Kopia GA, Kopaciewicz LJ, Ohlstein EH, Horohonich S, Storer BL, Shebuski RJ. Combinations of the thromboxane receptor antagonist, sulotroban, with streptokinase: demonstration of thrombolytic synergy. *J Pharmacol Exp Ther* 1989;**250**:887.

24. Grover GJ, Parham CS, Schumacher WA. The combined anti-ischemic effects of the thromboxane receptor antagonist SQ 30741 and tissue tube plasminogen activator. *Am Heart J* 1991;**121**:426.

25. Tranchesi B, Caramelli B, Bebara O, Bellotti G, Pileggi F, Van de Werf F, et al. Efficacy and safety of ridogrel versus aspirin in coronary thrombolysis with alteplase for myocardial infarction. *J Am Coll Cardiol* 1992;**19**:92A [Abstract].

26. Golino P, Ashton JH, Glas-Greenwalt P, McNatt J, Buja LM, Willerson JT. Mediation of reocclusion by thromboxane A_2 and serotonin after thrombolysis with tissue-type plasminogen activator in a canine preparation of coronary thrombosis. *Circulation* 1988;**77**:678.

27. Hellem A. The adhesiveness of human blood platelets in vitro. *Scand J Clin Invest* 1960;**12**:1–17.

28. Gaarder A, Jonsen A, Laland S, Hellem AJ, Owren P. Adenosine diphosphate in red cells as a factor in the adhesiveness of human blood platelets. *Nature* 1961;**192**:531–2.

29. Burnstock G. *Purinergic Receptors*. (Chapman and Hall, London, 1981).

30. Burnstock G, Kennedy C. Is there a basis for distinguishing two types of P_2 purinoceptor? *Gen Pharm* 1985;**16**:433–40.

31. Fredholm B, Abbracchio MP, Burnstock G, Daly JW, Harden TK, Jacobson KA, et al. Nomenclature and classification of purinoceptors. *Pharm Rev* 1994;**46**:143–56.

32. Abbracchio MP, Burnstock G. Purinoceptors: are there three families of P_{2x} and P_{2y} purinoceptors? *Pharmacol Ther* 1994;**64**:445–75.

33. Nachman RL, Ferris B. Binding of adenosine diphosphate by isolated membranes from human platelets. *J Biol Chem* 1974;**249**:704–10.

34. Altieri DC, Mannucci PM, Capitaneo AM. Binding of fibrinogen to human monocytes. *J Clin Invest* 1986;**78**:968–76.

35. Feolde E, Vigne P, Breittmayer JP, Frelin C. ATP, a partial agonist of atypical P_{2y} purinoceptors in rat brain capillary endothelial cells. *Br J Pharmacol* 1995;**115**:1199–203.

36. Humphries RG, Tomlinson W, Ingall AH, Cage PA, Leff P. FPL 66096: a novel, highly potent and selective antagonist at human platelet P_{2T}-purinoceptors. *Br J Pharmacol* 1994;**113**:1057–63.

37. Humphries RG, Tomlinson W, Clegg JA, Ingall AH, Kindon ND, Leff P. Pharmacological profile of the novel P_{2T}-purinoceptor antagonist, FPL 67085 in vitro and in the anaesthetized rat in vivo. *Br J Pharmacol* 1995;**115**:1110–16.

38. Humphries, RG. A novel series of P_2T purinoceptor antagonists: definition of the role of ADP in arterial thrombosis. *Trends Pharm Sci* 1995;**16**:179–81.

39. Clegg JA, Fraser-Rae L, Humphries RG, Robertson MJ. The effect of FPL 67085 on ADP-induced platelet aggregation ex vivo in the urethane-anaesthetized rat: A comparison with oral aspirin and ticlopidine. *Br J Pharmacol* 1995;**114**(Suppl): 102P.

40. Humphries RG. Unpublished data.

41. Fitzgerald GA, Reilly LA, Pederson AK. The biochemical pharmacology of thromboxane synthase inhibition in man. *Circulation* 1985;**72**:1194–1201.

42. Mullane KM, Foinabaio D. Thromboxane synthetase inhibitors reduce infarct size by a platelet dependent, aspirin-sensitive mechanism. *Cric Res* 1988;**62**:668–78.

43. Evans RJ, Gordon JD. Mechanisms of the antithrombotic actions of dextran. *N Engl J Med* 1974;**290**:748–56.

44. Clubb FJ, Schmitz JM, Butler MM, et al. Effect of dietary omega-3 fatty acid on serum lipids, platelet function, and atherosclerosis in Watanable heritable hyperlipidemic rabbits. *Arteriosclerosis* 1989;**9**:529–37.

45. Spector AA, Kaduce TL, Figard PH, et al.

Eicosapentaenoic acid and prostacyclin production by cultured human endothelial cells. *J Lipid Res* 1983;24:1595–604.

46. Gries A, Bode C, Peter K, Herr A, Böhrer H, Motsch J, et al. Inhaled nitric oxide inhibits human platelet aggregation, P-selectin expression, and fibrinogen binding in vitro and in vivo. *Circulation* 1998;97:1481–7.

47. Lelchuk R, Radomski MW, Martin JF, Moncada S. Constitutive and inducible nitric oxide synthases in human megakaryoblastic cells. *J Pharmacol Exp Ther* 1992;262:1220–24.

48. Mellion BT, Ignarro LJ, Ohlstein EH, et al. Evidence for the inhibitory role for guanosine 3′, 5′-monophosphate in ADP-induced human platelet aggregation in the presence of nitric oxide and related vasodilators. *Blood* 1981;57:946–55.

49. Myers PR, Minor RL, Guerra R Jr et al. Vasorelaxant properties of endothelium derived relaxing factor more closely resemble S-nitrosocystein than nitric oxide. *Nature* 1990;345:161–3.

50. Wolf A, Zalpour C, Theilmeier G, Wang B-Y, Ma A, Anderson B, et al. arginine supplementation normalizes platelet aggregation in hypercholesterolemic humans. *JACC* 1997;29:479–85.

51. Adams MR, Jessup W, Hailstones D, Celermajer DS. L-Arginine reduces human monocyte adhesion to vascular endothelium and endothelial expression of cell adhesion molecules. *Circulation* 1997;95:662–8.

52. Loscalzo J. Antiplatelet and antithrombotic effects of organic nitrates. *Am J Cardiol* 1992;70(**Suppl.**):18B–22B.

53. Marks DM, Vita JA, Folts JD, Keaney JF Jr, Welch GN, Loscalzo J. Inhibition of neointimal proliferation in rabbits after vascular injury by a single treatment with a protein adduct of nitric oxide. *J Clin Invest* 1995;96:2630–8.

54. Loscalzo J. N-Acetylcysteine potentiates inhibition of platelet aggregatio by nitroglycerin. *J Clin Invest* 1985;76:703–708.

55. Mendelsohn M, O'Neill S, George D, Loscalzo J. Inhibition of fibrinogen binding to human platelets by S-nitroso-N-acetylcysteine. *J Biol Chem* 1990;265:19 028–34.

56. Langford EJ, Wainwright RJ, Martin JF. Platelet activation in acute myocardial infarction and unstable angina is inhibited by nitric oxide donors. *Arterioscler Thromb Vasc Biol* 1996;16:51–5.

57. Kubes P, Kurose I, Granger DN. NO donors prevent intergrin-induced leukocyte adhesion but not P-selectin-dependent rolling in post-ischemic venules. *Am J Physiol* 1994;267:H931–H937.

58. Delyani JA, Nossuli TO, Scalia R, Thomas G, Garvey DS, Lefer AM. S-nitrosylated tissue-plasminogen activator protects against myocardial ischemia-reperfusion injury in cats: role of the endothelium. *J Pharmacol Exp Ther* 1996;279:1174–80.

59. Morley D, Maragos CM, Zhang X-Y, Boignon M, Wink DA, Keefer LK. Mechanism of vascular relaxation induced by the nitric oxide (NO/nucleophile complexes, a new class of NO-based vasodilators. *J Cardiovasc Pharmacol* 1993;21:670–76.

60. Diodati JG, Quyyumi AA, Hussain N, Keefer LK. Complexes of nitric oxide with nucleophiles as agents for the controlled biological release of nitric oxide: antiplatelet effect. *Thromb Haemost* 1993;70:654–8.

61. Saavedra JE, Southan GJ, Davies KM, et al. Localizing antithrombotic and vasodilatory activity with a novel, ultrafast nitric oxide donor. *J Med Chem* 1996;39:4361–5.

62. Smith DJ, Chakravarthy D, Pulfer S, et al. Nitric oxide-releasing polymers containing the [N(O)NO]-group. *J Med Chem* 1996;39:1148–56.

63. Reden J. Molsidomine. *Blood Vessels* 1990;27:282–94.

64. The ESPRIM trial. Short-term treatment of acute myocardial infarction with molsidomine. European Study of Prevention of Infarct with Molsidomine. *Lancet* 1994;344:91–7.

65. Messin R, Boxho G, De Smedt J, Buntinx IM. Acute and chronic effect of molsidomine on exercise capacity in patients with stable angina, a double-blind cross-over clinical trial versus placebo. *J Cardiovasc Pharmacol* 1995;25:558–63.

66. Lablanche JM, Grollier G, Lusson JR, et al. Effect of the direct nitric oxide donors linsidomine and molsidomine on angiographic restenosis after coronary balloon angioplasty.

The ACCORD Study. *Circulation* 1997;**95**: 83–9.

67. Wainwright CL, Martorana PA. Pirsidomine, a novel nitric oxide donor suppresses ischemic arrhythmias in anesthetized pigs. *J Cardiovasc Pharmacol* 1993;**22**:S44–S50.

68. Kita Y, Ohkubo K, Hirasawa Y, et al. FR 144420, a novel, slow, nitric oxide-releasing agent. *Eur J Pharmacol* 1995;**275**:125–30.

69. Rossoni G, Bert F, Bermareggi M, et al. Protective effects of ITF 296 in the isolated rabbit heart subjected to global ischemia. *J Cardiovasc Pharmacol* 1995;**26**:S44–S52.

70. Lefer DJ, Nakanishi K, Johnston WE, Vinten-Johansen J. Antineutrophil and myocardial protecting actions of a novel nitric oxide donor after acute myocardial ischemia and reperfusion of dogs. *Circulation* 1993;**88**:2337–50.

71. Schneider DJ, Tracy PB, Mann KG, Sobel BE. Differential effects of anticoagulants on the activation of platelets ex vivo. *Circulation* 1997;**96**:2877–83.

72. Legrand C, Morandi V, Mendelovitz, et al. Selective inhibition of platelet macroaggregate formation by a recombinant heparin-binding domain of human thrombospondin. *Arterioscler Thromb* 1994;**14**:1784–91.

73. Kelton JG, Smith JW, Warkentin TE, et al. Immunoglobulin G from patients with heparin-induced thrombocytopenia binds to a complex of heparin and platelet factor 4. *Blood* 1994;**83**:3232–9.

74. Spencer F, Liu L, Zxhang Q, Ball SP, Becker, RC. Enoxaparin suppresses platelet-dependent thrombin generation in vivo among patients with unstable angina or non-ST segment elevation MI. *J Am Coll Cardiol* 1997;**29**(**Suppl. A**):185A [Abstract].

75. Moliterno DJ, Califf RM, Aquirre FV, et al. Effect of platelet GPIIb/IIIa integrin blockade on activated clotting time during PTCA or directional atherectomy: the EPIC trial. *Am J Cardiol* 1995;**75**:559–62.

Section III:

Clinical applications

12

Overview of the clinical applications of antiplatelet therapy

Eric Garbarz, Michel Vayssairat, Sonia Alamowitch, Etienne Roullet and Alec Vahanian

Introduction

Atherosclerosis is the first cause of death in the industrialized world. It is a general disorder with manifestations in several vascular beds. Atherosclerosis arises from a multifactorial process, where platelets play a major role in thrombus formation;[1] this explains the wide and successful use of antiplatelet agents, particularly aspirin, in its treatment.[2] In this chapter, the general clinical applications of antiplatelet therapy in the treatment of cardiac, cerebral and peripheral disease will be reviewed, as well as the applications of antiplatelet agents in preventative therapy. Current practice, largely based on the use of aspirin, will be emphasized but possible new developments arising from trials of new therapeutic agents will be considered.

Cardiac disease
Acute coronary syndromes

The presence of platelet-rich coronary thrombi in unstable angina and myocardial infarction (MI) has been demonstrated using coronary angiography, angioscopy and pathological studies,[3] and the benefit of antiplatelet treatment been proven in several randomized trials.

| | n | Death/MI (%) | |
		Treatment	Placebo
Cairns et al[7]	278	12.2	25.9
Lewis et al[8]	1266	5	10
Risc group[9]	796	6.5	17.1
Theroux et al[10]	239	3.3	13.6
Total	2579	6.1	14.3

Table 12.1
Efficacy of aspirin in unstable angina.

Unstable angina

Of the treatments for unstable angina, aspirin is the one that has shown the greatest effect.[4-6] Several studies (Table 12.1) have shown consistently that aspirin reduces mortality and MI by 50%[8-11] and the Antiplatelet Trialist's Collaboration[11] showed that it reduces for over 2 years both non-fatal stroke and MI by one-third and vascular deaths also by one-third.

It follows from this that aspirin should be given as soon as possible during the course of unstable angina and continued thereafter. The initial dose should be 150–325 mg, while the maintenance dose should be between 80 mg and 160 mg. Nevertheless, aspirin is only a weak platelet inhibitor, several patients are non-responders or cannot tolerate it, and it also increases the risk of bleeding. Although ticlopidine is not usually recommended, because of its delay in action and toxicity, it could be used in cases where there is an allergy to aspirin.

Recent clinical trials have shown that GPIIb/IIIa blockers consistently reduce the incidence of death and MI in patients with unstable angina or non-QMI when compared with aspirin.[12-14] This benefit is very significant when these agents are used before or during angioplasty, and also to a lesser, but still significant extent, when they are part of medical treatment alone. Their use in reinforcing medical treatment should be explored further, particularly as regards the selection of ideal candidates.

Myocardial infarction

The validation of the use of aspirin in acute MI is largely derived from the ISIS-2 trial[15] (Figure 12.1) which showed that patients randomized for aspirin administration had a 20% reduction in mortality at 30 days, in addition to thrombolysis. In a meta-analysis of trials in which patients underwent acute and follow-up angiography and either were or were not treated systematically with aspirin, Roux[16]

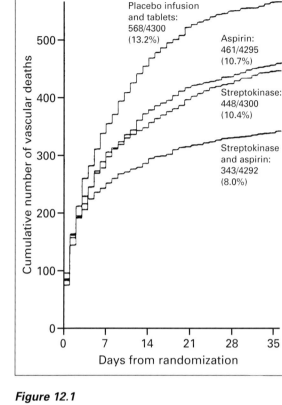

Figure 12.1
Use of Aspirin in acute MI. Cumulative vascular mortality in Days 0–35. Redrawn from ISIS-2 trial[15] with permission.

showed that regardless of the thrombolytic used, the frequency of angiographically demonstrated reocclusion was reduced by aspirin. Since then there has been strong evidence to suggest that aspirin should be used as soon as possible in the treatment of patients with acute MI. This is especially true of reperfusion using thrombolysis or percutaneous coronary angioplasty. The initial dose usually recommended is 160 mg by oral (chewable) administration or 325 mg orally, the maintenance dose being 325 mg per day.[17] In the CAPRIE trial there was no apparent benefit of clopidogrel over aspirin in patients with recent MI. The relative efficacy of low-dose aspirin combined with low-dose oral anticoagulants compared with either of these drugs used alone has yet to be answered.

Platelet aggregation and residual thrombus may contribute to the failure of thrombolysis and percutaneous coronary angioplasty. This raises therapeutic interest in using GPIIb/IIIa blockers. A subgroup of the EPIC study and the recently reported RAPPORT trial consistently showed that abciximab reduces acute ischemic complications during primary percutaneous coronary angioplasty. These findings appear to justify the use of these new agents during primary percutaneous coronary angioplasty and probably also during rescue percutaneous coronary angioplasty after failed thrombolysis. A combination of these potent agents with low-dose thrombolytics to increase the reperfusion efficacy, to reduce the reocclusion rates, and decrease the risk of bleeding has been suggested. The efficacy of this combination is currently being tested in angiographic trials and will be evaluated in large clinical trials to assess the risk:benefit ratio.[188]

Patients with a history of MI have a risk of recurrent ischemic events arising from recurrent thrombotic complications—these being the main cause of cardiac death and morbidity. In an overview of all trials available, the Antiplatelet Trialists' Collaboration[11] showed that long-term aspirin resulted in a reduction of 36% in the risk of any vascular events with large and significant reductions in non-fatal MI (20–30%) and vascular death (10–15%). Total mortality was also significantly reduced and there was a smaller but still significant reduction in non-fatal stroke. It is therefore recommended that chronic aspirin be continued indefinitely in all patients unless there are contraindications.

Chronic stable angina

Patients with chronic stable angina, like those with acute coronary syndromes, are at risk of recurrent ischemic events. Aspirin has, however, been found to produce a highly significant benefit in these patients: namely, a 35% decrease in MI and sudden death and a 32% reduction in secondary vascular events for at least 2 years.[11,19,20]

These patients should therefore receive antiplatelet therapy unless it is contraindicated. Trials are planned to see if the new agents GPIIb/IIIa inhibitors can improve the risk efficacy in this setting.

Coronary revascularization

Coronary angioplasty

Endothelial denudation, platelet deposition, and thrombus formation occur immediately after angioplasty and, among other things (e.g. dissection) may lead to acute occlusion.

Several studies have shown consistently that pretreatment with antiplatelet agents reduces the incidence of periprocedural ischemic complications.[21] Antiplatelet agents should therefore be administered before angioplasty. Since platelets play a central role in vascular response to injury, they are logical targets for the prevention of restenosis after percutaneous coronary angioplasty. No study to date, however, has shown a clear effect of antiplatelet therapy on restenosis. Nevertheless a significant reduction of vascular events after percutaneous coronary angioplasty, using antiplatelet agents has been shown[11], leading to interest in the long-term use of these agents in this setting.

In comparison with aspirin, prophylactic use of GPIIb/IIIa inhibitors significantly reduces the incidence of acute complications after angioplasty. This favorable effect is observed not only in high-risk patients, but also in low risk subgroups[22]. Although the literature supports the use of these new agents in almost all percutaneous coronary angioplasty patients, in practice their use is limited by economic considerations.[23] Despite their efficacy in acute settings, these new agents do not appear to reduce the incidence of restenosis. Further studies are planned with long-term administration of oral GPIIb/IIIa blockers that can also block vitronectin receptors.

Coronary stenting

Coronary stenting reduces the incidence of both acute complications and late restenosis after coronary angioplasty. Currently, 60–70% of angioplasty patients receive stents. Despite a high rate of procedural success, however, the early experience of stenting, using oral anticoagulants as antithrombotic treatment was marred by an unacceptably high rate of stent thrombosis and bleeding.

Since platelets have been shown to play a pivotal role in stent thrombosis, it has been suggested that a combination of antiplatelet agents be used instead of oral anticoagulants and aspirin to prevent thrombosis.[24] Several randomized trials have together shown that the risk–benefit ratio for stenting is improved with the use of aspirin plus ticlopidine for 15–30 days,[25] and this has now become the standard treatment (Table 12.2). The use of abciximab in comparison with standard treatment further reduces the incidence of acute ischemic complications after elective or bail out stenting, suggesting a role for this new agent in this setting too.[23]

Bypass grafts

The deterioration of saphenous coronary bypass grafts is the result of several mechanisms: thrombotic occlusion; intimal proliferation; and atherosclerosis. Platelet activation plays a role in each of these mechanisms; indeed antiplatelet agents have shown a beneficial effect in preventing graft occlusion up to 1 year.[29] In the same way, no treatment has

Treatment	ISAR[26]		FANTASTIC[27]		STARS[28]		
	OA	A+T	OA	A+T	OA	A+T	A
n	260	257	230	246	555	553	544
Subacute thrombosis (%)	5.4	0.8	9.5	0.4	2.4	0.6	3.6

*OA, Oral anticoagulation A, Aspirin; T, Ticlopidine.

Table 12.2
Subacute thrombosis after stent implantation. *

proved superior to ASA (aspirin) in preventing occlusion of arterial grafts.

In bypass graft patients, antiplatelet therapy not only prevents graft occlusion, but also provides a continued reduction in the number of vascular events.[11] Aspirin use should therefore be started immediately after surgery, and continued indefinitely, together with the control of risk factors.

Valve prostheses

Patients with prosthetic valve replacements have an increased immediate and long-term, risk of thromboembolic events whose origin is multifactorial and connected with the characteristics of the valve and of the patient.[30] Antiplatelet therapy alone does not give adequate protection against thromboembolism in patients with mechanical prostheses. These agents have been evaluated in combination with oral anticoagulants: there is no benefit but a significantly higher risk of hemorrhage with the use of high doses of aspirin in patients taking oral anticoagulants. Nevertheless, one study has demonstrated that low-dose aspirin given to patients with a target INR (International Normalised Ratio) of 3–4.5, reduced the risk of death and thromboembolic events without increasing the risk of major bleeding. The reduction in mortality in the aspirin-treated patients may, however, be related to the prevention of MI in patients with coronary artery disease, which was the case in 35% of the patients in this study;[31] further studies are necessary.

It is reasonable to assume that aspirin may be useful in patients with concomitant arterial disease. To minimize the risk of bleeding in these patients it should be used in low doses in combination with low-intensity anticoagulation—the prosthesis and characteristics of the patient permitting. Antiplatelet agents are often used in patients who have suffered a thromboembolic complication but there have as yet been no trials to support this. In addition, there is no evidence to support the long-term use of aspirin in patients with bioprostheses who do not have non-prosthetic risk factors.[32]

Atrial fibrillation

In the genesis of thromboembolism in atrial fibrillation, blood stasis seems to predominate over endothelial lesions of the heart or vessels. Oral anticoagulants would therefore appear to be superior to aspirin in the prevention of these events. Oral anticoagulants are justified in patients with atrial fibrillation of valvular origin. Moreover, in non-valvular atrial fibrillation, several randomized trials comparing aspirin, oral anticoagulants, and the combination of both for secondary prevention of stroke came to the conclusion that oral anticoagulants were superior in patients at high risk. The risk of embolism in patients with atrial fibrillation is increased in the presence of valvular disease, a history of embolism, advanced age, diabetes mellitus, and/or congestive heart failure. Aspirin is indicated in patients within the age range 60–75 years without other risk factors, and no treatment can be given to patients in the other categories.[33]

Lower limb arterial disease

Patients with lower limb arterial disease have a 2-fold increase of mortality, and a mean loss of 10 years in their life-expectancy.[34] Platelets play a key role in the development and progression of occlusive athrosclerotic lesions, and several trials have been devoted to the use of antiplatelet agents in such cases.[35]

In patients with lower limb arterial disease, prolonged drug-induced inhibition of platelet function affords valuable protection against fatal and non-fatal vascular events, and delays the progression of lower limb arterial disease. In 22 trials of 3395 patients with lower limb arterial disease, a statistically significant reduction of 2.1% in the absolute risk of vascular events and/or vascular deaths among patients taking antiplatelet agents was found.[11] In two placebo-controlled trials, one with aspirin and dypiridamole, and the other with ticlopidine, arteriography showed delayed progression of lower limb arterial disease.[36,37] A few other studies have indicated an improvement in walking distance,[38,39] and the authors of one study reported a reduced need for vascular leg surgery during long-term treatment of claudicant patients with ticlopidine.[40] Nevertheless, antiplatelet agents might not be equally efficacious in different subgroups of atherosclerotic patients. For example, diabetic patients with gangrene might not benefit from antiplatelet therapy, and there is no proof that antiplatelet agents reduce the amputation rate.[41]

Patients with lower limb arterial disease are possible candidates for lower limb revascularization by angioplasty, or by venous or prosthetic grafts. Thrombosis appears to be the final step common to various causes that lead to graft failure and justify the preventive long-term use of antiplatelet agents. This was investigated by the antiplatelet trialists' study which performed a meta-analysis of 14 trials, and in which maintenance of vascular graft or arterial patency by antiplatelet therapy was improved by 43%.[42] Both aspirin and ticlopidine[43] have been validated in such indications, while further studies of Clopidogrel and GPIIb/IIIa blockers are necessary.

Non-atherosclerotic peripheral disease

The effects of antiplatelet agents in the prophylaxis of venous thromboembolism, have been reviewed by the Antiplatelet Trialists' Collaboration, which grouped together 53 trials concerning a total of 8400 patients.[41] Antiplatelet agents are effective for such prophylaxis but less so than other anticoagulants.[44] Aspirin therefore cannot be recommended for the prevention of venous thromboembolism.

Another possible application for antiplatelet agents is hemodialysis, where antiplatelet therapy substantially reduces the occlusion of arteriovenous fistulae or shunts established for hemodialysis access.[41] It could also reduce the high incidence of major vascular events in such patients.

Cerebrovascular disease

Ischemic strokes are a major cause of death and morbidity in the industrialized world. The role of platelet-fibrin emboli was identified in patients with transient ischemic ocular and cerebral events. Antiplatelet therapy has since been evaluated in numerous trials in the treatment of ischemic stroke.

In two studies[45,46] of early aspirin use (within 48 h) in patients suffering acute ischemic stroke the respective results were: a small but significant benefit with 13 fewer dead or dependant patients per 1000 patients treated on follow-up; and a significant reduction in the risk of death or non-fatal recurrent stroke within 14 days with no significant benefit at 6 months. It is difficult to determine if aspirin is effective in acute cerebral infarction, or if the benefit results from its action in early prevention. Both studies, however, suggested that aspirin should be started as soon as

	% Variations resulting from aspirin		
	Non-fatal MI	Non-fatal stroke	Treatment total mortality
US physicians[53]	(−) 39 ± 9	(+) 19 ± 15	(−) 2 ± 15
British doctors[54]	(−) 3 ± 19	(+) 13 ± 24	(−) 7 ± 14
Total	(−) 32 ± 8	(+) 18 ± 13	(−) 5 ± 10

Table 12.3
Antiplatelet therapy in primary prevention.

possible after the onset of ischemic stroke.[45,46]

Since the Canadian Co-operative Study in 1978,[47] over 50 trials have shown the benefit of aspirin in patients with previous stroke. Indeed antiplatelet therapy has been found to significantly reduce the risk of non-fatal stroke in high-risk patients to a similar degree as in MI patients.[11] The information available also showed that antiplatelet therapy reduced the incidence of both disabling or fatal stroke and non-disabling stroke. Antiplatelet therapy also leads to a reduction in other vascular events, which are reduced by 37% (−9 per 1000 non-fatal MI and −11 per 1000 vascular deaths), the improvement being comparable in patients with or without completed stroke.

There is therefore a clear indication for antiplatelet therapy in stroke patients. Aspirin is still the most important component of medical treatment and remains the agent of choice. There is a large and continuing debate concerning the optimum dose of aspirin for stroke prevention and this deserves further investigation.[48–51] Any dose over 30 mg seems to be equally effective as a high dose. Ticlopidine is similarly effective as aspirin but it is far more toxic.[52–54] Post-hoc subgroup analyses have,

however, suggested that Ticlopidine might be more effective than aspirin in patients with completed stroke, in women and in patients with ischemia in the posterior circulation. Clopidogrel might be considered in patients with severe[53] and diffuse cardiovascular disease, or where there is an allergy to aspirin. Doubts exist regarding the interest of a combination of aspirin plus dipyridamole.[55] The GPIIb/IIIa blockers have not yet been tested in large trials of patients with cerebrovascular disease. Particularly in patients with atrial fibrillation and cerebral ischemia, the preferred treatment is oral anticoagulation with a target INR of 2–3, aspirin being given only when oral anticoagulants are contraindicated.

Prevention

Patients with a localized atherosclerotic disease often present with other co-morbid diseases because of the common underlying pathology. This explains why the treatment of the atherosclerotic disease at one site may also treat and prevent manifestations elsewhere. A review of 70 000 patients in over 174 trials, (Figure 12.3) has confirmed the value of

Category of trial	No. of trials with data	MI, stroke, or vascular death		Stratified statistics		Odds ratio and confidence interval (antiplatelet: control)	% Odds reduction (SD)
		Antiplatelet	Adjusted controls[†]	O-E	Variance		
Prior MI	11	1331/9877	1693/9914	−158.5	561.6		25% (4)
Acute MI	9	992/9388	1348/9385	−177.9	510.3		29% (4)
Prior stroke/TIA	18	1076/5837	1301/5870	−98.5	386.5		22% (4)
Acute stroke	1	2/15	3/14	−0.6	1.1		
Other cardiac disease:							
Unstable angina	7	182/1991	285/2027	−49.1	89.7		
Post-CABG	19	124/2529	127/2546	−4.1	38.0		
Post-PTCA	4	32/663	61/669	−13.0	18.2		
Stable angina/CAD	5	27/278	42/273	−7.5	14.6		
Atrial fibrillation	2	82/888	113/904	−14.6	43.5		
Rheumatic valve disease	1	9/78	17/76	−4.2	5.4		
Valve surgery	6	46/602	79/642	−13.8	27.3		
Perhiperal vascular disease:							
Intermittent claudication	22	160/1646	195/1649	−15.7	63.6		
Peripheral grafts	9	65/771	69/768	−4.6	27.3		
Peripheral angioplasty	2	5/194	8/195	−1.0	1.9		
Other high-risk patients:							
Renal dialysis	10	2/256	6/269	−1.8	1.9		
Diabetes	7	34/687	30/678	0.9	12.1		
Other	9	14/836	23/832	−5.0	7.9		
All trials[†]	142	4183/36 536 (11.4%)	5400/36 711 (14.7%)	−568.8	1810.9		27% (2)

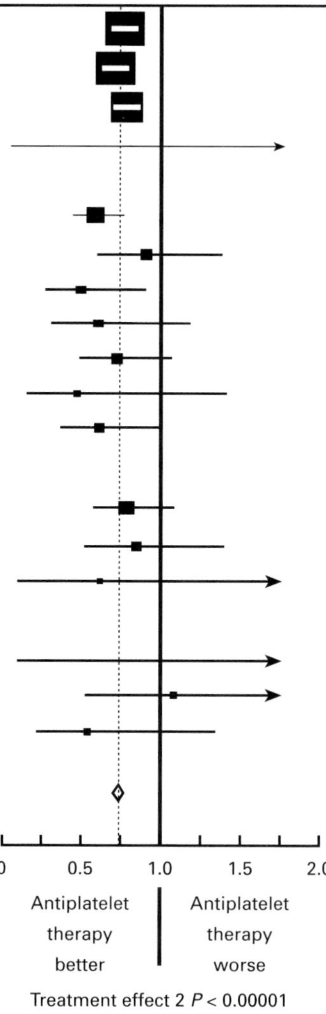

Test for heterogeneity: χ^2_{16} = 18.9; $p > 0.1$; NS

[†]Crude, unadjusted control total = 4706/32 278

Odds ratio scale: 0 0.5 1.0 1.5 2.0

Antiplatelet therapy better | Antiplatelet therapy worse

Treatment effect 2 $P < 0.00001$

Figure 12.3
Proportional effects of antiplatelet therapy in secondary prevention. CABG, coronary artery bypass grafting; PTCA, percutaneous translational coronary angioplasty; CAD, coronary artery disease. Redrawn from the Antiplatelet Trialist Collaboration[11] with permission.

antiplatelet therapy for the secondary prevention of vascular events (e.g. vascular deaths, MI infarction, non-fatal stroke) in traditionally high-risk patients.[11] It also showed, however, that this benefit was extended to other high-risk patients such as those with atrial fibrillation, valve surgery, or peripheral disease. Moreover, the benefit was observed across different subgroups: younger and older, women and men, hypertensive or not, diabetic or non-diabetic patients. Consequently, unless contraindicated, aspirin should clearly be given to all patients with prior manifestations of overt atherosclerotic disease.

Compelling data derived from large-scale trials has established that a median dose of aspirin of 75–325 mg per day affords the best cost–efficacy–risk benefit, and there is no evidence that higher doses are more effective, although they increase the risk of side-effects. For patients taking aspirin, biological monitoring is unnecessary; while in patients taking ticlopidine or clopidogrel, hematological toxicity must be checked.

The optimal duration of antiplatelet therapy is unknown, but prolonged therapy is probably beneficial for secondary prevention since additional benefit has been demonstrated when the therapy lasts from 1–3 years.

Data concerning primary prevention is far more limited and comes to us from two randomized trials in healthy individuals.[56,57] It shows the benefit to be much smaller than in secondary prevention and must be weighed against the risk. Globally, these trials showed a smaller but significant reduction in the risk of non-fatal myocardial infarction but were unable to demonstrate any effect on mortality. The existing data shows that aspirin produces an excess of hemorrhagic and ischemic stroke in low-risk patients but this cannot yet be considered conclusive because of the low event rate. Based on these findings, antiplatelet agents cannot routinely be recommended for all patients without overt cardiovascular disease.

The indications of antiplatelet agents should balance the risk–benefit ratio for each individual. Treatment might well benefit patients with several risk factors, while the risk might outweigh the benefits in other patients. Trials are planned to evaluate the benefit of antiplatelet agents in primary prevention in patients with or without risk factors, and also in women, who were excluded from the initial trials.

Conclusions

Antiplatelet therapy, mainly aspirin, unless contraindicated, is clearly indicated in almost all patients suffering acute manifestations of atherosclerotic disease. It also provides a very significant benefit in secondary prevention in a wide range of patients who have suffered a prior cardiovascular event. Its beneficial use in primary prevention is unproven; thus it should be given only on an individual basis in this setting.

Despite their well-established efficacy, antiplatelet agents are nevertheless presently under-used.[58] The general public should be better informed of their importance. Expansion of indications for antiplatelet use will depend on improved tolerance, which might be achieved with the use of new agents (e.g. clopidogrel) and also on greater efficacy, which may be achieved by using a combination of agents such as aspirin plus clopidogrel, or new compounds such as GPIIb/IIIa blockers.

In conclusion, antiplatelet therapy in addition to the other medical treatments, has an important part to play in the treatment of atherosclerotic disease, revascularization, and overall control of risk factors.

References

1. Stein B, Fuster V, Halperin JL, et al. Antithrombotic therapy in cardiac disease: an emerging approach based on pathogenesis and risk. *Circulation* 1989;**80**:1501–13.
2. Fuster V. Mechanisms leading to myocardial infarction: insights from studies of vascular biology. *Circulation* 1994;**90**:2126–46.
3. Mizuno K, Satomura K, Miyamoto A, et al. Angioscopic evaluation of coronary-artery thrombi in acute coronary syndromes. *N Engl J Med* 1992;**326**:287–91.
4. Granger CB, Califf RM. Stabilizing the unstable artery. In: Califf R, Mark D, Wagner G (eds). *Acute Coronary Care*, 2nd edn (St Louis, Mosby 1995) 525–41.
5. Fuster V, Badimon L, Badimon JJ, et al. The pathogenesis of coronary artery disease and the acute coronary syndromes (part I), *N Engl J Med* 1992;**326**:242–50.
6. Fuster V, Badimon L, Badimon JJ, et al. The pathogenesis of coronary artery disease and the acute coronary syndromes (part II). *N Engl J Med* 1992;**326**:310–18.
7. Cairns JA, Gent M, Singer J, et al. Aspirin, sulfinpyrazone, or both in unstable angina. *N Engl J Med* 1985;**313**:1369–75.
8. Lewis HDJ, Davis JW, Archibald DG, et al. Protective effects of aspirin against acute myocardial infarction and death in men with unstable angina. *N Engl J Med* 1983; **309**:396–403.
9. The RISC Group. Risk of myocardial infarction and death during treatment with low dose aspirin and intravenous heparin in men with unstable coronary artery disease. *Lancet* 1990;**336**:827–30.
10. Theroux P, Quimet H, McCans J, et al. Aspirin, heparin, or both to treat acute unstable angina. *N Engl J Med* 1998;**319**: 1105–11.
11. Antiplatelet Trialists' Collaboration. Collaborative overview of randomized trials of antiplatelet therapy—I: Prevention of death, myocardial infarction, and stroke by prolonged antiplatelet therapy in various categories of patients, *Br Med J* 1994; **308**:81–106.
12. Braunwald E, Maseri A, Armstrong PW, et al. Rationale and clinical evidence for the use of GPIIb/IIIa inhibitors in acute coronary syndromes. *Eur Heart J* 1998;**19**(**Suppl. D**): D22–D30.
13. The CAPTURE Investigators. Randomised placebo-controlled trial of abciximab before and during coronary intervention refractory unstable angina: the CAPTURE study. *Lancet* 1997;**349**:1429–35.
14. Moliterno DJ, Topol EJ. Meta analysis of platelet GPIIb/IIIa antagonist randomized clinical trials in ischemic heart disease. Consistent, durable, salutary effects. *Circulation* 1997;**96**: I-475.
15. ISIS-2 (Second International Study of Infarct Survival) Collaborative Group. Randomised trial of intravenous streptokinase, oral aspirin, both, or neither among 17 187 cases of suspected acute myocardial infarction: ISIS-2. *Lancet* 1988;**ii**:349–60.
16. Roux S, Christeller S, Ludin E. Effects of aspirin on coronary reocclusion and recurrent ischemia after thrombolysis: a meta-analysis. *J Am Coll Cardiol* 1992; **19**:671–77.
17. CAPRIE Steering Committee. A randomised, blinded, trial of clopidogrel versus aspirin in patients at risk of ischemic events (CAPRIE). *Lancet* 1996;**348**:1329–39.
18. Topol E. Toward a new frontier in myocardial reperfusion therapy. Emerging platelet preeminence. *Circulation* 1998;**97**:211–18.
19. Juul-Möller S, Edvardsson N, Jahnmatz B, et al for the Swedish Angina Pectoris Aspirin Trial (SAPAT) Group. Double-blind trial of aspirin in primary prevention of myocardial infarction in patients with stable chronic angina pectoris. *Lancet* 1992;**340**:1421–5.
20. Ridker PM, Manson JE, Gaziano JM, et al. Low-dose aspirin therapy for chronic stable angina. A randomized, placebo-controlled clinical trial. *Ann Intern Med* 1991;**114**:835–9.
21. Kuntz RE, Piana R, Pomerantz RM, et al.

Changing incidence and management of abrupt closure following coronary intervention in the new device era, *Cathet Cardiovasc Diagn* 1992;**27**:183–90.

22. EPILOG Investigators. Platelet glycoprotein IIB/IIIA receptor blockade and low-dose heparin during percutaneous coronary revascularization. *N Engl J Med* 1997;**336**:1689–96.

23. Chronos N, Vahanian A, Betriu A, et al. Use of abciximab in interventional cardiology. *Eur Heart J* 1998;**19**(Suppl. D):D31–D39.

24. Lablanche JM, McFadden EP, Bonnet JL, et al. Combined antiplatelet therapy with ticlopidine and aspirin: a simplified approach to intracoronary stent management. *Eur Heart J* 1996;**17**: 1373–80.

25. Schomig A, Neumann FJ, Kastrati A, et al. A randomized comparison of antiplatelet and anticoagulant therapy after the placement of coronary artery stents. *N Engl J Med* 1996;**334**:1084–9.

26. Schomig A, Neumann FJ, Kastrati A, Schuhler H, Blasini R, Hadamitzky M, Walter H, et al. A randomized comparison of antiplatelet and anticoagulant therapy after the placement of coronary artery stents. *N Engl J Med* 1996; **334**:1084–9.

27. Bertrand M, Legrand V, Boland J, Fleck E, Bonnier J, Emmanuelson H, Vrolix, et al. Randomized multicenter comparison of conventional anticoagulation versus antiplatelet therapy in unplanned and elective coronary stenting. *Circulation* 1998;**98**:1597–603.

28. Leon MB, Baim DS, Popma JJ, Gordon PC, Cutlip DE, Ho KK, Giambartolomei A, et al. A clinical trial comparing three antithrombotic drug regimens after coronary artery stenting. *N Engl J Med* 1998;**339**:1665–71.

29. Motwani JG, Topol EJ. Aortocoronary saphenous vein graft disease. Pathogenesis, predisposition, and prevention. *Circulation* 1998;**97**: 916–31.

30. Butchart EG. Thrombogenesis and its management. In: Acar J, Bodnar E (eds) *Textbook of Acquired Heart Value Disease.* (London, ICR, 1995) 1048–20

31. Turpie AGG, Gent M, Laupacis A, et al. A comparison of Aspirin with placebo in patients treated with warfarin after heart valve replacement. *N Engl J Med* 1993;**329**:524–9.

32. Gohlke-Barwolf C, Acar J, Burckhardt D, et al. Guidelines for prevention of thromboembolic events in valvular heart disease. *J Heart Valve Dis* 1993;**2**:398–410.

33. Halperin JL, Petersen P. Thrombosis in the cardiac chambers: ventricular dysfunction and atrial fibrillation. In: *Cardiovascular Thrombosis and Thromboneurology*, 2nd edn (1998) Chapter 23: (Town, Publisher, Year) 415–38.

34. Smith GD, Shipley MJ, Rose G. Intermittent claudication, heart disease risk factors, and mortality: The Whitehall Study. *Circulation* 1990;**82**:1925–31.

35. Ross R, Glomset JA. The pathogenesis of atherosclerosis. *N Engl J Med* 1976; **295**: 369–77, 420–25.

36. Hess H, Mietaschk A, Diechsel G. Drug-induced inhibition of platelet function delays progression of peripheral occlusive arterial disease. *Lancet* 1985;**i**:415–19.

37. Stiegler H, Hess H, Mietaschk A, et al. Einfluss von Ticlopidin auf die periphere obliterierende Arteriopathie. *Dentsch Med Wochenschr* 1984;**109**:1240–43.

38. Arcan JC, Blanchard J, Boissel JP, et al. Multicenter double-blind study of ticlopidine in the treatment of intermittent claudication and the prevention of its complications. *Angiology* 1988;**39**:802–11.

39. Libretti A, Catalano M. Treatment of claudication with dipyridamole and aspirin. *Int J Clin Pharma Res* 1988;**6**:59–60.

40. Berqvist D, Almgren B, Dickinson JP. Reduction of requirement for leg vascular surgery during long-term treatment of claudicant patients with ticlopidine: results from the Swedish Ticlopidine Multicentre Study (STIMS). *Eur J Vasc Endovasc Surg* 1995;**10**: 69–76.

41. Colwell JA, Bingham SF, Abraira C, et al. Veterans Administration Co-operative study on antiplatelet agents in diabetic patients after amputation for gangrene: II. Effects of aspirin and dipyridamole on atherosclerotic vascular disease rates. *Diabetes Care* 1986;**9**:140–48.

42. Antiplatelet Trialists' Collaboration. Collaborative overview of randomised trials of antiplatelet therapy—II: Maintenance of vascular graft or arterial patency by antiplatelet therapy. *Br Med J* 1994;**308**:159–68.

43. Becquemin JP, and the Etude de la Ticlopidine Après Pontage Femoro-poplité and the Association Universitaire de Recherche en Chirurgie. Effect of ticlopidine on the long-term patency of saphenous-vein bypass grafts in the legs. *N Engl J Med* 1997;**337**:1726–31.
44. Antiplatelet Trialists' Collaboration. Collaborative overview of randomised trials of antiplatelet therapy—III: reduction in venous thrombosis and pulmonary embolism by antiplatelet prophylaxis among surgical and medical patients. *Br Med J* 1994;**308**:235–46.
45. International Stroke Trial Collaborative Group. The international stroke trial (IST): a randomised trial of aspirin, subcutaneous heparin, both or neither among 19435 patients with acute ischemic stroke. *Lancet* 1997:**349**:1569–81.
46. CAST (Chinese Acute Stroke Trial) Collaborative Group. CAST randomised controlled trial of early aspirin use in 20 000 patients with acute ischemic stroke. *Lancet* 1997;**349**:1641–9.
47. The Canadian Co-operative Study Group. A randomized trial of aspirin and sulfinpyrazone in the threatened stroke. *N Engl J Med* 1978;**299**:53–9.
48. Patrono C, Roth GJ. Aspirin in ischemic cerebrovascular disease. How strong is the case for a different dosing regimen? *Stroke* 1996;**27**:756–60.
49. UK–TIA Study Group. United Kingdom transient ischemic attack (UK–TIA) aspirin trial: final results. *J Neurol Neurosurg Psychiatr* 1991;**54**:1044–54.
50. The Dutch TIA Trial Study Group. A comparison of two doses of Aspirin (30 mg versus 283 mg a day) in patients after a transient ischemic attack or minor ischemic events. *N Engl J Med* 1991;**325**:1261–6.
51. The SALT Collaborative Group. Swedish Aspirin Low dose Trial (SALT) of 75 mg aspirin as secondary prophylaxis after cerebrovascular ischaemic events, *Lancet* 1991;**338**:1345–9.
52. Hass WK, Easton JD, Adams HP, et al. A randomized trial comparing ticlopidine hydrochloride with aspirin for the prevention of stroke in high-risk patients. *N Engl J Med* 1989;**321**:501–7.
53. Hershey LA. Stroke prevention in women: role of aspirin versus ticlopidine. *Am J Med* 1991;**91**:288–92.
54. Harbison JW. Ticlopidine versus aspirin for the prevention of recurrent stroke: analysis of patients with minor stroke from the Ticlopidine Aspirin Stroke Study. *Stroke* 1992;**23**:1723–7.
55. Diener HC, Cunha L, Forbes C, et al. European Stroke Prevention Study 2. Dipyridamole and acetylsalicylic acid in the secondary prevention of stroke. *J Neurol Sci* 1997;**151** (**Suppl.**):S1–S77.
56. The Steering Committee of the Physicians Health Study Research Group. Final report on the aspirin component of the Physicians' Health Study. *N Engl J Med* 1989;**321**:129–35.
57. Peto R, Gray R, Collins R, et al. A randomised trial of the effects of prophylactic daily Aspirin in British male doctors. *Br Med J* 1988;**296**:313–16.
58. Grambow DW, Topol EJ. Effect of maximal medical therapy on refractoriness of unstable angina pectoris. *Am J Cardiol* 1992;**70**:577–81.

13

Antiplatelet therapy in the peripheral vascular system

Scott M Surowiec, Victor J Weiss and Alan B Lumsden

Introduction

Patients who have undergone prior peripheral arterial interventions or who have peripheral vascular disease (i.e. 'high-risk patients') are at increased risk of 'vascular' events (e.g. non-fatal myocardial infarction (MI), non-fatal stroke, or vascular death). Antiplatelet therapy has been shown to be effective in reducing these events. Furthermore, many peripheral vascular interventions fail at some point in their natural history: technical errors or hypotension during or after the operation cause early graft failures; intimal hyperplasia produces mid-term failures; and recurrent atherosclerosis causes very late graft failures. Platelets play an important role in all of these processes. It is hoped that by inhibiting platelet responses, antiplatelet agents could prolong the life of a vascular intervention.

Several antiplatelet agents are used commonly in vascular patients. Aspirin is the prototype antiplatelet agent. It has been studied the most and its effects and mechanism of action are well described. Questions arise as to the efficacy of antiplatelet agents in decreasing cardiovascular events (e.g. stroke, MI, or limb loss), prolonging graft patency, and decreasing intimal hyperplasia. There is also controversy over the use of single or multiple agents. Many of the clinical trials that evaluated the effects of aspirin after peripheral vascular procedures included the concomitant use of dipyridamole.

It is now clear that no increase in efficacy is added to aspirin by using dipyridamole.[1] Ticlopidine and clopidogrel appear to offer some increased protection compared with aspirin but with increased side-effects and cost.

The specific antiplatelet agents and their mechanisms of action have been detailed in Section II of this book. The purpose of this chapter is to outline the current evidence regarding the use of antiplatelet therapy in several areas pertinent to vascular surgery. Specific recommendations are given at the end of the chapter regarding the use of these antiplatelet agents.

Platelets and the formation of intimal hyperplasia

Intimal hyperplasia is a process that threatens all vascular interventions. This includes the insertion of all types of vascular grafts or the ultimate effectiveness of balloon angioplasty, surgical endarterectomy, or stent implantation. Direct and indirect evidence demonstrates that platelets contribute substantially to intimal hyperplasia formation; however, these interactions are complex. It is believed currently that platelets act in concert with several other factors when producing intimal hyperplasia.[2] The role of platelets is thought to result from either the induction of smooth muscle cell *replication* in intimal lesions[3] or by the *migration* of smooth muscle cells into the intima (with their proliferation mediated by other factors).[4,5]

Platelets play a role in the formation of intimal hyperplasia arising from the injury and reparative processes inherent in the creation of a new vascular anastomosis, the breakage of a plaque during angioplasty, the stripping of the intima during endarterectomy, or the placement of an intraluminal stent. Flowing blood exposed to an injured vessel or foreign material causes an immediate cascade of blood proteins to attach to the vessel wall and subsequent platelet adhesion to this surface. These platelets begin the sequence of events leading to clotting or to intimal hyperplasia. Exaggerated platelet responses are seen with several clinical risk factors common to 'vascular patients'. Increased age,[6] heavy smoking,[2] diabetes mellitus,[7] and hyperlipidemia[8] all tend to increase platelet aggregability or to cause platelet hyperactivity. These patients are prone not only to develop atherosclerosis and to need a vascular procedure but they are also prone to develop intimal hyperplasia and subsequent graft failure once the vascular procedure is complete.

Antiplatelet agents may be useful in decreasing intimal hyperplasia in humans but direct morphometric studies of the effects of antiplatelet agents on intimal hyperplasia in human grafts are difficult to obtain. Several animal studies have evaluated antiplatelet agents and the prevention of intimal hyperplasia in peripheral vascular surgery. Six studies have been performed on dogs; three[9–11] found no decrease in intimal hyperplasia with ibuprofen, aspirin, dipyridamole, or cod liver oil, while three studies[12–14] showed decreased intimal hyperplasia with these same agents. One study of rabbits showed no decrease in intimal hyperplasia when the rabbits were given aspirin[15] and had autologous, small-caliber, arterial end-to-side anastomosis. Two studies of primates[16,17] have shown that both aspirin and dipyridamole decrease intimal hyperplasia in vein bypass and small-caliber PTFE grafts at 4 months. A recent study by Mawatari and colleagues[18] evaluated the efficacy of new agent 4-cyano-5, 5-*bis*[methoxyphenyl]-4-pentenoic acid (E5510) on intimal hyperplasia in a poor distal runoff canine model. They found that E5510 significantly reduced intimal hyperplasia at 1 and 4 weeks compared with aspirin, and that aspirin had no effect compared with controls. Thus, antiplatelet therapy has shown mixed results in several animal models. Indirect evidence is available that these agents may be useful in decreasing intimal hyperplasia in humans, based on several trials that look at patency of vein and prosthetic bypasses (see next section). It appears certain that, while platelets play some role in the formation of intimal hyperplasia, other factors are involved in this process.

Peripheral vascular reconstructive surgery

Intermittent claudication occurs in 3–5% of men over the age of 50 years, and non-invasive testing has revealed femoropopliteal occlusive disease in 12–36% of the population. It is estimated that symptomatic occlusive peripheral vascular disease occurs in 2–3% of men and 1% of women over age 50–65 years.[19] Femoropopliteal bypass is indicated for those patients with disabling claudication, gangrene, rest pain, or a threatened limb when the superficial femoral or popliteal artery is continuous with any of its three terminal branches. A more distal bypass is indicated if the isolated popliteal artery is occluded. Combined, 4-year cumulative patency of a reversed saphenous vein graft averages 69–77% for an above-knee popliteal graft and 62% for a below-knee graft. With PTFE at 4 years, these patencies decrease to 40–60% for an above-knee graft and to 21% for a tibial PTFE graft.[20] Considering these patency rates, even under ideal conditions, a need for adjunctive pharmacologic therapy to increase patency is evident.

Platelets also play a role in the immediate failure of peripheral arterial bypass grafts. Platelet interactions and adhesion to a disrupted intimal surface (between 10 min and 48 h after intimal injury) lead to thrombosis and this process mediates many early graft failures. Multiple clinical trials have been conducted to study the effect of aspirin, dipyridamole, and ticlopidine on the patency of vein and prosthetic arterial bypass grafts in the lower extremities.

Several early studies have looked at platelet uptake and adherence to various vascular graft materials in animal and human models. Oblath and colleagues[21] studied the effect of aspirin (325 mg per day) and dipyridamole (50 mg twice a day) on platelet adherence in knitted Dacron internal velour and polytetrafluoroethylene (PTFE) femoral artery bypass grafts in dogs. Twice as many platelets adhered to the Dacron grafts compared with the PTFE grafts. Dogs treated preoperatively with aspirin and dipyridamole had reduced platelet adherence by 62% for Dacron and 63% for PTFE at 2 hours following placement. These results were statistically significant. Pumphrey and colleagues[22] studied the effects of dipyridamole (75 mg three times a day) and aspirin (325 mg three times a day) on the adherence of indium[111]-labeled autologous platelets in Dacron aortofemoral grafts and PTFE femoropopliteal grafts in humans. They found decreased platelet deposition on the Dacron grafts in those patients treated with

aspirin and dipyridamole, but no effect was seen in the PTFE grafts. Goldman and colleagues[23] studied the effects of aspirin (300 mg three times a day) and dipyridamole (75 mg three times a day) on Dacron, PTFE, and saphenous vein grafts in humans. Again, a significant reduction in platelet adherence was seen with the use of aspirin and dipyridamole (given together) in the Dacron and PTFE grafts. They noted, however, that vein grafts accumulated few, if any, labeled platelets and aspirin and dipyridamole had no further influence. This same group[24] compared retrospectively the group of patients that occluded their bypass graft with those that maintained a patent graft (both at 1-year follow-up). They found that those patients who had a patent graft had an initial 63% reduction in platelet adherence 1-week after the graft was placed. When the analysis was restricted to prosthetic grafts, those patients who maintained an open graft had a 55% reduction in platelet adherence during the first week of the life of the graft. Overall, these studies have led to disfavor in the use of Dacron for smaller-diameter arterial bypass operations, a preference for the use of native vein, and the use of aspirin adjunctively when PTFE has to be used for lower-extremity femoropopliteal bypass operations.

Other authors have tried to establish whether aspirin is more effective if given before or after a vascular procedure. Mackey and colleagues[25] studied platelet function and uptake after a single dose of aspirin given during interposition grafting of a baboon carotid artery with a 4 mm Dacron graft. They found that a single 5.4–7.4 mg/kg dose of aspirin decreased platelet uptake and improved 2-h patencies in these grafts. Stratton and Ritchie[26] tried to determine whether aspirin and dipyridamole could inhibit platelet deposition on older grafts in humans. They administered aspirin (325 mg three times a day) and dipyridamole (75 mg three times a day) to 18 patients with Dacron aortic bifurcation grafts in place for a mean of 43 months. They noted a 13% reduction in platelet deposition in the treatment group, which was statistically significant. They concluded that the effects of aspirin and dipyridamole are more pronounced in recently implanted grafts, which accumulate more platelets than older grafts.[27] It appears that aspirin has its greatest effect (and needs to be 'onboard') at the time of graft placement, especially in Dacron large-diameter grafts, when platelet deposition is at its greatest. However, with large-caliber aortoiliac grafts this benefit may be of limited clinical significance.

Many clinical trials have evaluated the clinical efficacy of antiplatelet agents on extending the patency of lower-extremity peripheral arterial bypass grafts. A collaborative overview of all such trials up until 1994 has been published.[28] The authors found 39 trials of antiplatelet therapy versus control for patients with peripheral vascular procedures. Only those trials that were properly randomized and that systematically evaluated vascular graft and arterial occlusion were included in the report. Only 11 trials[29–41] of these 39 trials met the authors' criteria. Eight of these trials evaluated some combination of aspirin and dipyridamole, two evaluated sulphinpyrazone, and one trial evaluated ticlopidine. The results for vein bypasses and prosthetic bypasses were not differentiated. Mean follow-up (for all 11 trials) was 13.8 months, and 1318 patients were in the composite study. A 33% gross reduction in graft occlusion was seen for those patients taking antiplatelet therapy (193 occlusions were seen in the antiplatelet therapy group, and 288 occlusions were seen in the control group). This result was highly statistically significant for this large composite patient group. The authors found that no single antiplatelet agent or regimen was more effective than any other and that there was a trend (which was not statistically significant) towards a slightly better effect with somewhat lower doses of aspirin.

Data in regards to the use of antiplatelet agents in saphenous vein bypasses has been conflicting.[42–44] McCollum and colleagues[30] studied the effects of aspirin 600 mg per day and dipyridamole 300 mg per day on 549 patients undergoing only saphenous vein bypasses at a mean follow-up of 3 years. They found an improved patency of 6% (78% versus 72%) at 1 year, 8% (70% versus 62%) at 2 years, and 1.0% (61% versus 60%) at 3 years, but none of these results achieved statistical significance. Patients in the aspirin and dipyridamole group, however, had a significantly lower incidence of MI or cerebrovascular accident at 3 years. A more recent multicenter clinical trial[45] has compared the effect of ticlopidine on the long-term patency of saphenous vein bypass grafts in 243 patients. Patients received either 500 mg of ticlopidine a day or placebo for 2 years after operation. The 2-year cumulative patency was improved 19% (82% versus 63%) for those patients on ticlopidine, and these results achieved statistical significance ($p = 0.002$). The weight of evidence appears to support the use of antiplatelet therapy in saphenous vein reconstructions. Newer agents (such as ticlopidine) need to be compared with the current standard, aspirin, prior to widespread recommendation for their use.

The benefits of antiplatelet therapy must, nevertheless, be balanced against the risk of bleeding. Possible bleeding complications can occur before, during, or after any vascular procedure. In the Antiplatelet Trialists' Collaboration,[28] in patients having peripheral vascular treatment, the gross incidence of fatal bleeding was 0.15% in those patients taking antiplatelet agents and 0.03% in the control patients, and this result was almost statistically significant ($p = 0.06$). The incidence of non-fatal major bleeds before the procedure (2.2% versus 0.91%) and the incidence of reoperation, hematoma, or infection due to bleed before the procedures (5.5% versus 3.6%) were, however, greater and statistically significant. Thus there is an increased risk of bleeding complications in patients who are undergoing vascular procedures and who are taking antiplatelet therapy.

Hemodialysis access

The autogenous radial-cephalic arteriovenous fistula has remained the gold standard for long-term hemodialysis since its introduction in 1966. Unfortunately, many older patients in need of dialysis have vessels that are unsuitable for direct fistula creation. In 1976, expanded polytetrafluoroethylene (PTFE) was introduced[46] and is now the preferred prosthetic material used for long-term hemodialysis. Hirth[47] reports that, in 1990, 65% of patients beginning dialysis had a PTFE graft. Despite widespread use, however, there has been no improvement in their patency since they were first introduced. Graft failure occurs, on average, 18 months following implantation, generally as a consequence of venous anastomotic neointimal hyperplasia.[48–50] Graft thrombectomy adds a paltry 3 months to the life of the graft. Again, questions arise as to the role of platelets in the failure of these grafts and to the possibility that the life of these conduits could be prolonged with antiplatelet therapy.

The effects of hemodialysis on platelets are not, however, completely understood. Platelets are thought to become activated by the artificial surfaces present in the dialysis circuit or

by the high shear forces and turbulent flow present in the arteriovenous graft. Windus and colleagues[51] performed a time-course study of indium[111]-labeled platelets in PTFE loop grafts. They found that a marked dialysis-associated enhancement of platelet deposition occurred in the arterial side of the loop near the dialysis needle. The authors found almost no deposition of platelets in the two patients with native vein fistulas that they studied. In another study,[52] these same authors tried to determine if aspirin and ticlopidine could modify this response. They found that in this same region of high platelet deposition, aspirin resulted in a 33% reduction in deposition, and ticlopidine resulted in a 44% reduction in platelet deposition. These studies suggest that antiplatelet agents can partially inhibit platelet deposition in a PTFE dialysis graft, and that native vein fistulas have much less platelet deposition during the course of dialysis.

Several clinical trials have been published evaluating the efficacy of antiplatelet therapy in extending the life of a hemodialysis access graft. The Antiplatelet Trialists' Collaboration addressed some of these studies in 1994[28] by compiling nine trials[53–62] that systemically monitored vascular occlusion as an endpoint. Five trials utilized ticlopidine, two trials utilized aspirin, and two trials utilized sulphinpyrazone. In all, 418 patients (206 receiving antiplatelet therapy and 212 controls) were randomized for a mean of only 2.4 months' treatment. Vascular occlusion was seen in 34/206 (17%) patients in the antiplatelet group, and in 82/212 (39%) in the control group. This result was highly statistically significant, even when considering separately those patients with PTFE grafts and those patients with fistulas. Clearly, trials with longer follow-up periods are needed in this area.

In another study,[63] 107 patients with PTFE

grafts were randomized to receive aspirin, dipyridamole, placebo, or aspirin and dipyridamole over 18 months. Of those patients with new PTFE grafts ($n = 73$), a statistically significant benefit was seen for those patients in the dipyridamole group (79% patency at 18 months versus 60% patency for placebo); however, patients taking aspirin alone had the highest risk of thrombosis (20% patency at 18 months). The authors attributed the increased thrombosis rate in the aspirin therapy group to the fact that cyclo-oxygenase inhibition by aspirin may shift platelet arachidonic acid metabolism in the direction of 12-HETE, which has been shown to mediate the PDGF-induced chemoattraction of vascular smooth muscle cells. This would paradoxically increase the rate of neointimal hyperplasia and increase the rate of graft thrombosis. No morphometric data were provided in this study.

Considering the available data, it is surprising that few hemodialysis patients at our institution are on some form of antiplatelet therapy. The effects of antiplatelet agents are more complex in these uremic patients, however, and the choice of agent is still debatable. Few studies have addressed these issues, perhaps because of the transient nature of the grafts in dialysis patients. The accelerated nature of intimal hyperplasia seen in these conduits makes hemodialysis access a unique human model to study.

Carotid endarterectomy

Carotid endarterectomy is accepted[64] for the treatment of *symptomatic* patients with recent, non-disabling carotid artery ischemic events and ipsilateral (70–99%) carotid artery stenosis. It is not beneficial, however, for symptomatic patients with 0–29% stenosis. There is uncertainty about the potential benefits for symptomatic patients with 30–69% stenosis.

For those patients with *asymptomatic* disease, the indications for carotid endarterectomy are more complex. For patients with a surgical risk (of stroke or death) of less than 3% and a life-expectancy of at least 5 years, ipsilateral carotid endarterectomy is acceptable for stenotic lesions ($\geq 60\%$) irrespective of contralateral artery status. For patients with a surgical risk greater than 3%, no absolute indications for carotid endarterectomy exist. Platelets adhere to the endarterectomy surface immediately after carotid flow is restored and can lead to thrombosis or restenosis at the endarterectomy site.

Antiplatelet agents 'on board' the patient at the time of endarterectomy can decrease platelet accumulation at the time of surgery. Platelet deposition at carotid endarterectomy sites in humans has been studied[65] by injecting autogenous indium[111]-labeled platelets less than 30 min after carotid endarterectomy. A 35% increase in platelet deposition was seen in endarterectomized carotid arteries compared with controls in the early postoperative period, which reduced to baseline over time. A similar study was performed[66] with the addition of daily 990 mg aspirin and 225 mg dipyridamole in one-half of the study subjects. The antiplatelet agents were started 5 days preoperatively and continued 5 days postoperatively, with measurements taken 24 h after surgery. A 43% reduction in labeled platelet accumulation at the endarterectomy site in the aspirin/dipyridamole treated group was seen.

The clinical implications of reducing platelet accumulation at the time of endarterectomy are still being evaluated, however. Antiplatelet therapy could decrease the perioperative stroke/MI rate, the risk of early postoperative thrombosis, or the risk of late restenosis. In a controlled trial of aspirin (1300 mg/day) versus placebo after carotid endarterectomy, there were fewer strokes or death in the aspirin group, but few patients were studied and few events took place.[67] In another study[68] patients that received 1000 mg aspirin per day after carotid endarterectomy had a higher probability of survival postoperatively than those receiving placebo. A similar study[69] compared low-dose aspirin with placebo in 301 patients who had recently undergone carotid endarterectomy. At 21 months postoperatively, aspirin reduced the risk of transient ischemic attack (TIA), stroke, acute myocardial infarction, and vascular death by 11%, but this result was not statistically significant. Another study[70] evaluated 232 patients who were randomized to receive either 75 mg aspirin (started preoperatively and continuing for 6 months) or placebo. The patients in the aspirin group had significant reductions in the numbers of strokes and a trend towards decreased mortality. Harker and colleagues[71] administered 975 mg aspirin and 225 mg dipyridamole to evaluate restenosis following carotid endarterectomy. No significant benefit utilizing aspirin and dipyridamole was seen on serial duplex examination to detect restenosis at a 12-month follow-up.

Patients with a history of TIAs or prior stroke are at high-risk for non-fatal MI, non-fatal stroke, and vascular death. The Antiplatelet Trialists' Collaboration[72] showed a 22% odds reduction for these events with antiplatelet therapy in this group of patients, and unlike previous studies, results were independent of gender. Likewise, the Mayo Asymptomatic Carotid Endarterectomy Study[73] compared the effects of low-dose aspirin with carotid endarterectomy in patients with asymptomatic carotid stenosis. The patients in the surgical group were not given aspirin, and the trial had to be terminated early because of significantly more MIs and TIAs occurred in the surgical group. Most

events were unrelated to the surgery but were ascribed to an absence of aspirin. The results of the above two studies support the use of aspirin in the preoperative and postoperative periods in patients with carotid stenosis who undergo carotid endarterectomy.

Endovascular interventions: percutaneous transluminal angioplasty and stenting

The recent explosion in catheter-based technologies has led to an increasing use of percutaneous transluminal angioplasty (PTA) and the insertion of stents into the vascular system to treat atherosclerotic occlusive disease. Compared with conventional bypass techniques, common iliac angioplasty has a 10–20% lower overall patency rate.[74] The patency of aortoiliac bypass is 65–95% at 5 years; at 10 years it is 62–78%.[75] Considering the intimal appearance of an angioplastied blood vessel, it is remarkable that these patency rates are comparable at all. Transluminal angioplasty produces endothelial desquamation, splitting of the atheromatous plaque, and frequent intimal dissection of the recipient vessel.[76] Platelets can adhere to this ragged intimal surface and lead to acute clot formation. Platelets may also play a role in intimal hyperplasia mediated restenosis (through PDGF-mediated stimulation of vascular smooth muscle cells) and late failure of these interventions.

Several authors have studied platelet deposition after peripheral angioplasty and the effects of antiplatelet agents in altering this process. The effects of pre-procedure aspirin (variable doses) compared with no aspirin on indium[111]-platelet deposition 2 hours after peripheral arterial angioplasty were observed retrospectively.[77] Not surprisingly, less platelet deposition was found in the men ($n = 9$) who had received aspirin within the 4 days prior to angioplasty than in the men ($n = 8$) who had not received aspirin for at least 2 weeks prior to angioplasty. Platelet deposition after angioplasty was also studied[78] in 92 patients who underwent PTA of iliac artery stenoses ($n = 20$), femoropopliteal artery stenoses ($n = 41$), or femoropopliteal occlusions ($n = 31$). The significant increase in platelet accumulation at 4–6 hours after angioplasty (compared to 1 or 2 days after the procedure) was similar between the group receiving high-dose (1000 mg) aspirin compared with those receiving low doses (100 mg). Platelet accumulation tended to occur in segments with more severe dissection. Interestingly, of the 22 patients that developed angiographically verified recurrences after PTA (at 4.5 months median follow-up), 21 were from the femoropopliteal segment and platelet accumulation was found to be significantly *less* ($p < 0.05$) in patients with recurrence than those without recurrent stenosis or obstruction. These data suggest that the use of antiplatelet agents to prevent platelet deposition after PTA may not be useful for prevention of restenosis, especially for femoropopliteal stenoses.

The significance of acute platelet accumulation at peripheral angioplasty sites was also studied[79] in 30 patients with stenoses and 8 patients with occlusions. Daily aspirin (75 mg) was given to all patients after angioplasty. Two acute occlusions were seen, and five patients developed clinical angioplasty failure at 9-month follow-up. A significant increase in platelet accumulation was found in the patients with acute occlusion ($n = 2$), and a trend toward higher accumulation found in patients who developed restenosis. Acute platelet accumulation thus plays a role in acute angioplasty failure, and antiplatelet agents seem to be effective in reducing these occlusions.

Antiplatelet agents may also be useful in increasing primary patency after peripheral arterial PTA.

In 223 patients undergoing PTA of the common iliac, external iliac, femoral, and popliteal arteries, those given aspirin (25 mg) and dipyridamole (200 mg) twice-daily the day before PTA for 3 months had no difference in patency (as assessed by the surgeon) or lifestyle status (as assessed by the patients) over a 12 month follow-up period between the two groups was found.[80] Unfortunately, in this study follow-up angiography was not obtained, and the dose of aspirin used was quite low.[81] In another study of 160 patients who underwent femoropopliteal PTA[81] the effect of 25 mg aspirin and 200 mg dipyridamole both twice a day (started 24–48 h before PTA) was compared with phenprocoumon oral anticoagulation. Angiographic patency of the stenotic/occluded segment was used as the endpoint in the study. In the patients treated with phenprocoumon anticoagulation, 53% had a patent segment at the end of their follow-up compared with 69% of patients treated with aspirin and dipyridamole. These differences were not statistically significant ($p = 0.18$) but show a slightly better performance of aspirin and dipyridamole. The dose of aspirin used in this study was again quite low. In another randomized study, patency after successful femoropopliteal PTA and in patients taking 330 mg aspirin combined with 75 mg dipyridamole three times daily was significantly better than in those taking placebo.[82] In a more recent study,[83] reocclusions at the site of peripheral angioplasty occurred exclusively in patients in whom aspirin failed to inhibit ADP and collagen-induced platelet aggregation using whole-blood aggregometry. This suggests that it may be possible and important to predict those patients who are at an elevated risk of reocclusion following peripheral PTA. Antiplatelet therapy appears to offer some benefit in prolonging primary patency of angioplastied vessels, although larger studies may be needed to achieve statistical significance.

No controlled clinical trials exist with regard to the use of antiplatelet agents and the insertion of peripheral arterial stents. Numerous coronary stent trials are available, however, and it appears that *combined* antiplatelet therapy (aspirin plus ticlopidine) is associated with a significant reduction in ischemic complications within the first 4 weeks of stent implantation.[84] In addition, it appears that combined antiplatelet therapy is important in reducing acute and subacute thrombotic occlusions of the stents, especially in high-risk patients.[85] It is uncertain if this data can be applied to the larger stents used in the peripheral arterial system, and studies in this area are needed.

Antiplatelet agents and the venous system

Venous disease can generally be divided into two types: obstructive or refluxive. Obstructive venous disease in the lower extremities classically results from deep venous thrombosis in the deep veins in the leg, with resultant pain, dependent edema, varicosity formation, and possible leg ulceration from cutaneous venous hypertension. Apart from the role of antiplatelet therapy in high-risk patients and preventing vascular events, little is known about the role of antiplatelet therapy in preventing the complications of venous insufficiency. Most available data pertain to the prevention of deep venous thrombosis in the perioperative period.

The prevention of deep venous thrombosis is of prime importance to the surgeon. Approximately one-quarter of general surgical patients and about one-half of orthopedic surgical patients develop deep venous thrombosis in the perioperative period.[86] These thromboses can produce vascular damage and chronic venous insufficiency in the lower extremities and some may embolize to the lungs. The Antiplatelet Trialists' Collaboration compiled a meta-analysis of clinical trials comparing all forms of antiplatelet therapy versus controls in patients undergoing general surgical, traumatic orthopedic, or elective orthopedic cases.[87] Thromboses were sought prospectively by venography or radiolabelled fibrinogen uptake testing, and outcome measures were undertaken for deep venous thrombosis, pulmonary embolism, and mortality. The antiplatelet agents used in these studies were heterogeneous (variable doses and combinations of aspirin, dipyridamole, ticlopidine, sulphinpyrazone, suloctidil, and hydroxychloroquine), were begun for several days preoperatively, and they were continued for 1–3 weeks postoperatively. Of 45 surgical trials totaling 4654 patients, antiplatelet therapy was associated with a 25% gross reduction in deep venous thrombosis and a 63% gross reduction in pulmonary embolus. These results were highly statistically significant considering the large number of patients compiled.

Classically, antiplatelet agents have been discontinued at least 2 weeks prior to any surgical procedure for avoidance of intraoperative or postoperative bleeding. The above data suggest that, for major general surgical and orthopedic procedures, this plan may be detrimental and lead to an increased risk of deep venous thromboses and pulmonary embolus. The Antiplatelet Trialists noted that there was no significant difference in fatal bleeding between the two groups of patients but that there was a significant excess of major bleeding, reoperation, wound hematoma, or infection from bleeding (7.8% antiplatelet therapy versus 5.6% controls). This data is similar to that seen in the peripheral arterial reconstruction series, and indicates that the use of antiplatelet agents in the perioperative period is not without risk.

Conclusions and recommendations

Current evidence suggests that patients with peripheral arterial insufficiency, carotid disease, or renal failure should be taking low-dose aspirin (80–325 mg/day), unless contraindicated. This recommendation is based on the repeated findings that antiplatelet therapy is effective in reducing the rates of vascular events (non-fatal MI, non-fatal stroke, or vascular death) in high-risk patients. This low-dose aspirin should be continued for as long as the patient can tolerate it.

For patients undergoing peripheral arterial bypass surgery, aspirin should be given preoperatively and continued for at least 1 year (for patients with vein grafts) or indefinitely (for patients with prosthetic grafts). It is still too early to recommend higher doses of aspirin (or the other newer antiplatelet agents) for more

specific indications in vascular surgery until more data become available. For patients undergoing dialysis with a PTFE graft, the data supports the use of antiplatelet therapy (dipyridamole over aspirin) but further studies are certainly needed in this area. Patients undergoing angioplasty or stenting should be covered with 1–2 weeks' antiplatelet therapy before and after the procedure. Patients undergoing major abdominal surgery or orthopedic surgery should also be covered with antiplatelet therapy both in the pre- and postoperative periods.

The (modified) adage, 'an aspirin a day keeps the vascular surgeon away' seems to ring true with the current data presented here. Our knowledge about the effects of platelets and their influence on intimal hyperplasia and the patency of vascular interventions is still in its infancy. As more information about specific molecular interactions becomes available, the vascular surgeon may then possess agents to interrupt (and not just slow down) the processes that lead to graft failure. To date, no such agents exist, and our final recommendations are tempered by the hope that soon this will be possible.

References

1. Edwards JM, Taylor LM, Porter JM. Drugs in vascular disease. In: Sidaway AN, Sumpio BE, DePalma RG (eds), *The Basic Science of Vascular Disease* (Armonk, NY: Futura, 1997).

2. Schwarcz TH, Dobrin PB Role of platelets in the formation of intimal hyperplasia. In: Dobrin PB (ed.) *Intimal Hyperplasia* (Austin, TX: RG Landes, 1994) 177–92.

3. Friedman RJ, Stemerman MB, Wenz B, et al. The effect of thrombocytopenia on experimental arteriosclerotic lesion formation in rabbits. Smooth muscle cell proliferation and re-endothelialization *J Clin Invest* 1977;**60**:1191–201.

4. Fingerle J, Johnson R, Clowes AW, Majesky MW, Reidy MA. Role of platelets in smooth muscle cell proliferation and migration after vascular injury in the rat carotid artery. *Proc Natl Acad Sci* 1989;**86**:8412–16.

5. Reidy MA, Fingerle J, Lindner V. Factors controlling the development of arterial lesions after injury, *Circulation* 1993;**86**:III-43–III-46.

6. Vilen L, Jacobsson S, Wadenvik H, Kutti J. ADP-induced platelet aggregation as a function of age in healthy humans. *Thromb Haemost* 1989;**61**:490–92.

7. Davi G, Catalano I, Averna M, Notarbartolo A, Strano A. Thromboxane biosynthesis and platelet function in type II diabetes mellitus. *N Engl J Med* 1990;**322**:1769–74.

8. Stuart MJ, Gerrard JM, White JG. Effect of cholesterol on production of thromboxane B_2 by platelets in vitro. *N Engl J Med* 1987;**302**:6–10.

9. McCready RA, Price MA, Kryscio RJ, Hyde GL, Mattingly SS, Griffen WO. Failure of antiplatelet therapy with ibuprofen (Motrin) to prevent neointimal fibrous hyperplasia. *J Vasc Surg* 1985;**2**:205–13.

10. DeCampli WM, Kosek JC, Mitchell RS, Handen CE, Miller DC. Effects of aspirin, dipyridamole, and cod liver oil on accelerated myointimal proliferation in canine venoarterial allografts. *Ann Surg* 1988;**208**:746–54.

11. Landymore RW, MacAulay MA, Fris J. Effect of aspirin on intimal proliferation and tissue cholesterol in long-term experimental bypass grafts, *Eur J Cardiothorac Surg* 1992;**6**:422–6.

12. Dobrin PB, Golan J, Fareed J, Blakeman B, Littoy FN. Pre- vs postoperative pharmacologic inhibition of platelets: effect on intimal hyperplasia in canine autogenous vein grafts. *J Cardiovasc Surg* 1992;**33**:705–9.

13. Landymore RW, Karmazyn M, MacAulay MA, Sheridan B, Cameron CA. Correlation between the effects of aspirin and dipyridamole on platelet function and prevention of intimal hyperplasia in autologous vein grafts. *Can J Cardiol* 1988;**4**:56–9.

14. Landymore RW, MacAulay M, Sheridan B, Cameron C. Comparison of cod-liver oil and aspirin-dipyridamole for the prevention of intimal hyperplasia in autologous vein grafts. *Ann Thor Surg* 1986;**41**:54–7.

15. Quinones-Baldrich WJ, Ziomed S, Henderson T, Moore WS. Patency and intimal hyperplasia: the effect of aspirin on small arterial anastomosis. *Ann Vasc Surg* 1988;**2**:50–56.

16. Hagen PO, Wang ZG, Mikat EM, Hackel DB. Antiplatelet therapy reduces aortic intimal hyperplasia distal to small diameter vascular prostheses (PTFE) in nonhuman primates. *Ann Surg* 1982;**195**:328–39.

17. McCann RL, Hagen PO, Fuchs JCA. Aspirin and dipyridamole decrease intimal hyperplasia in experimental vein grafts. *Ann Surg* 1980;**191**:238–43.

18. Mawatari K, Komori K, Kuma S, et al. The inhibition of canine vein graft intimal thickening using a newly developed antiplatelet agent. *J Cardiovasc Surg* 1997;**38**:359–65.

19. Boobis LH, Bell PR. Can drugs help patients with lower limb ischemia? *Br J Surg* 1982;**69**:S-17.

20. Dalman RL, Taylor LM. Basic data related to infrainguinal revascularization procedures. *Ann Vasc Surg* 1990;**4**:309–12.

21. Oblath RW, Buckley FO, Green RM, Schwartz

SI, DeWeese JA. Prevention of platelet aggregation and adherence to prosthetic vascular grafts by aspirin and dipyridamole. *Surgery* 1978; **84**:37–44.

22. Pumphrey CW, Chesebro JH, Dewanjee MK, et al. In vivo quantitation of platelet deposition on human peripheral arterial bypass grafts using indium[111]-labeled platelets. Effect of dipyridamole and aspirin. *Am J Cardiol* 1983;**51**:796–801.

23. Goldman MD, Simpson D, Hawker RJ, Norcott HC, McCollum CN. Aspirin and dipyridamole reduce platelet deposition on prosthetic femoro-popliteal grafts in man. *Ann Surg* 1983;**198**:713–16.

24. Goldman M, Hall C, Dykes J, Hawker RJ, McCollum CN. Does [111]indium-platelet deposition predict patency in prosthetic arterial grafts? *Br J Surg* 1983;**70**:635–8.

25. Mackey WC, Connolly RJ, Callow AD, et al. Aspirin decreases platelet uptake on Dacron vascular grafts in baboons. *Ann Surg* 1984;**200**:93–9.

26. Stratton JR, Ritchie JL. Reduction of indium[111]-platelet deposition on dacron vascular grafts in humans by aspirin plus dipyridamole. *Circulation* 1986;**73**:325–30.

27. Stratton JR, Thiele BL, Ritchie JL. Natural history of platelet deposition on Dacron aortic bifurcation grafts in the first year after implantation in man. *Am J Cardiol* 1983;**52**:371.

28. Antiplatelet Trialists' Collaboration. Collaborative overview of randomised trials of antiplatelet therapy—II: maintenance of vascular graft or arterial patency by antiplatelet therapy. *Br Med J* 1994;**304**:159–68.

29. Green RM, Roedersheimer LR, DeWeese JA. Effects of aspirin and dipyridamole on expanded polytetrafluoroethylene graft patency. *Surgery* 1982;**92**:1016–26.

30. McCollum C, Alexander C, Kenchington G, Franks PJ, Greenhalgh R. Antiplatelet drugs in femoropopliteal vein bypasses: a multicentre trial. *J Vasc Surg* 1991;**13**:150–62.

31. Donaldson DR, Salter MCP, Kester RC, Rajah SM, Kester RC. The influence of platelet inhibition on the patency of femoro-popliteal Dacron bypass grafts. *Vascular Surgery* 1985;**19**:224–30.

32. Sheehan SJ, Salter MCP, Donaldson DR, Rajah SM, Kester RC. Five-year follow-up of long-term aspirin/dipyridamole in femoropopliteal Dacron bypass grafts. *Br J Surg* 1987;**74**:330.

33. Boehme K, Loew, Artik N. Planung, durchfuhrung und biometrische auswertung einer langzeitstudie mit azetysalizylsaure. *Med Welt* 1977;**28**:1163–6.

34. Ehresmann U, Alemany J, Loew D. Prophylaxe von rezidivverschlussen nach revaskularisationseingriffen mit acetylsalicylsaure. *Med Welt* 1977;**28**:1157–62.

35. Comberg HU, Janssen EJ, Diehm C, et al. Sulphinpyrazone versus placebo nach operativer rekonstruktion der oberschenkeletage bei arterieller verschlusskrankheit. *Vasa* 1983;**12**:172–8.

36. Blakely JA, Pogoriler G. A prospective trial of sulphinpyrazone after peripheral vascular surgery. *Thromb Haemost* 1977;**38**:238.

37. Castelli P, Basellini A, Agus GB, et al. Thrombosis prevention with ticlopidine after femoropopliteal thromboendarterectomy. *Int Surg* 1986;**71**:252–5.

38. Goldman MR, McCollum C. A prospective randomized study to examine the effect of aspirin plus dipyridamole on the patency of prosthetic femoro-popliteal grafts. *Vasc Surg* 1984;**18**:217–21.

39. Goldman MR, Hall C, Dykes J, Hawker RJ. Does [111]Indium-platelet deposition predict patency in prosthetic arterial grafts? *Br J Surg* 1983;**70**:635–8.

40. Zekert F. Klinische anwendung von aggregationshemmern bei arterieller verschlusskrankheit. In: Zekert F (ed.) *Thrombosen, Embolien und Aggregationshemmer in der Chirurgie*, (Stuttgart, Schattauer, 1975) 68–72.

41. Harjola P, Meurala H, Frick HH. Prevention of early reocclusion by dipyridamole and ASA in arterial reconstructive surgery. *J Cardiovasc Surg* 1981;**22**:141–4.

42. Kohler TR, Kaufman JL, Kacoyanis G, et al. Effect of aspirin and dipyridamole on the patency of lower extremity bypass grafts. *Surgery* 1984;**96**:462–6.

43. Sheehan SJ, Salter MCP, Donaldson DR, Rajah SM, Kester RC. Five-year follow-up of long-term aspirin/dipyridamole in femoropopliteal Dacron bypass grafts. *Br J Surg* 1987;**74**:330 [Abstract].

44. Rosenthal D, Mittenthal MJ, Ruben DM, et al. The effects of aspirin, dipyridamole, and warfarin in femorodistal reconstruction: long-term results. *Am Surg* 1987;**53**:477–81.

45. Becquemin JP. Effect of ticlopidine on the long-term patency of saphenous vein bypass grafts in the legs. *N Engl J Med* 1997;**337**: 1726–31.

46. Baker LD, Johnson JM, Goldfarb D. Expanded polytetrafluoroethylene (ePTFE) subcutaneous arteriovenous conduit: an improved vascular access for chronic hemodialysis. *TASAIO* 1976; **22**:382–7.

47. Hirth RA, Turenne MN, Woods JD, et al. Geographic and demographic variations in vascular access. In: Henry ML, Ferguson RM (eds), *Vascular Access for Hemodialysis—V*, (Tucson AZ: Precept Press, 1997) 22–31.

48. Palder SB, Kirkman RL, Whittemore AD, Hakim RM, Lazarus JM, Tilney NL. Vascular access for hemodialysis. *Ann Surg* 1986;**202**: 235–9.

49. Zibari GB, Rohr MS, Landreneau MD, et al. Complications from permanent hemodialysis vascular access. *Surgery* 1988;**104**:681–6.

50. Bell DD, Rosenthal JJ. Arteriovenous graft life in chronic hemodialysis. *Arch Surg* 1988;**123**: 1169–72.

51. Windus DW, Santoro S, Royal HD. The effects of hemodialysis on platelet deposition in prosthetic graft fistulas. *Am J Kidney Dis* 1995;**26**: 614–21.

52. Windus DW, Santoro SA, Atkinson R, Royal HD. Effects of antiplatelet drugs on dialysis-associated platelet deposition in polytetrafluoroethylene grafts. *Am J Kidney Dis* 1997;**29**: 560–4.

53. Kaegi A, Pineo GF, Shimizu A, Trivedi H, Hirsh J, Gent M. Arteriovenous shunt thrombosis, prevention by sulphinpyrazone. *N Engl J Med* 1974;**290**:304–6.

54. Kaegi A, Pineo GF, Shimizu A, Trivedi H, Hirsh J, Gent M. The role of sulphinpyrazone in the prevention of arterio-venous shunt thrombosis. *Circulation* 1975;**52**:497–9.

55. Harter H, Burch J, Majerus P, et al. Prevention of thrombosis in patients on hemodialysis by low-dose aspirin. *N Engl J Med* 1979; **301**:577–9.

56. Andrassy K, Malluche H, Barnefield H, et al. Prevention of p.o. clotting of av cimino fistula with acetylsalicyl acid. Result of a prospective double blind study. *Klin Wochenschr* 1974; **52**:348–9.

57. Ell S, Mihindukulasuriya JCL, O'Brien JR, Polak A, Vernham G. Ticlopidine in the prevention of blockage of fistulae and shunts. *Haemostasis* 1982;**12**:180 [Abstract 322].

58. Fiskerstrand CE, Thompson IW, Burnet ME, Williams P, Anderton JL. Double-blind randomized trial of the effect of ticlopidine in arteriovenous fistulas for hemodialysis, *Artif Organs* 1985;**9**:61.

59. Dodd NJ, Turney JH, Weston MJ. Ticlopidine preserves vascular access for hemodialysis. In: *Proceedings of the VI International Congress of Mediterranean League against Thrombosis*, Monte Carlo: 1980. [Abstract 326F].

60. Grontoft K, Mulec H, Gutierrez A, Olander R. Thromboprophylactic effect of ticlopidine in arteriovenous fistulas. *Scand J Urol Nephrol* 1985;**19**:55–7.

61. Schnitker J, Koch HF. Multizentrische studie ticlopidin thromboseprophylaxe in der hamodialyse (Munich, Labaz, 1983) [Labaz internal report].

62. Michie DD, Womboldt DG. Use of sulphinpyrazone to prevent thrombus formation in arteriovenous fistulas and bovine grafts of patients on hemodialysis. *Curr Ther Res* 1977;**22**:196–204.

63. Sreedhara R, Himmelfarb J, Lazarus JM, Hakim R. Anti-platelet therapy in graft thrombosis: results of a prospective, randomized, double-blind study. *Kidney Int* 1994; **45**:1477–83.

64. Biller J, Feinberg WM, Castaldo JE et al. Guidelines for carotid endarterectomy: a statement for healthcare professionals from a Special Writing Group of the Stroke Council, American Heart Association. *Circulation* 1998;**97**:501–9.

65. Stratton JR, Zierler RE, Kazmers A. Platelet deposition at carotid endarterectomy sites in humans. *Stroke* 1987;**18**:722–7.

66. Findlay JM, Lougheed WM, Gentili F, Walker PM, Glynn MF, Houle S. Effect of perioperative platelet inhibition on postcarotid endarterectomy mural thrombus formation. *J Neurosurg* 1985;**63**:693–8.

67. Fields WS, Lemak NA, Frankowski RF, Hardy RJ. Controlled trial of aspirin in cerebral ischemia, Part II: surgical group. *Stroke* 1978; **9**:309–19.

68. Kretschmer G, Pratschner T, Prager M, et al. Antiplatelet treatment prolongs survival after carotid bifurcation endarterectomy. Analysis of the clinical series followed by a controlled trial, *Ann Surg* 1990;**211**:317–22.

69. Boysen G, Sorensen PS, Juhler M, et al. Danish very-low-dose aspirin after carotid endarterectomy. *Stroke* 1988;**19**:1211–15.

70. Lindblad B, Persson NH, Takolander R, Bergqvist D. Does low-dose acetylsalicylic acid prevent stroke after carotid surgery? A double-blind, placebo-controlled randomized trial. *Stroke* 1993;**24**:1125–8.

71. Harker LA, Bernstein EF, Dilley RB, et al. Failure of aspirin plus dipyridamole to prevent restenosis after carotid endarterectomy. *Ann Int Med* 1992;**116**:731–6.

72. Antiplatelet Trialists' Collaboration. Collaborative overview of randomized trials of antiplatelet therapy—I: Prevention of death, myocardial infarction, and stroke by prolonged antiplatelet therapy in various categories of patients. *Br Med J* 1994;**308**:81–106.

73. Mayo Asymptomatic Carotid Endarterectomy Study Group. Results of a randomized controlled trial of carotid endarterectomy for asymptomatic carotid stenosis. *Mayo Clin Proc* 1992; **67**:513–18.

74. Kotb MM, Kadir S, Bennett JD, Beam CA. Aortoiliac angioplasty: is there a need for other types of percutaneous intervention? *J Vasc Interv Radiol* 1992;**3**:67.

75. Brothers TE, Greenfield LJ. Long-term results of aortoiliac reconstruction, *J Vasc Interv Radiol* 1990;**1**:49.

76. Block PC, Myler RK, Stertzner S, Fallon JT. Morphology after transluminal angioplasty in human beings. *New Engl J Med* 1981; **305**:382–5.

77. Cunningham DA, Kumar B, Siegel BA, Gilula LA, Totty WG, Welch MJ. Aspirin inhibition of platelet deposition at angioplasty sites: demonstration by platelet scintigraphy. *Radiology* 1984;**151**:487–90.

78. Minar E, Ehringer H, Ahmadi R, et al. Platelet deposition at angioplasty sites and its relation to restenosis in human iliac and femoropopliteal arteries. *Radiology* 1989;**170**: 767–72.

79. Nyamekye I, Costa D, Raphael M, Bishop CR: Thrombosis and restenosis after peripheral angioplasty: does acute [111]Indium-platelet accumulation predict angioplasty outcome? *Eur J Vasc Endovasc Surg* 1997;**13**:388–93.

80. Study group on pharmacologic treatment after PTA. Platelet inhibition with ASA/dipyridamole after percutaneous balloon angioplasty in patients with symptomatic lower limb arterial disease. A prospective double-blind trial. *Eur J Vasc Surg* 1994;**8**:83–8.

81. Dai-Do D, Mahler F. Low-dose aspirin combined with dipyridamole versus anticoagulants after femoropopliteal percutaneous transluminal angioplasty. *Radiology* 1994;**193**:567–71.

82. Heiss HW, Just H, Middleto D, Deichsel G. Reocclusion prophylaxis with dipyridamole combined with acetylsalicylic acid following PTA. *Angiology* 1990;**9**:263–9.

83. Mueller MR, Salat A, Stangl P, et al. Variable platelet response to low-dose ASA and the risk of limb deterioration in patients submitted to peripheral arterial angioplasty. *Thromb Haemost* 1997;**78**:1003–7.

84. Kastrati A, Schuhlen H, Hausleiter J, et al. Restenosis after coronary stent placement and randomization to a 4-week combined antiplatelet or anticoagulant therapy: six-month angiographic follow-up of the Intracoronary Stenting and Antithrombotic Regimen (ISAR) trail. *Circulation* 1997;**96**: 462–7.

85. Schuhlen H, Hadamitzky M, Walter H, Ulm K, Schomig A. Major benefit from antiplatelet therapy for patients at high risk for adverse cardiac events after coronary Palmaz-Schatz stent placement: analysis of a prospective risk stratification protocol in the intracoronary stenting and antithrombotic regimen (ISAR) trial. *Circulation* 1997;**95**:2015–21.

86. Kakkar VV. Prevention of venous thromboembolism. *Clin Haematol* 1981;**10**:543–82.

87. Antiplatelet Trialists' Collaboration. Collaborative overview of randomized trials of antiplatelet therapy—III: reduction in venous thrombosis and pulmonary embolism by antiplatelet prophylaxis among surgical and medical patients. *Brit Med J* 1994;**308**:235–46.

14

Atrial fibrillation

Stephen L Kopecky

Introduction

Atrial fibrillation is present in less than 1% of the general population, but its prevalence increases with age to approximately 2–5% in those over 60 years of age.[1-3] In a population-based study, non-valvular atrial fibrillation (non-rheumatic) has been associated with a 5-fold increase in the risk of stroke, and up to 35% of all patients with non-valvular atrial fibrillation eventually suffer a stroke.[4,5] The yearly risk of stroke in all non-valvular atrial fibrillation patients varies depending on coexisting diseases but, in general, is approximately 5%. In many of the patients that develop a stroke, the underlying etiology is cardiogenic embolism from thrombus originating in the left atrium and especially the left atrial appendage;[6] because of this the prevention of the formation of thrombus is one of the cornerstones in the treatment of patients with atrial fibrillation.

It is believed that there are different patho-physiologic sources of cardiogenic emboli in patients with stasis, and that those having a large left ventricle with a low ejection fraction, or those with a large left atrium, may be best benefited by anticoagulation. Patients that may have structural abnormalities, however, such as mitral annular calcification, mitral valve prolapse, or aortic atherosclerosis in which platelet activation may play a larger role in the initiation of thrombus formation, may derive adequate stroke reduction from antiplatelet agents such as aspirin. The role atrial fibrillation plays in the formation of thromboemboli was elucidated by the population based Mayo Clinic study of patients under 60 years of age with lone atrial fibrillation. This study showed that atrial fibrillation, per se, is not a significant risk factor for stroke.[7] In this cohort of 97 patients followed over three decades, the incidence of stroke without anticoagulation was less than 1% per year. This was a well-defined group of patients; specifically, the following comorbid diseases and conditions were excluded: coronary artery disease according to clinical or laboratory criteria; hyperthyroidism; valvular heart disease including mitral valve prolapse; congestive heart failure; cardiomyopathy; chronic obstructive pulmonary disease; cardiomegaly apparent on the chest radiograph; hypertension on medication, or an average systolic pressure above 140 mmHg or diastolic pressure above 90 mmHg on three separate occasions; age over 60 years at the time of diagnosis; lack of electrocardiographic (ECG) documentation of atrial fibrillation; identifiable and potentially life-shortening non-cardiac disease (including insulin-dependent diabetes); and the occurrence of atrial fibrillation only during trauma, surgery, or an acute medical illness. What this study showed convincingly was that atrial fibrillation without the above comorbid diseases did not place patients at high risk for stroke. Only when other diseases are present that promote stasis of blood flow (such as left ventricular systolic failure) or structural changes that possibly promote platelet activation (such as valvular disease) are patients at significantly increased risk for cardiogenic thromboemboli.

Risk factors for stroke

When deciding which antiplatelet or anticoagulant strategy for stroke reduction, it is important to understand which comorbid conditions increase the patient's risk for stroke. In the SPAF I (Stroke Prevention in Atrial Fibrillation) study, clinical and echocardiographic risk factors for stroke were delineated.[8] The clinical risk factor predictors for stroke were: history of hypertension, prior history of arterial thromboembolism, or congestive heart failure in the last 3 months.[9] The echocardiographic risk factors for stroke were found to be left atrial enlargement over 2.5 cm/m^2 of body surface area and fractional shortening 25% or lower.[10] When none of these risk factors were present, the thromboembolic rate per year was 1%; with one or two risk factors present, 6%; and when three risk factors or more were present, patients had an 18.6% thromboembolic rate per year. Clearly, this data supported the notion that there were certain clinical and echocardiographic risk factors that are predictors of subsequent thromboembolic events. Subsequently, the Atrial Fibrillation Investigators pooled the data from the five major randomized studies available at the time.[8,11–14] This pooling of data of almost 4000 patients was not just a meta-analysis in that similar risk factors were compared with the same definition (i.e. hypertension defined as systolic blood pressure over 160 mmHg). This combined effort showed that risk for stroke rose in patients

with prior stroke or TIA, a history of diabetes, a history of hypertension, a history of congestive heart failure in the last 100 days, or increasing age. Patients with coronary artery disease without congestive heart failure, however, were not at increased risk for stroke. Also, the type of atrial fibrillation, for example, paroxysmal compared with chronic, or the duration of the arrhythmia, for example new-onset compared with long-standing atrial fibrillation, were not found to increase a patient's risk for stroke. This data indicated that there were clearly patients who may not warrant long-term anticoagulation because of the inherently low risk for stroke if their atrial fibrillation was not accompanied by certain comorbidities. Buttressing this argument are the approximately 200 patients with lone atrial fibrillation in the abovementioned studies who have never suffered a stroke throughout follow-up. Subsequent studies, including the SPAF II[15] and SPAF III[16] trials, have not randomized lone atrial fibrillation patients below 60 years of age in their cohort owing to their low risk for stroke. The issue, however, is what is the definition of lone atrial fibrillation and which patients are adequately prophylaxed against stroke using an antiplatelet agent such as aspirin.

The Stroke Prevention in Atrial Fibrillation III study was designed to follow prospectively patients with atrial fibrillation at low risk for stroke, while giving them enteric-coated aspirin (325 mg/day).[17] Patients were excluded if they had the following:

(1) Impaired left ventricular function manifested by congestive heart failure in the last 100 days or fractional shortening to 25% or less using M-mode echo;
(2) Systolic blood pressure over 160 mmHg at entry on two blood pressure measurements taken on separate days or one blood pres-

sure measurement over 160 mmHg and either the other over 150 mmHg or documented systolic blood pressure over 160 mmHg in the last 3 months;

(3) Prior ischemic stroke, TIA, or systemic embolus;

(4) Female over age 75 (this elderly female group was found in earlier SPAF studies to be at an increased risk for stroke, purely on the basis of age without concomitant comorbidities).

The primary endpoint was ischemic stroke or systemic emboli. In all, 892 patients, of which 78% were male, were followed for a mean of 2.0 years. The mean age was 67 years and 16% of patients were over age 75 years at the time of entry (none of these were female). Of interest, 28% of patients had intermittent atrial fibrillation, 45% had a history of hypertension, 13% had a history of diabetes, 7% had a history of myocardial infarction and 9% had a history of congestive heart failure. One-third of the patients were on anticoagulants at the time of entering the study and were taken off this drug and placed on aspirin. The mean left atrial diameter on echo was 4.6 cm and 25% of patients had left atrial size over 5 cm. In all patients, the primary event rate was 2.2% per year (95% conference interval (CI) 1.6–3.0) with an ischemic stroke rate of 2.0% per year (95% CI 1.5–2.8) and a disabling ischemic stroke rate of 0.8% per year (95% CI 0.5–1.3). In the patients without a history of hypertension (55%), the primary event rate was only 1.1% per year (95% CI 0.6–2.0) and the disabling stroke rate was 0.4% (95% CI 0.2–1.1). This study clearly showed that patients could be prospectively identified as being at low risk for stroke with atrial fibrillation and given adequate prophylaxis against stroke with the use of enteric-coated aspirin (325 mg/day).

Benefit from antiplatelet agents in randomized clinical trials

It is important to review many of the excellent randomized clinical trials that have been done to evaluate the risk factors for stroke and the benefit from antiplatelet agents. The only antiplatelet agent that has been studied in randomized trials against placebo for primary prevention of stroke is aspirin.

The three studies of the effects of aspirin on stroke are the AFASAK,[11] SPAF I,[8] and BAATAF.[12] In the AFASAK study, 1007 patients with chronic atrial fibrillation were randomized to either aspirin (80 mg/day), anticoagulation, or placebo. The embolic rate per year in the placebo group, aspirin group, and anticoagulation group was 6.3%, 5.9%, and 1.5%, respectively. There was a significant reduction of 75% in the embolic rate per year in the anticoagulation group. From this study, the conclusion was made that the antiplatelet agent, aspirin, was unable to reduce the thromboembolic stroke rate and that it was no more effective than placebo. In the SPAF I study, 1244 patients, of which one-third had paroxysmal atrial fibrillation, were also randomized to placebo, enteric-coated aspirin (325 mg), or warfarin. The embolic rate per year was very similar to the AFASAK study with a rate of 6.3%, 3.2% and 1.6% in the placebo, aspirin, and warfarin groups respectively. This resulted in an 81% risk reduction for emboli using anticoagulation but also over a 40% reduction in the embolic rate of patients taking aspirin compared with placebo. Finally, in the BAATAF study, 420 patients in which approximately one-third had paroxysmal atrial fibrillation, were randomized to either placebo or anticoagulation. However, approximately half of the patients on placebo were taking aspirin. The embolic rate was 3% per year in the placebo group versus 0.4% per year in the anticoagulation group with a significant reduction of 86%.

These studies indicated that the aspirin as an antiplatelet stroke reduction agent was inferior to anticoagulation in a general population of patients with atrial fibrillation. Nevertheless, aspirin was shown to reduce the embolic rate when compared to placebo. The efficacy of aspirin in these studies, however, was not consistent in that in the SPAF study there was a 40% reduction with embolic rates in patients given 325 mg of enteric-coated aspirin per day compared with placebo ($p < 0.02$). In the AFASAK study, there was an 18% reduction with 75 mg per day of aspirin when compared with placebo. The differential effects may be accounted for because the AFASAK study included patients with a higher rate of heart failure, which may have led to stasis and thereby less benefit from aspirin compared with warfarin therapy. In the BAATAF study, there was no reduction in embolic rates by p.r.n. aspirin. The aspirin efficacy in these three studies was not uniform and was found to be better in patients with atrial fibrillation who were under 75 years of age. Finally, the Antiplatelet Trialist Collaboration found that pooling multiple trials showed a significant reduction in stroke with oral anticoagulants compared with aspirin.[18] In the SPAF II study, the rate of thromboembolism was different in low- and high-risk patients. The differential benefit of aspirin in patients grouped by risk criteria and age is shown in Figure 14.1.

Lone atrial fibrillation

The SPAF III and the Mayo Clinic studies differed in their approach to patients with lone

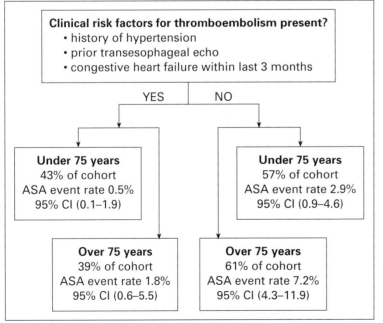

Figure 14.1
Rate of thromboembolism in low- and high-risk patients in the SPAF II study.

atrial fibrillation. In the SPAF III study, patients with lone atrial fibrillation were excluded from the low-risk cohort. Lone atrial fibrillation as defined in the Mayo Clinic study was, however, a more restrictive group and accounted for approximately 3% of all patients in Olmsted County, Minnesota with atrial fibrillation. The group of patients with atrial fibrillation at low risk for stroke as defined by the SPAF III study contained approximately 25% of all atrial fibrillation patients.

It has been recommended that patients with lone atrial fibrillation either receive aspirin or no therapy; however, no matter which low-risk group of patients are being treated, there is approximately a 5% incidence per year of the patient developing high-risk criteria. Therefore, these patients should be checked annually, at least, for evaluation of the development of comorbidities that may increase their risk for stroke.

Risk of bleeding

The risk of intracranial hemorrhage in patients treated with antiplatelet agents (aspirin) in the randomized trials is low, at less than 0.5% per year. This is important since the risk of intracranial hemorrhage and a major bleed in patients on anticoagulants is higher than with aspirin and, in some patients, the risk of major bleed on anticoagulation is greater than the risk of thromboemboli. Risk factors for hemorrhage on anticoagulation therapy are as follows:

Increasing age;
Dementia;
Alcoholism;
Unstable gait;
Occupational hazards;
Uncontrolled hypertension (>180/100 mmHg);
Prior severe hemorrhage (on therapeutic INR);
Requirement for non-steroidal anti-inflammatory drugs (NSAIDs);
Gastrointestinal/genitourinary bleeding.

In a study by Hylek and Singer,[19] the odds ratio of intracranial hemorrhage increased with advancing age: the odds ratio for patients under 65 years was 1.0; in those between 65 and 79 years it was 1.6; and in patients 80 years or more the odds ratio was 2.8. The average age of atrial fibrillation in the USA is 75 years; therefore, almost half of patients with atrial fibrillation are at risk for significant bleeds, simply because of their age. In the six randomized trials (SPAF I, SPINAF, EAFT, CAFA, AFASAK, BAATAF) over 38 000 patients were screened but only approximately 4000 patients were enrolled into the studies (Table 14.1). Therefore, almost 90% of patients were excluded from these randomized trials of anticoagulants, and the primary reasons were contraindications to anticoagulation or inability to give informed consent. Therefore, the issue of antiplatelet therapy in patients with atrial fibrillation gains importance since many patients with this disease are unable to safely take or self-monitor this chronic medication. In addition, all patients with significant bleeding risk factors were excluded from the randomized trials in which oral anticoagulant therapy was a treatment arm.

Combined anticoagulant and antiplatelet therapy

The SPAF investigators also evaluated the possibility of combining low-dose warfarin with aspirin in an attempt to decrease stroke rates while lowering the bleeding complication rate. In the SPAF III study,[16] a group at high risk for stroke was defined as females over 75

Study	Screened	Excluded	Contraindications to anticoagulants	Enrolled
SPAF I[8]	18 376	17 046	7267	1330
SPINAF[14]	7982	7444	3206	528
EAFT[6]	4007	3338	2338	669
CAFA[13]	5384	5006	2961	378
AFASAK[11]	2546	1539	505	1007
BAATAF[12]				428
Total	38 295	34 373	16 277	4340

Table 14.1
Percentage of patients with atrial fibrillation who have contraindications to anticoagulants.

years of age, patients with prior history of stroke or TIA, congestive heart failure in the last 3 months, or systolic blood pressure over 160 mmHg. Patients were randomized to either warfarin (with an INR of 2–3), or warfarin (with an INR of 1.2–1.5) plus enteric-coated aspirin (325 mg/day). The primary event rate of stroke and thromboemboli was significantly higher in the combined arm than in the warfarin only arm. The study was stopped early after interim analysis showed that in 1011 patients, the primary event rate

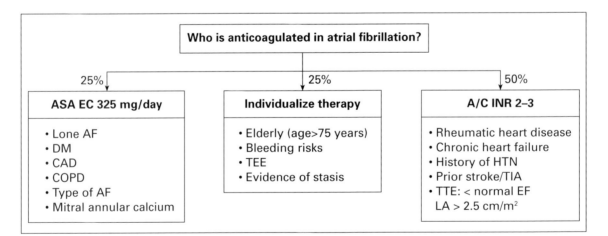

Figure 14.2
Diagram showing percentage of patients in given categories given anti-coagulation therapy. AF, atrial fibrillation, DM, diabetes mellitus; CAD, chronic arterial disease; COPD, chronic obstructive pulmonary disease; TEE, transesophageal echo; HTN, hypertension; TIA, transient ischemic attack; TTE, transthoracic echo; EF, ejection fraction; LA, left atrium.

was 8.6% in the aspirin/low-dose warfarin arm compared with 2.6% in the standard-dose warfarin arm. Of interest, the bleeding rates between the two groups were not significantly different; comparing aspirin plus warfarin with warfarin only groups the annual major bleeding rate was 2.5% versus 2%, the annual intracranial bleed rate was 0.6% versus 0.4% and, in a subgroup of patients over age 75 years, the annual major bleed rate was 3.6% versus 2.4%. The study indicated that combination therapy, at least with an INR in the rate of 1.2–1.5, when combined with aspirin is ineffective in lowering the thromboembolic

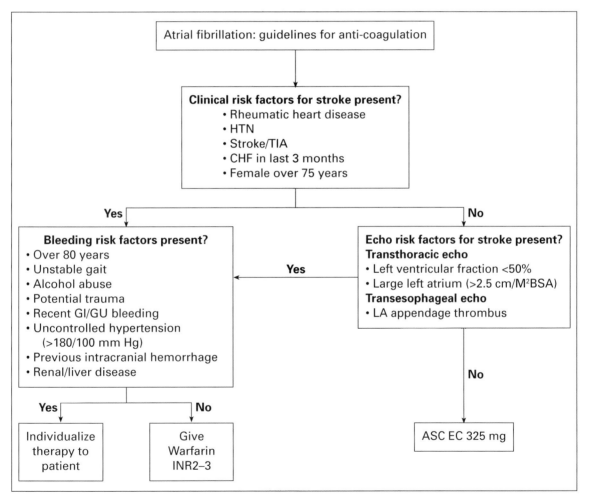

Figure 14.3
Diagram showing criteria for anticoagulation therapy in those with atrial fibrillation. CHF, chronic heart failure; HTN, hypertension; GI, gastrointestinal; GU, genitourinary; LA, left atrium; INR, international normalized ratio; TIA, transient ischemic attack.

rate; there actually being a trend towards an increase in significant bleed rate in elderly patients. It may be, however, that aspirin combined with warfarin with a higher INR rate in the 1.7–2.0 range may be beneficial, but other studies will need to be performed.

Summary

In summary, the lessons that have been learned from patients with lone atrial fibrillation and those at low risk for stroke, as determined by the Atrial Fibrillation Investigators, indicate that these subgroups may be treated safely with antiplatelet agents for stroke prophylaxis (Figure 14.2). It is always important to risk-stratify patients not only for stroke but also for bleeding risk factors since a significant portion of the patients with atrial fibrillation are aged over 75 years and therefore, have an increased intrinsic risk for bleeding with any stroke prophylactic regimen, especially full-dose anticoagulation. Patients that have rheumatic heart disease, a recent history of congestive heart failure, a history of hypertension, prior stroke or TIA, or echo risk factors for stroke (lowered normal ejection fraction or left atrial size more than 2.5 cm/m^2 body surface area) are at an increased risk for stroke and should be treated with anticoagulants with an INR of 2 to 3 if no bleeding con-

Predictor	Thromboembolism rate (%/year)
No risk factors	1.0
1 or 2 risk factors	6.0
≥ 3 risk factors	18.6

Table 14.2
Risk stratification using clinical and transthoracic echo predictors.

traindications are present. Patients that are aged over 75 years, have bleeding risks with, or have transesophageal echo evidence of stasis should be given tailored therapy with either anticoagulants or aspirin. Finally, approximately 25% of patients with atrial fibrillation can be safely given prophylaxis using enteric-coated aspirin (325 mg/day). A suggested algorithm for thromboemboli and bleeding-risk stratification is shown in Figure 14.3 and a risk predictor of thromboembolism in Table 14.2. No other antiplatelet agent has been specifically studied in clinical trials but future efforts need to be planned with other antiplatelet agents, for example clopidogrel and the oral GP IIb/IIIa platelet inhibitors.

References

1. Kannel WB, Abbott RD, Savage DD, Macnamara PM. Epidemiologic features or chronic atrial fibrillation: The Framingham Study. *N Engl J Med* 1982;**306**:1018–22.
2. Ostrander LD, Brandt RL, Kjelsberg MO, Epstein FH. Electrocardiographic findings among the adult population of a total natural community. Tecumseh, Michigan. *Circulation* 1965;**31**:888–98.
3. Martin A. Atrial fibrillation in the elderly. *Br Med J* 1977;**1**:712–16.
4. Wolf PA, Dawber TR, Thamer HE, Kannel WB. Epidemiologic assessment of chronic atrial fibrillation in risk of stroke: The Framingham Study. *Neurology (NY)* 1978; **28**: 973–7.
5. Sherman DG, Goldman L, Whiting RB, Jurgensen K, Kaste M, Easton D. Thromboembolism in patients with atrial fibrillation. *Arch Neurol* 1984;**41**:708–10.
6. Aberg H. Atrial fibrillation: a study of atrial thrombosis and systemic embolism in a necropsy material. *Acta Med Scandinavia* 1969;**185**:373–9.
7. Kopecky SL, Gersh BJ, McGoon MD, Whisnant JP, Holmes DR, Jr, Ilstrup DM, et al. The natural history of lone atrial fibrillation: a population-based study over three decades. *N Engl J Med* 1987;**317**(11):669–74.
8. Stroke Prevention in Atrial Fibrillation Investigators. Stroke Prevention in Atrial Fibrillation study: final results. *Circulation* 1991;**84**: 527–39.
9. SPAF Investigators. Predictors of thromboembolism in atrial fibrillation: I. Clinical features of patients at risk. *Ann Intern Med* 1992; **116**:1–5.
10. Stroke Prevention in Atrial Fibrillation Investigators. Predictors of thromboembolism in atrial fibrillation: II, Echocardiographic features—the patients at risk. *Ann Intern Med* 1992;**116**:6–12.
11. Petersen P, Boysen G, Godtfredsen J, et al. Placebo-controlled randomized trial of warfarin and aspirin for prevention of thromboembolic complications in chronic atrial fibrillation: the Copenhagen AFASAK Study. *Lancet* 1989;**1**:175–9.
12. The Boston Area Anticoagulation Trial for Atrial Fibrillation Investigators. The effect of low-dose warfarin on the risk of stroke in patients with non-rheumatic atrial fibrillation. *N Engl J Med* 1990;**323**:1505–11.
13. Connolly SJ, Laupacis A, Gent M, et al. Canadian Atrial Fibrillation Anticoagulation (CAFA) study. *J Am Coll Cardiol* 1991;**18**: 349–55.
14. Ezekowitz MD, Bridgers SL, James KE, et al. Warfarin in the prevention of stroke associated with nonrheumatic atrial fibrillation. *N Engl J Med* 1992;**327**:1406–12.
15. Stroke Prevention in Atrial Fibrillation Investigators. Warfarin versus aspirin for prevention of thromboembolism in atrial fibrillation: Stroke Prevention in Atrial Fibrillation II study. *Lancet* 1994;**343**:687–91.
16. The Stroke Prevention in Atrial Fibrillation Investigators. Adjusted dose warfarin versus low-intensity fixed-dose warfarin plus aspirin for high-risk patients with atrial fibrillation: Stroke Prevention in Atrial Fibrillation III Randomized Clinical Trial. *Lancet* 1996; **348**:633–8.
17. The SPAF III Writing Committee for the Stroke Prevention in Atrial Fibrillation Investigators. Patient with nonvalvular atrial fibrillation at low risk of stroke during treatment with aspirin. Stroke Prevention in Atrial Fibrillation III Study. *J Am Med Assoc* 1998; **279**: 1273–7.
18. Collaboration overview of randomised trials of antiplatelet therapy–I: Prevention of death, myocardial infarction and stroke by prolonged antiplatelet therapy in various categories of patients. Antiplatet Trialists' Collaboration. *Br Med J* 1994;**308**:81–106.
19. Hylek EM and Singer DE. Risk factors for intracranial hemorrhage in outpatients taking warfarin. *Ann Intern Med* 1994;**120**:897–902.

15

The use of antiplatelet therapy in interventional cardiology

Mahomed Salame, Spencer B King III and Nicolas Chronos

Introduction

Atheromatous plaque rupture, platelet activation with consequent thrombus formation and impairment of coronary arterial blood flow is a common theme linking acute coronary syndromes (ACS).[1–4] The importance of antiplatelet therapy in the treatment of acute myocardial infarction (MI) was amply demonstrated in the second International Study of Infarct Survival (ISIS-2).[5] At present, aspirin and, to a lesser extent, heparin, are used in nearly all patients with ACS. In spite of the improvements in prognosis using these treatments, the incidence of adverse events in patients with ACS remains significant[6–9] and demonstrates the need for further improvement.

Aspirin is a relatively weak antiplatelet agent. The documented beneficial coronary effects include the primary prevention of coronary artery disease,[10] improvement of outcome in chronic stable angina,[11,12] unstable angina,[13–15] and acute MI.[5] Aspirin therapy also improves saphenous vein graft patency rate after coronary artery bypass grafting.[16] In the field of percutaneous coronary intervention, preprocedural administration of aspirin reduces the risk of abrupt coronary closure by 50–75%.[17,18] It works by irreversibly acetylating and, thus inactivating, prostaglandin synthetase/cyclo-oxygenase[19] and results in the decreased formation of thromboxane A$_2$,[20] a potent agonist of platelet aggregation.[21] Nevertheless, platelets are able to undergo aggregation by several thromboxane A$_2$-independent pathways (via platelet activators such as thrombin, ADP, adrenaline, and subendothelial collagen)[22–24] thus limiting the antithrombotic effect of aspirin. In addition, cyclo-oxygenase is also needed for the synthesis of several antithrombotic prostaglandins by endothelial cells, including prostacyclin,[25] a potent platelet inhibitor. Apart from these pharmacodynamic limitations, aspirin causes the side-effect of gastritis, which results in a significant proportion of patients being non-compliant with the medication.

There has been a rapid expansion of trial data on the use of glycoprotein IIb-IIIa (GPIIb/IIIa) receptor antagonists across the full spectra of acute coronary syndromes. This is, in part, related to a recognition of the limitations of other antiplatelet agents and a better understanding of the mechanisms of platelet activation and aggregation. The realization that the GPIIb/IIIa platelet receptor is the final common pathway through which all the platelet agonists exhibit their effects on platelet aggregation, makes this receptor a promising target for antiplatelet therapy.[26]

Whilst there are several receptors involved in platelet activation and adhesion to the plaque surface, the GPIIb/IIIa receptor is the

Study	GPIIb/IIIa Antagonist	Clinical Setting	Composite Events Measured at 30 Days	Effect at 30 days
EPIC[27,28] (n = 2099)	Abciximab	High risk coronary angioplasty or atherectomy	Death, MI, urgent revascularization	Placebo : 12.8% Bolus : 11.4% Bolus 1 infusion : 8.3% (P = 0.008)
EPILOG[29] (n = 2792)	Abciximab	Coronary intervention	Death, MI, urgent revascularization	Placebo : 11.7% Std dose heparin : 5.2% Low dose heparin : 5.4% (P < 0.001)
CAPTURE[30] (n = 1265)	Abciximab	Refactory unstable angina undergoing intervention	Death, MI, urgent revascularization	Placebo : 15.9% Abciximab : 11.3% (P = 0.012)
EPISTENT[31] (n = 2399)	Abciximab	Stent-eligible coronary intervention	Death, MI, urgent revascularization	Stent alone : 10.8% PTCA + abciximab : 6.9% Stent + abciximab : 5.3% (P < 0.001)
RAPPORT[32] (n = 483)	Abciximab	Acute MI undergoing primary PTCA	Death, MI, or any revascularization	Placebo : 16.1% Abciximab : 13.3% (P = 0.32)
ERASER[33] (n = 225)	Abciximab	Elective stents	In-stent restenosis (% IVUS volume obstruction at 6 months)	Placebo : 32.4% 12 hr abciximab Rx : 37.7% 24 hr abciximab Rx : 34.2% (P = NS)
IMPACT-II[34] (n = 4010)	Eptifibatide	Coronary intervention	Death, MI, or urgent revascularization	Placebo : 11.4% Low dose Integrilin : 9.2% (P = .062) High dose Integrilin : 9.2% (P = 0.22)

RESTORE[35] (n = 2141)	Tirofiban	Unstable angina patients undergoing coronary intervention	Death, MI, or any revascularization	Placebo : 12.2% Abciximab : 10.3% (P = 0.160)
PURSUIT[36] (n = 10984)	Eptifibatide	Acute coronary syndromes (not necessarily intervened on)	Death, MI at 30 days	Placebo : 15.7% Eptifibatide : 14.2% (P = 0.04)
PRISM-PLUS[37] (n = 1915)	Tirofiban	Higher risk acute coronary syndromes (not necessarily intervened on)	Death, MI, or recurrent ischemia at 30 days	Placebo : 22.3% Tirofiban : 18.5% (P = 0.03)
ADMIRAL (n = 299)	Abciximab	Acute MI undergoing stent (85%)	Death, MI, ischemia-driven TVR	Placebo : 20% Abciximab : 10.7% (P = 0.03)

Table 15.1
Major clinical trials of intravenous GP IIb/IIIa antagonists for coronary intervention: clinical setting and 30-day results.

most numerous platelet receptor (with approximately 70 000 per platelet) and is the only one that mediates platelet aggregation. The GPIIb/IIIa receptor belongs to the integrin family of adhesion molecules and binds fibrinogen, von Willebrand factor, and vitronectin and is therefore able to form crossbridges between adjacent activated platelets. Platelet activation results in the exposure of the fibrinogen (RGD) binding site of the GPIIb/IIIa receptor on the cell surface.

The GPIIb/IIIa inhibitors are a relatively new class of compounds that offer several potential advantages to other currently available therapies. They are specific to platelets, inhibit platelet aggregation induced by all platelet agonists while not affecting platelet adhesion. Coller et al developed the murine 7E3 monoclonal antibody to the GPIIb/IIIa receptor[38] and this was further refined to a chimeric antibody (abciximab) in order to minimize the immune reaction to the foreign protein.[39] Likewise, several peptides and non-peptides that either contain or mimic the arginine-glycine-asparagine (RGD) necessary for the GPIIb/IIIa receptor–ligand binding have been developed. The small-molecule (either peptidic or non-peptidic) GPIIb/IIIa inhibitors (e.g. tirofiban (Aggrastat) and eptifibatide (Integrilin) are designed to avoid antibody-induced disadvantages such as immunogenicity, and to have rapid onset of action and rapid off-rate with cessation of drug delivery.

Ticlopidine is an orally active inhibitor of ADP-induced platelet aggregation.[40] Its use in interventional cardiology is presently restricted to patients receiving coronary stent implantation and its major limitation is the significant side-effect of neutropaenia.[41] Recently, the ticlopidine analogue, clopidogrel, was evaluated in the CAPRIE trial in over 19 000 patients, showing that it decreased ischemic events in patients with atherosclerotic vascular disease.[42] Recent data have also become available suggesting that clopidogrel may be superior to ticlopidine (from a safety standpoint) in patients undergoing coronary stenting.

In the fast-growing arena of antiplatelet therapy and with the wealth of data that is currently amassing, a contextual framework is needed by the practising cardiologist/physician, firstly to help in decisions on the optimum treatment for a given patient, and secondly, to provide a structure into which new trial data can be easily assimilated. In this chapter, both the efficacy and safety data from the clinical trials on GPIIb/IIIa antagonists are examined in the context of patients undergoing percutaneous coronary intervention across the full spectrum of coronary syndromes. A patient-orientated approach is taken rather than simply a drug or trial based-approach. In addition the data supporting the use of ticlopidine in coronary stenting are discussed.

Patients with unstable angina/non-Q-wave MI undergoing PCI

The prognostic benefit of using antiplatelet therapy in patients with unstable angina/non-Q-wave MI has been known for some time.[5] However, in spite of the use of aspirin and heparin, the morbidity and mortality of patients in this group remains significant.[43,44] The hope that an incremental prognostic benefit in patients with unstable angina/non-Q-wave MI could be obtained with the use of thrombolytic therapy[45] or coronary intervention[46] has not yet been observed. Possible causes for this lack of prognostic benefit of fibrinolytic therapy alone or intervention alone could have been insufficient efficacy of the antiplatelet therapy; since platelets are able to undergo aggregation through activation of several thromboxane A_2-independent pathways, the antithrombotic effect of aspirin is limited. It is not unreasonable therefore to postulate that GPIIb/IIIa inhibitors may improve outcome especially with the concomitant use of percutaneous intervention in this subgroup of patients.

Efficacy data on the use of adjunctive GPIIb/IIIa inhibitors

The EPIC study[27] was the first large trial to test the hypothesis that blocking the platelet GPIIb/IIIa receptor could prevent postprocedural ischemic complications in 'high-risk' patients undergoing PTCA or atherectomy. This was a prospective, randomized, double-blind trial in approximately 2100 patients using the chimeric monoclonal-antibody Fab fragment (c7E3 Fab) directed against the GPIIb/IIIa receptor. Patients were considered to be at high risk if they were: scheduled to undergo PTCA or atherectomy and had unstable angina with ECG changes despite medical therapy, were undergoing direct or rescue intervention within 12 h of an acute MI, or had high-risk lesion angiographic characteristics. Patients were randomized to receive a bolus and infusion of placebo, or a bolus of c7E3 Fab and an infusion of placebo, or a bolus and an infusion of c7E3 Fab and all patients received oral aspirin (325 mg) and intravenous heparin (non-weight-adjusted). The bolus of abciximab was started at least 10 min before the procedure whilst the infusion was continued for a 12-h period. The subgroup of patients ($n = 489$) with unstable angina or non-Q-wave myocardial infarction underwent PTCA or atherectomy within 1 h of the initiation of c7E3 Fab administration. Of all the EPIC subgroups, this subgroup had the greatest benefit of the treatment; the 30-day composite endpoint of death, acute MI or urgent revascularization in the patients randomized to bolus followed by infusion of the drug was reduced by 62% and by over 70% when the 470 patients who actually received the drug were analysed and compared to placebo. For death and MI at 30 days there was a striking 94% relative risk reduction. The 6-month composite end point of death or MI continued to show a significant 88% relative risk reduction (16.6% versus 2.0%; $p < 0.001$).[47] This reduction in the event rate at 6 months mainly reflected a decreased need for CABG or repeat percutaneous intervention. Most importantly, at 3 years, in the subgroup with highest risk (i.e in those with an evolving MI or unstable angina), there was a significant 60% reduction in mortality in the treated group compared with placebo (5.1% versus 12.7%).[28] The long-term prognostic advantage has been attributed to the prevention of periprocedural MI by abciximab on the basis of a correlation noted between periprocedural CK rises and risk of late cardiac death.

In view of the clear efficacy seen with the bolus plus infusion of abciximab in the EPIC trial at the expense of a doubling of major bleeding complications when compared to placebo, the EPILOG trial was designed to test the hypothesis that the benefit of abciximab could be extended to patients regarded to be at a 'lower risk' of post-angioplasty complications and also to evaluate whether the incidence of hemorrhage could be reduced without loss of efficacy by using weight-adjusted heparin (standard or low) dosing.

In EPILOG trial of patients undergoing urgent or elective PTCA, the trial was terminated by the data safety monitoring board owing to the clear superiority of the treatment for patients receiving abciximab; at 30 days, the primary composite endpoint being 5.4% (abciximab + 100 U/kg heparin), 5.2%

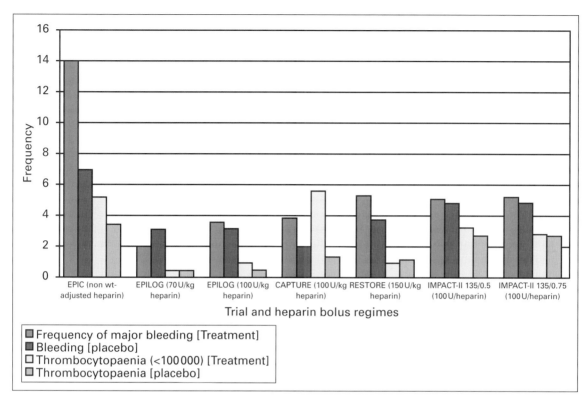

Figure 15.1
Frequency of major bleeding and thrombocytopaenia in the trials of adjunctive GPIIb/IIIa inhibitors in patients mandated for percutaneous coronary intervention.

(abciximab + 70 U/kg heparin) and 11.7% (placebo + standard-dose heparin) with an approximately 55% relative reduction for both abciximab arms compared with placebo. The benefits of abciximab were consistent irrespective of age, sex, body weight and perceived coronary risk.

Subgroup analysis of the EPILOG data reveals that patients who had clinical unstable angina at randomization treated with abciximab plus standard-dose heparin or abciximab plus low-dose heparin had a composite endpoint at 30 days of 5.0% and 4.8% respectively compared with placebo 12.2%. Similarly, patients with recent MI (less than 7

days prior to randomization) also benefited at 30 days; the corresponding figures being 4.2%, 7.5% and 11.1% respectively (Figure 15.1). At 6 months a significant reduction (>40%) in the composite end point of death, MI or *urgent* revascularization in both abciximab arms compared to placebo was seen. However, unlike the EPIC trial, there was an attenuation of the risk reduction for the composite end point of death, MI or *any* revascularization.

The CAPTURE trial also examined the use of abciximab in high-risk patients mandated to receive percutaneous intervention. This trial was designed to assess whether abciximab, given to patients with refractory unstable angina (documented by ECG, recurrent ischemia despite treatment with aspirin, nitrates and heparin), could improve outcome. The primary endpoints were death, MI or urgent revascularization. The CAPTURE study differed from the other studies in this group in that the patients had more severe refractory unstable angina and also the abciximab infusion was started 18–24 h before the percutaneous intervention and continued for only 1 h after PTCA. Abciximab resulted in a 29% reduction of composite primary endpoint at 30 days (11.3% versus 15.9%, $p = 0.012$) primarily by reducing the incidence of Q-wave MI ($p = 0.067$) and non-Q-wave MI, $p = 0.036$). Subgroup analyses of patients by risk showed similar results. Of interest, not only was the incidence of MI significantly reduced (by 53%) during and 24 h after the intervention (2.6% versus 5.5% for placebo); but so was the incidence of MI pre-intervention by 71% (0.6% versus 2.1%, $p = 0.029$), perhaps demonstrating that abciximab stabilized or passivated the plaque. In contrast to the EPIC results at 6 months, the composite outcome did not differ significantly between abciximab and placebo.

The efficacy and safety of tirofiban (a non-peptide inhibitor of the GPIIb/IIIa receptor), was evaluated in approximately 2100 patients receiving aspirin and heparin and undergoing coronary interventions using balloon angioplasty or directional atherectomy within 72 h of presentation of an episode of unstable angina or acute MI in the RESTORE trial. Patients in the treatment arm of RESTORE received a bolus (10 µg/kg body weight over 3 min) followed by a 36-h infusion (0.15 µg/kg/min) of tirofiban. During the period of drug effect the composite and the components of this endpoint, excluding death, were substantially reduced. At Day 2 post-intervention, there was a 38% reduction in composite end point of death, MI or *any form* of revascularization of the target-vessel noted (8.7% versus 5.4%; $p > 0.005$). Benefit was still present at 7 days with the reduction in composite endpoint being 27% (10.4% versus 7.6%; $p = 0.022$). However at 30 days, the relative reduction of the primary composite endpoint was reduced to half (16% relative reduction, $p = 0.16$) that seen at 24 h; tirofiban and placebo groups being 10.3% versus 12.2% respectively. The effect was, however, consistent across all the components of the composite endpoints as well as the relative benefit to all subgroups of patients treated.

A re-analysis of the RESTORE data according to the definitions used in EPIC study (thus re-defining the composite endpoint as death, MI or *urgent* revascularization) yielded a 24% relative reduction in composite endpoint at 30 days ($p = 0.052$). The data at Days 2 and 7 were similarly re-analysed showed a 40% ($p = 0.002$) and 30% ($p = 0.016$) relative reduction in the frequency of the re-defined composite endpoint. The 6-month follow up showed that the composite end point of death from any cause, new MI or target vessel revascularization was 24.1% in the tirofiban arm versus 27.1% in the placebo group ($p = 0.11$). It is important to note that the absolute reduction in events was 3% at 6 months, similar to the absolute reduction in the EPILOG study at 6 months. Coronary angiography in a subset at the 6-month follow-up showed that tirofiban did not reduce the incidence of restenosis, which was around 50% in each arm.[48] The angiographic restenosis rate is probably a reflection of both the trial-mandated low use of stents and the fact that patients who were re-studied were the symptomatic ones.

A study of over 4000 patients undergoing elective, urgent or emergency percutaneous revascularization has been undertaken in the IMPACT-II trial.[34] Although the study enrolled a broad cross-section of patients with coronary syndromes, it is relevant to the discussion on unstable angina/non-Q-wave MI because approximately 40% of the patients in the trial fell into this group. At 30 days, the primary composite endpoint of death, MI, repeat revascularization, was 11.4% in the placebo group, 9.2% in the 135/0.5 eptifibatide (135 µg/kg bolus + 0.5 µg/kg/min infusion) group ($p = 0.063$) and 9.9% in the eptifibatide (135 mg/kg − 0.75 µg/kg/min) group ($p = 0.22$). However, when analysed by treatment-analysis, the 135/0.5 regimen produced a significant reduction in the composite endpoint (11.6% versus 9.1%) ($p = 0.035$). Subgroup analyses by risk strata showed treatment effects to be similar to the primary analysis.

PRISM-PLUS,[37] although not primarily an interventional trial, is also discussed in this chapter as approximately 30% of the patients underwent percutaneous coronary intervention. This trial therefore give us an insight of 'real world' use of PTCA after trial of medical therapy for treating unstable angina/non-Q-wave MI. This randomized prospective double-blind trial evaluated tirofiban alone, heparin alone and tirofiban plus heparin in over 1900 patients with unstable angina/non-Q-wave MI. At 7 days, the combination of heparin and tirofiban significantly reduced the incidence of the composite endpoint of death, MI or refractory ischemia by 28% (17.9% versus 12.9%). Although the 475 patients that progressed to percutaneous intervention were not based on a randomized cohort, patients who underwent angioplasty appeared to derive a 43% reduction in the composite endpoint of death or MI from 48 h of pretreatment with tirofiban and heparin.

The largest clinical trial to date of any GPIIb/IIIa inhibitor, the PURSUIT trial,[36] evaluated bolus plus up to 72 h eptifibatide infusion (96-h infusion if coronary intervention was performed near the end of the 72-h period) versus placebo bolus and infusion in over 10 900 patients presenting with unstable angina or non-Q-wave MI. Approximately 60% of patients in each arm of this large trial went on to undergo cardiac catheterization and percutaneous coronary intervention at the discretion of the treating doctor. Although the progression on to percutaneous intervention was not subject to randomization, it is interesting to observe the outcomes of patients with unstable angina/non-ST-elevation-MI patients according to whether or not they underwent percutaneous coronary intervention (Table 15.2).

This finding in the placebo group, is in keeping with the VANQWISH trial[46] in that patients receiving aspirin and heparin for unstable angina, do not receive incremental benefit by undergoing PTCA. In patients receiving eptifibatide, however, there appears to be a lower incidence of the primary composite endpoint in those undergoing PTCA. This reopens the debate as to whether percutaneous intervention is preferable to conservative medical management for unstable angina in the new era of GPIIb/IIIa inhibitors.

Comparative efficacy of the different GPIIb/IIIa inhibitors in patients with unstable angina/non-Q-wave MI undergoing PCI

The efficacy of the various GPIIb/IIIa inhibitors in these trials is measured in terms of the frequency of endpoints (single or composite). The endpoint definitions in RESTORE differed subtly from those of the other interventional trials in this group (EPIC, EPILOG, CAPTURE and IMPACT-II). The

	Placebo	Eptifibatide	Absolute risk reduction	Relative risk reduction
Percutaneous coronary Intervention	16.7%	11.6%	5.1%	31%
No percutaneous coronary intervention	15.6%	14.5%	1.1%	7%

Table 15.2
The incidence of the primary composite end point of death or myocardial infarction in patients in the PURSUIT trial.

latter trials included in the composite endpoint only those repeat revascularization procedures (CABG and repeat angioplasty), which were performed on an urgent/emergency basis. The 30-day follow up efficacy data on the use of adjunctive GPIIb/IIIa with coronary intervention in acute MI/non-Q-wave MI, showed a significant drug-related benefit over placebo in EPIC, EPILOG, CAPTURE, and IMPACT-II. The re-analysis of the 30-day data from the RESTORE trial also showed drug-related benefit, demonstrating, the importance of endpoint definitions when comparing drug efficacy between trials. At 6 months, the EPIC data continued to show benefit of abciximab. Whilst the 6-month EPILOG efficacy data showed a similar significant reduction (over 40%) in the composite end point of death, MI or *urgent* revascularization in both abciximab arms compared with placebo (approx. 8.3% versus 14.7%; $p < 0.001$), however, there was an attenuation of the risk reduction for the composite end point of death, MI or *any* revascularization.

The reasons for the disparate effects on non-urgent revascularization rates between the EPIC trial, and the EPILOG and CAPTURE trials (which also used abciximab) are unknown.

In common with EPILOG, CAPTURE and IMPACT-II, the RESTORE did not show a statistically significant benefit at 6 months despite showing a 11% relative reduction in composite endpoint. Nevertheless, it is possible that the erosion of benefit by 6 months between EPIC trial and the RESTORE and IMPACT-II trials may in part be explained by the pharmacodynamics or pharmacokinetics of the agents used. It may be pertinent that the drugs used in IMPACT-II (eptifibatide) and RESTORE (tirofiban), both have short half-lives compared with abciximab. Although the details of the pharmacokinetics of abciximab appear complex, it is clear that the drug avidly binds to platelets, and that platelet-bound drug is still detectable using flow cytometry 2 weeks after administration. Platelet survival remains normal at around 10 days and this therefore implies that abciximab is transferred to newly released platelets. This redistribution phenomenon may result in prolonged biological effects even when the degree of platelet receptor occupancy falls below the 80% necessary for complete inhibition of platelet aggregation. Another possible reason for the smaller reduction in relative risk in the IMPACT-II trial compared with the EPIC trial may be a reflection of less than 50% platelet inhibition of aggregation achieved during the trial.[49] It is therefore tempting to speculate whether longer treatment periods for the peptide and non-peptide GPIIb/IIIa inhibitors with optimized dosing protocols may yield added benefit.

The major pharmacodynamic difference between abciximab and the smaller peptide and non-peptide inhibitors lies in the selectivity of these agents for the GPIIb/IIIa receptors. Abciximab is able to bind to other receptors including the $\alpha_v\beta_3$ (vitronectin)[50] receptor present on platelets, endothelial cells and vascular smooth muscle cells. Furthermore, platelet-leukocyte and leukocyte-endothelial interactions may be inhibited by the interference of abciximab with CD11/CD18 complex.[51] The importance of these binding characteristics of abciximab are presently unknown, although inhibition of the vitronectin receptor ($\alpha_v\beta_3$) has been shown to reduce neointimal hyperplasia in primate balloon injured vessels.[52] The 6 months' follow-up data from the EPIC trial reported 26% reduction in repeat target vessel revascularization with the curves remaining parallel after 30 days; this was interpreted to suggest that the use of GPIIb/IIIa inhibitors may reduce the incidence of restenosis. However, an angiographic substudy was not performed in that trial to assess restenosis rates. This effect of abciximab has not been reproduced in the subsequent trials of angioplasty with adjunctive GPIIb/IIIa inhibitors. Indeed, in the ERASER study, which evaluated abciximab in coronary stenting, volumetric assessment of neointimal proliferation using intracoronary ultrasound, did not demonstrate a significant difference in neointimal volume between patients receiving abciximab and those that did not.[33]

Important or unresolved efficacy issues of GPIIb/IIIa inhibitors in unstable angina/non-ST-elevation MI patients

How long before intervention should the GPIIb/IIIa inhibitor therapy begin?

The CAPTURE trial demonstrated that starting abciximab 18–24 h prior to percutaneous coronary intervention resulted in a reduction of adverse events prior to the intervention. This 'passivation' of the culprit lesion may have occurred by the disaggregation of intracoronary thrombus limiting platelet accumulation to an adherent monolayer on the baro-traumatized subendothelial structures. The use of GPIIb/IIIa inhibitors may therefore be beneficial in preventing further adverse thrombotic events in patients with unstable angina while they are waiting for a more definitive coronary intervention. This may have particular relevance to patients in hospitals without immediate access to invasive cardiology or coronary surgery. It is presently unclear, however, whether the strategy of using GPIIb/IIIa inhibitors in patients with unstable angina will be successful in preventing coronary intervention altogether. Some initial information on this point may be gleaned from the PRISM-PLUS and PURSUIT trials in which intervention was not mandated by the protocols, but a significant proportion of patients went on to receive percutaneous coronary intervention. These two trials evaluated GPIIb/IIIa inhibitors in a comprehensive treatment strategy of medical stabilization followed by angiography and angioplasty as was felt to be indicated by the doctor for patients with unstable angina/non-Q-wave MI. In PRISM-PLUS, of the patients on heparin and aspirin alone, 89.4% went on to be revascularized, whereas only 67.6% of patients randomized to receive tirofiban plus heparin were revascularized (risk ratio 0.76; 95% CI, 0.59–0.97). In the PURSUIT trial, 69% of patients in each arm progressed to require percutaneous coronary intervention. The decision to revascularize the 475 patients in PRISM-PLUS and the 1228 patients in the PURSUIT trial by percutaneous intervention, however, was not based solely on the patients' clinical course (e.g. ongoing instability) but also on the angiographic findings.

Given the ability of GPIIb/IIIa inhibitors in passivating the culprit lesion and thus prevent adverse outcomes in patients awaiting revascularization, as shown in the CAPTURE and PRISM-PLUS data, these agents clearly have relevance to centres lacking interventional facilities. A treatment paradigm might exist, in which patients with unstable angina/non-Q-wave MI, receive traditional heparin, aspirin, nitrates and a GPIIb/IIIa inhibitor for an initial period of time (yet to be determined), and are then triaged to angiography and subsequently to intervention (PTCA or CABG) through use of an ECG exercise test or pharmacological stress SPECT. This might represent a potentially more cost-effective strategy in managing patients with unstable angina/non-Q-MI.

How long should GPIIb/IIIa treatment continue after intervention for unstable angina?

With percutaneous coronary intervention there is further loss of the coronary endothelium and exposure of highly thrombogenic subendothelial elements (e.g. collagen, cholesterol rich plaque) resulting in additional platelet activation, which may lead to acute or subacute thrombosis. While most procedure-related subacute thrombotic events occurs within the first 24 h of percutaneous coronary intervention, some can occur even after 2 weeks. While abciximab is known to exist on platelets

2 weeks after administration, this is at a level that would not inhibit platelet aggregation and would thus be subtherapeutic. The use of intravenous agents for prolonged therapy would be costly and less than practical. Investigation of the potential role of longer-term therapy using oral GPIIb/IIIa inhibitors in the setting of unstable angina/non-Q-wave MI with or without percutaneous coronary intervention seems desirable. The effects of *prolonged* GPIIb/IIIa blockade on the restenotic process after percutaneous intervention is also presently unknown and may be answered in coming years with the use of oral agents.

Patients with acute MI undergoing primary angioplasty

Acute myocardial infarction (AMI) typically results from the rupture of an atheromatous plaque with consequent platelet activation and localized thrombus formation resulting in the total occlusion of the coronary artery.[53] Primary angioplasty has been shown to be superior to fibrinolytic therapy both angiographically and clinically; TIMI Grade III flow at 90 min post-AMI has higher prognostic benefit[54] with lower recurrence of ischemic events.[55] Nevertheless, the incidence of periprocedural adverse events in primary angioplasty AMI is still significant.[56] Intuitively this is perhaps not surprising, as the procedure of primary angioplasty, while relieving the obstruction, merely compresses the thrombus into the vessel wall and thus the latter is able to act as a nidus for further thrombosis or embolization, resulting in further ischemic events. The clinical scenario of an AMI in which the treatment modality of primary intervention is to be performed would therefore seem an ideal one to test the hypothesis that intravenous anti GPIIb/IIIa agents reduce the peri-procedural complications in this setting.

Efficacy of adjunctive GPIIb/IIIa inhibitors in these patients

Post-hoc subgroup analysis of the EPIC study, provided early evidence for the possible benefits of GPIIb/IIIa antagonist adjunctive therapy in patients with acute MI undergoing primary or rescue PTCA.[39] In the subgroup of patients with acute MI ($n = 64$) in the EPIC study, 42 patients underwent direct PTCA while 22 patients had rescue PTCA. Analysis of the pooled data on the 64 patients revealed an 83% reduction in the primary efficacy composite end point of death, reinfarction, percutaneous or surgical revascularization (26.1% placebo versus 4.5% abciximab bolus and infusion, $p = 0.06$). At 6 months, the benefit of abciximab remained with the composite end point in the abciximab bolus plus infusion arm of 4.5%, while that of the placebo was 47.8%, which was a relative reduction of 91%; $p = 0.002$.

In the RAPPORT trial,[32] 483 patients undergoing primary PTCA within 12 h of onset of acute MI were randomized to receive a bolus plus infusion of abciximab started before intervention and continued for 12 h. There was no difference in the incidence of the primary 6-month endpoint of death, re-infarction and *any* target vessel revascularization, between treatment and placebo group (28.1% versus 28.2%). However, when the composite end-point of death, reinfarction and *urgent* target vessel revascularization was used, abciximab was associated with a significant benefit at 7 days (3.3% versus 9.9%, $p = 0.003$); at 30 days (5.8% versus 11.2%, $p = 0.03$); and at 6 months (11.6% versus 17.8%, $p = 0.05$).

The recently reported ADMIRAL study has also suggested that adjunctive abciximab may be significantly beneficial in acute MI patients undergoing coronary stenting (Chapter 8).

The other interventional trials evaluating adjunctive GPIIb/IIIa inhibitors that included patients with acute MI are IMPACT-II, RESTORE and recently EPISTENT. While patients with acute MI made up 33% of the sample population in the RESTORE study, an analysis of this subgroup has not been reported. In the IMPACT-II study the number of patients with acute MI was approximately 3% only. Patients with acute MI undergoing elective primary stenting in the EPISTENT trial, had a 30-day composite endpoint of death, reinfarction or urgent revascularization of 4.5% in the stent plus abciximab group compared with 9.6% for stent plus placebo. Similarly, patients with acute MI undergoing primary balloon angioplasty with adjunctive abciximab had a composite endpoint of 5.3% versus 9.6% in the group undergoing primary stenting without adjunctive abciximab, suggesting that balloon angioplasty with abciximab is safer than stenting without abciximab.

Unresolved issues with the use of adjunctive GPIIb/IIIa inhibitors in acute MI patients

On the evidence of the RAPPORT and ADMIRAL trials and the subgroup analyses of EPIC and EPISTENT, it would appear that the use of abciximab in patients undergoing primary angioplasty or primary stenting for acute MI, improves the clinical outcome at 30 days. Beyond 30 days, the EPIC subgroup analysis and the ADMIRAL trial demonstrated a significant benefit, while the RAPPORT study failed to show a significant difference between abciximab and placebo. While encouraging, however, the efficacy evidence is based on relatively few patients and needs to be confirmed in larger trials.

The optimal duration of GPIIb/IIIa inhibitor therapy after percutaneous intervention for acute MI also needs to be defined. The CADILLAC trial[57] of the use of GPIIb/IIIa inhibitors in stenting in acute MI was studied and it will be interesting to compare these results with those of the Percutaneous Intervention in Acute Myocardial Infarction (PAMI)[56] and PAMI-STENT trials.[58]

Another area that needs further study is in the use of GPIIb/IIIa inhibitors as a rescue therapy in patients with acute MI having failed treatment with fibrinolytic therapy and rescue angioplasty. In the GUSTO-III trial, analysis of 387 patients with acute MI undergoing rescue percutaneous coronary intervention, showed that there was a mortality rate at 30 days of 3.7% in the 81 patients receiving abciximab, while the mortality rate was 9.8% in the 306 patients that did not receive abciximab, $p = 0.04$.[59]

Patients with chronic stable angina

The coronary artery lesion causing chronic stable angina is likely to be a flow-limiting unruptured plaque without predominant fresh thrombus. This may account for the lower incidence of acute periprocedural adverse ischemic coronary events compared with patients with unstable angina or postinfarction angina.[60] Nevertheless, percutaneous coronary intervention results in vessel wall injury and exposure of the subendothelium, with consequent activation of platelets and the coagulation cascade. Indeed, some types of coronary intervention procedures are associated with increased complications (for example, directional and rotational atherectomy and bailout stenting discussed later. In addition, certain types of lesions are known to be associated with increased acute ischemic complications such as thrombus-containing lesions,[61] chronic total occlusions,[62,63] or long lesions.[64] Within the clinical group of stable angina therefore, patients may be risk-stratified according to their pre-intervention angiographic findings, the device strategy to be used and the periprocedural adverse signs of complications.

No trial has been designed to test the hypothesis that GPIIb/IIIa inhibitors improve outcome in percutaneous coronary intervention specifically in patients with chronic stable ischemia. Nevertheless supportive data comes from subgroup analysis in the EPILOG and IMPACT-II trials, trials in which the proportion of patients with chronic stable angina made up approximately 33% and 59% of the study population respectively. In the EPILOG trial, which compared placebo plus standard-dose heparin with abciximab plus low- or high-dose heparin, roughly 300 patients with stable ischemia were randomized to each of the three arms. Hazard ratios for the 30-day efficacy endpoint in prespecified subgroups defined according to risk, revealed that not only did patients with unstable ischemia benefit from abciximab, so did patients with stable ischemia (Figure 15.1). Similarly, in IMPACT-II, the subgroup of patients with chronic stable angina also demonstrated benefit from a GPIIb/IIIa inhibitor (see Figure 15.1).

Discussion

The absence of data from a trial specifically designed to evaluate the use of adjunctive GPIIb/IIIa inhibitors in patients with chronic stable angina, the limitations of subgroup analyses of EPILOG and IMPACT-II, and the difficulties in stratifying risk according to the clinical label of chronic stable angina, makes it difficult to come to a definitive conclusion that GPIIb/IIIa inhibitors be used in all patients undergoing coronary intervention. Some prefer the strategy of selective use of GPIIb/IIIa inhibitors in patients with chronic stable angina undergoing percutaneous coronary intervention, for example with bailout stenting or in the presence of poor flow. Prospective randomized trials supporting this strategy are, however, presently lacking.

Efficacy of antiplatelet therapy in specific coronary interventions

Antiplatelet therapy and coronary stenting

In the early days of coronary stenting, subacute thrombotic closure was a major problem, occurring in 3.5–8.6% of patients[65–74] and often resulting in a major clinical event such as death, Q-wave infarction or emergency revascularization. This encouraged the experimentation of aggressive anticoagulation regimes with warfarin, dextran, aspirin, dipyridamole, aspirin and heparin, which resulted in little change in the thrombotic rate[75] and in significant increase in the incidence of haemorrhages and longer hospitalization.[68,69] Colombo and colleagues[76,77] made a major contribution by demonstrating that high-pressure inflation resulted in better vessel wall apposition of the stent struts and that intravascular ultrasound-guided stent deployment with higher inflation pressures resulted in the diminution of the thrombogenic dead-spaces between the stent and the vessel wall. At the same time of this change in stent deployment technique, combination therapy of aspirin and ticlopidine was being evaluated and it is therefore difficult to determine the relative contributions of the concurrent changes in stenting practice. However, as a result the incidence of stent thrombosis fell from greater than 15% to less than 2% and high-pressure stent deployment with aspirin plus ticlopidine rapidly became the widely used antiplatelet regimen with coronary stenting. This initial acceptance of the regimen was confirmed by three prospective, randomized trials, ISAR,[78] STARS[79] and FANTASTIC,[80] which demonstrated the superiority of antiplatelet therapy with ticlopidine plus aspirin compared to anticoagulation and aspirin for stented patients, see Table 15.3 (see Chapter 7).

The low incidence of ischemic events to 30 days in these trials may be a reflection of the patients enrolled being of low risk, that is elective stenting with 'optimal' stent deployment. The danger of extrapolating this data to higher-risk groups of stented patients is demonstrated by subgroup analysis of patients in the STARS registry with less than optimal stent deployment that showed a 7-fold increase (i.e. 3.5%) in subacute stent thrombosis.[81] Similarly, in the MATTIS trial,[82] the incidence of the composite endpoint of death, MI or urgent revascularization was 5.6% in the ticlopidine plus aspirin group.

More recent data from the CLASSICS trial have demonstrated that clopidogrel may be significantly better tolerated than ticlopidine in patients undergoing stent placement. The ongoing CREDO trial will also examine whether loading with clopidogrel and/or extended oral therapy convey any benefit.

The early clinical interventional trials with adjunctive GPIIb/IIIa inhibitors provided initial evidence that these agents not only reduced the requirement for unplanned stenting but also improved the outcome in patients who received unplanned stenting. In the EPILOG trial, the requirement for unplanned stent deployment was reduced significantly in patients receiving prophylactic abciximab plus low-dose weight-adjusted heparin compared with placebo plus standard-dose heparin (9.0% versus 13.7% respectively, $p < 0.001$).[83,84] Similarly, in the setting of primary angioplasty, the RAPPORT trial demonstrated that abciximab reduced the requirement for bailout stenting by 41% ($p = 0.02$).[78]

Subgroup analyses of IMPACT-II[79] and EPI-LOG trials[76,77] as well as a meta-analysis of EPIC, EPILOG and CAPTURE trials[80] demonstrated that the use of adjunctive GPIIb/IIIa inhibitors improved the clinical outcomes in patients who underwent bailout coronary stenting. In IMPACT-II, the use of eptifibatide was associated with a reduction in periprocedural MI ($p = 0.017$) and in the composite end point of death, MI or urgent revascularization ($p = 0.002$) at 30 days in patients who received an unplanned stent. In the EPILOG study, clinical outcomes were compared in the 326 patients with unplanned stenting receiving abciximab or placebo on a randomized basis. The hazard ratio for the composite endpoint of death, MI or urgent intervention was 0.39 at 30 days and 0.46 at 6 months. Likewise the hazard ratio for the composite endpoint of death, MI or urgent intervention in the meta-analysis (EPIC, EPI-LOG and CAPTURE trials) was 0.36 (CI 0.22-0.58) at 30 days and 0.46 (CI 0.28–0.77) at 6 months.

Prospective randomized data on the evaluation of a GPIIb/IIIa inhibitor in elective stenting was first provided in the ERASER trial.[33] 'Optimal' stenting was performed under IVUS-guidance. Abciximab reduced the composite endpoint of death, MI or target vessel revascularization by 53% compared with placebo (aspirin and ticlopidine) but did not reduce the incidence of restenosis. The most conclusive data on the benefit of GPIIb/IIIa inhibitors in elective stenting comes from the recently published multicenter, prospective, randomized, controlled, EPILOG-STENT (EPISTENT) trial.[31] Approximately 2400 patients were randomized into three groups; stent plus placebo, stent plus abciximab, and

angioplasty plus abciximab and the primary composite endpoint of death, MI or urgent revascularization at 30 days were 10.8%, 5.3% and 6.9% respectively. There were significant differences in the incidence of composite endpoints between the stent plus placebo group compared with the stent plus abciximab group ($p < 0.001$) and the angioplasty plus abciximab group ($p < 0.007$). The relatively high event rate in the stent plus placebo arm was ascribed to the diverse population of patients with higher-risk lesions, for example long lesions and vein-graft disease.

GPIIb/IIIa inhibitors and atherectomy (directional and rotational)

Directional coronary atherectomy (DCA) is known to result in significantly more platelet activation[88] and more periprocedural non-Q-wave MI[89,90] compared with angioplasty. A meta-analysis of the EPIC and EPILOG trials demonstrated that in patients undergoing DCA, the use of prophylactic abciximab was associated with a reduction at 30 days in the composite endpoint of death, MI or urgent revascularization ($p = 0.008$), and in the incidence of MI ($p = 0.003$). Likewise, at 6 months, the incidence of death, MI or target vessel revascularization was reduced ($p = 0.02$) as well as the incidence of MI ($p = 0.002$).[91,92] However, subgroup analysis from the IMPACT-II trial on the 451 patients (11.2%) receiving DCA revealed that eptifibatide was not associated with a significant reduction in the composite endpoint of death, MI or repeat revascularization.

Rotational atherectomy (RA) is also associated with significant platelet activation[93,94] and periprocedural MI.[95,96] Platelet activation in RA has been shown to be speed dependent[95,96] and CKMB elevations are related to burr

Study	Drugs	Clinical Setting	Endpoints	Results
Ticlopidine trial ($n = 337$)	Placebo ASA/dipyridamole Ticlopidine	PTCA	Ischemic complications Restenosis	Ischemic complications: Placebo – 14% ASA/dip – 4% Ticlopidine – 3% ($P < .01$) No signif effect on restenosis
STARS[97] ($n = 1653$)	ASA Warfarin + ASA Ticlopidine + ASA	Successful stent (J&J)	Death, MI, TVR, or thrombosis at 30 days	ASA – 3.6% Warfarin + ASA – 2.7% Ticlopidine + ASA – 0.5% ($P = 0.001$)
ISAR[98, 99] ($n = 517$)	Warfarin + ASA Ticlopidine + ASA	Successful stent (J&J)	Cardiac death, MI, revasc at 30 days	Warfarin + ASA – 6.2% Ticlopidine + ASA – 1.6% ($P < 0.01$)
FANTASTIC[80] ($n = 236$)	Warfarin + ASA Ticlopidine + ASA	Elective and non-elective stent (Wiktor)	(1°) Bleeding (2°) Clinical events (Death, MI, occlusion at 6 months)	Bleeding Warfarin + ASA – 21% Ticlopidine + ASA – 13.5% ($P = 0.03$) Clinical events Warfarin + ASA – 15.5% Ticlopidine + ASA – 12.9% ($P = NS$)
MATTIS[83] ($n = 350$)	Warfarin + ASA Ticlopidine + ASA	High risk stents	Death, MI, repeat revasc at 30 days	Warfarin + ASA – 11% Ticlopidine + ASA – 5.6% ($P = 0.07$)
Albiero et al.[100] ($n = 801$)	ASA Ticlopidine + ASA	Successful, optimized stent (usually with IVUS)	Death, MI, repeat revasc, vascular complications at 30 days	ASA – 1.9% Ticlopidine + ASA – 2.0% ($P = NS$)

Study	Drugs	Clinical Setting	Endpoints	Results
Moussa et al.[101] (n = 1489)	ASA + Ticlopidine ASA + Clopidogrel (not randomized)	Stent	Clinical events Drug side effects	Clinical events ASA + Ticlopidine – 1.5% ASA + Clopidogrel – 1.4% (P = NS) Drug side effects ASA + Ticlopidine – 10.6% ASA + Clopidogrel – 5.3% (P = 0.006)
CLASSICS[102] (n = 1020)	ASA + Ticlopidine ASA + Clopidogrel ASA + Clopidogrel (loaded)	Successful stent	(1°) Safety bleeding neutropenia thrombocytopenia early drug D/C (2°) Clinical events (Death, MI, TVR at 6 months)	Safety ASA + Ticlopidine – 9.1% ASA + Clopid – 6.3% ASA + Clopid (load) – 2.9% (P = 0.005) Clinical events ASA + Ticlopidine – 0.9% ASA + Clopid – 1.5% ASA + Clopid (load) – 1.2% (P = NS)
CREDO	ASA + Clopidogrel ASA + Clopidogrel (loaded) Short vs. long term Rx	Stent	Clinical events	[Ongoing]
EXCITE[103] (n = 7232)	Xemilofiban Up to 6 months With procedural heparin and aspirin	Coronary Intervention	Death, MI, urgent intervention	30 days: placebo – 8.1% Xemilo (10 mg) – 8.1% Xemilo (20 mg) – 7.3% (P = NS) 6 months: placebo – 13.6% Xemilo (10 mg) – 14.1% Xemilo (20 mg) – 12.6% (P = NS) Trend towards *higher* mortality on low-dose Xemilofiban group

Table 15.3
Major clinical trials of oral antiplatelet agents for coronary intervention.

257

decelerations, prolong ablation times, and patient related factors such as lesion length and the presence of unstable angina.[95,96] Approximately 10% of the patients in each arm of the IMPACT-II trial went on to receive RA. Although the progression to RA was not a randomized step, but a decision based on angiographic findings, high-dose eptifibatide was associated with a reduced incidence of the composite endpoint (death, MI, repeat revascularization) compared with placebo (12.4% versus 19.9%, $p = 0.059$).[104]

Saphenous vein grafts

Elevations of cardiac enzymes (CK-MB) occur in up to 20% of patients undergoing percutaneous saphenous vein graft intervention and independent predictors of this include angiographic thrombus and large vessel diameter but not device type.[105] Subgroup analysis of the EPIC trial showed that the use of abciximab was associated with a reduced incidence of non-Q-wave MI and periprocedural distal embolization in patients undergoing saphenous vein graft intervention.[106,107] A meta-analysis of the EPIC and EPILOG trials revealed that abciximab was associated with a 41% reduction in the composite endpoint of death, MI and urgent revascularization to 30 days.[108] This suggests that the ischaemic complications associated with vein graft interventions are not solely due to distal embolization of atheromatous debris but may also be thrombus-mediated and thus potentially avoidable by the use of GPIIb/IIIa inhibitors.

Safety issues on the use of GPIIb/IIIa inhibitors in patients undergoing percutaneous coronary intervention

Although the EPIC study amply demonstrated the effectiveness of abciximab in decreasing ischemic complications in high-risk angioplasty or atherectomy, there was a significant incidence of bleeding complications. All patients were treated with 325 mg aspirin and heparin. The heparin was given to all patients as a bolus dose (10 000–12 000 units) at the start of the procedure and further boluses of 3000 units were given to keep the ACT at 300–500 s during the procedure. Heparin was then continued after the procedure as an infusion for 12 h and the arterial sheath removed 4 h after the end of the heparin infusion. Similarly, abciximab was infused for 12 h also in the abciximab infusion arm. The group given abciximab bolus plus infusion had a substantial incidence of major bleeding (14%) compared with the no abciximab group (7%) and abciximab bolus only group (11%). The rate of major bleeding in the no abciximab group was, however, high, implying that leaving the sheaths in for 12 h after angioplasty was a problem. It was also noted that the risk of bleeding increased in the lighter patients who received higher doses of heparin per kg body weight. This finding prompted the design of the EPILOG trial to incorporate the weight-adjusted heparin regimes.

The EPILOG study compared heparin at 'standard' and low doses. The adjustment of the heparin doses for body weight, even in the abciximab plus 'standard'-dose heparin arm resulted in less heparin being given compared with the EPIC patients. The actual absolute risk of haemorrhage in the EPILOG study was substantially less than in the EPIC study. There were no significant differences in the incidence of major haemorrhage between the three arms of the EPILOG trial, with the incidence of bleeding in the abciximab arms being similar to placebo. It is interesting to note that the incidence of major bleeding in the placebo arm was only 3.1%, substantially less than the

7% seen in EPIC reflecting the importance of the combination of weight-adjusted heparin and early sheath removal. However, the incidence of minor bleeding was significantly increased in the abciximab plus standard heparin arm compared with the other two treatment arms. Nevertheless, the EPILOG study demonstrated that the benefits of abciximab could be achieved without necessarily incurring the penalty of significant haemorrhage.

In the CAPTURE trial, patients received weight-adjusted heparin (bolus of 100 U/kg to a max of 10 000 U) with the target ACT of 300 s. Although the incidence of major bleeding was statistically significantly higher in the abciximab group (3.8%) compared with the placebo group (1.9%); $p = 0.043$, the incidence of major bleeding was similar to those in the EPILOG trial and much less than that in EPIC, thus again confirming the benefit of using heparin in a weight-adjusted manner.

The RESTORE study was designed in the pre-EPILOG era, and although heparin bolus was weight-adjusted, it was given at 150 U/kg but to a maximum of 10 000 U bolus before the procedure and more heparin given during the procedure to maintain an ACT of 300–400 s. The heparin was stopped at the end of the PTCA procedure and arterial sheath removed early (i.e. when ACT < 180 s or at 4 h after stopping heparin). Major bleeding, although not statistically significantly increased in the tirofiban group compared with the placebo treatment arm, was nevertheless relatively high at 5.3% in the tirofiban arm, which may be a reflection of the heparin bolus being as high as 150 U/kg.

In the IMPACT-II trial, weight-adjusted heparin bolus was given at a dose of 100 U/kg followed by infusion to maintain the ACT between 300–350 s. There was no statistical difference in the frequency of major bleeding between the treatment arms and placebo.

In the RAPPORT trial, which assessed the efficacy and safety of abciximab in primary angioplasty, heparin was given as a bolus 100 U/kg body weight with further heparin to keep the KCT > 300 s during the procedure. There was a significant increase in bleeding in the abciximab group compared with placebo (16.6% versus 9.5%; $p = 0.02$). The authors noted that this was a reflection of the relatively long interval between the angioplasty and sheath removal.

Recommendation on the heparin protocol in patients undergoing PCI *with adjunctive abciximab*

The EPILOG study data established the superior safety of a low-dose, weight-adjusted heparin regimen in conjunction with early sheath removal for patients undergoing percutaneous coronary intervention (PCI) with adjunctive abciximab. The initial heparin bolus was 70 U/kg followed by the administration of additional boluses as needed to achieve and maintain an activated clotting time (ACT) of over 200 s. Heparin was stopped immediately after the procedure and the vascular sheath was removed when the ACT reached less than 175 s, generally 4–6 h later. This modification of traditional heparin dosing eliminated the excess bleeding risk in patients treated with abciximab, bringing the incidence of bleeding events down to placebo levels. With confirmation of the safe use of GPIIb/IIIa antagonists in the presence of weight-adjusted heparin in several large trials, the recommendation for their clinical use has become based on a weight-adjusted heparin regime. There is a tendency for low-dose heparin to be used as the standard for all percutaneous coronary interventional procedures as bail-out GPIIb/IIIa antagonists may be considered during the procedure. It should be stated, however, that low-dose heparin has not been shown to be safe in PTCA without the use of GPIIb/IIIa inhibitors. The need for heparin when GPIIb/IIIa inhibitors are being used has been demonstrated by the result of the discontinued tirofiban/no heparin arm of PRISM-PLUS. Finally, it has become standard practice to remove the femoral artery sheaths early after the intervention once the activated clotting time has dropped below 150 s, with the GPIIb/IIIa antagonist infusion continuing during the sheath removal.

Oral IIb/IIIa blockers

The oral GPIIb/IIIa antagonists (see Chapter 10) have received a lot of recent attention. These compounds are pro-drug precursors of peptidomimetic IIb/IIIa antagonists, which can be administered orally, and given for extended periods of time. Initial clinical reports suggested a measureable dose-response effect in terms of platelet inhibition, and that these drugs could generally be administered safely (in terms of bleeding risk) for prolonged (up to 3 months) periods of time. However, the clinical efficacy of the oral IIb/IIIa antagonists has recently come into question with the recent results of the EXCITE and OPUS trials, in patients undergoing coronary intervention and patients with acute coronary syndromes, respectively.

In the EXCITE study, a total of 7232 qualifying patients undergoing percutaneous coronary intervention were randomized to recieve one or two doses of the oral GP IIb/IIIa antagonists xemilofiban (20 mg) 30–90 minutes prior to the procedure and subsequently either 10 mg TID, 20 mg TID or placebo. Follow-up continued for at least 6 months. The primary endpoint of the study was the composite of death, MI and urgent intervention. Stent were

utilized in approximately 71% of patients; abciximab use was discouraged. Approximately 17–20% of patients enrolled were diabetic. At 30 days, there were no significant differences among the three groups in composite events (placebo – 8.1%, xemilofiban 10 mg – 8.1%, xemilofiban 20 mg – 7.3%) although they tended to be somewhat less frequent in the higher dose xemilofiban group. A similar pattern was evident at 6 months (13.6%, 14.1%, 12.6%, respectively). Disturbingly, mortality tended to be slightly higher in the lower dose xemilofiban group, both at 30 days (placebo – 0.4%, xemilofiban 10 mg – 0.9%, xemilofiban 20 mg – 0.6%) and at 6 months (1.0%, 1.6%, 1.1%, respectively). Interestingly, there did appear to be significant benefit of xemilofiban in reducing clinical events in patients with diabetes, but no other clinical group showed any demonstrable benefit.

The OPUS-TIMI 16 Study[109] was a multicenter, randomized, placebo-controlled trail of the oral platelet GP IIb/IIIa antagonists orbofiban in patients with acute coronary syndromes. A total of 10 302 patients with unstable coronary syndromes were randomized to orbofiban 50 mg BID, orbofiban 50 mg BID × 30 days then 30 mg BID, or placebo. All patients received aspirin (150–162 mg/d). The primary endpoint was the composite of death, MI, recurrent ischemia leading to rehospitalization or urgent revascularization or stroke. Analysis were performed at 30 days and through subsequent follow-up (mean 7 months). Enrolment into the trial was halted early because of excess 30 day mortality in one of the treatment groups, and the trial was subsequently halted prior to the target enrolment of 12 000 patients. The 30 day mortality rate was 1.4% in the placebo group, 2.3% in the orbofiban 50/30 group, and 1.6% in the orbofiban 50/50 group. 30 day composite primary endpoints were 10.7% in the placebo group, 9.7% in the orbofiban 50/30 group, and 9.3% in the orbofiban 50/50 group. There was significant benefit of orbofiban in reducing recurrent ischemic events leading to revascularization (5.3% with placebo, 2.9% with orbofiban 50/30, 3.3% with orbofiban 50/50). Follow-up composite event rates (Kaplan-Meier through 300 days) were 20.5%, 20.2%, and 19.5%, respectively, death (3.2%, 4.7%, 4.0%) and recurrent ischemia leading to revascularization (7.9%, 5.9%, 5.8%) showed significant trends similar to those observed at 30 days. Severe or major bleeding was slightly, but significantly increased with orbofiban: 1.9% (0.4% severe) with placebo, 3.3% (1.2% severe) with orbofiban 50/30 and 3.7% (0.7% severe) with orbofiban 50/50. Thrombocytopenia was rare, but slightly more frequent with orbofiban. Interestingly, patients in OPUS-TIMI 16 who underwent percutaneous interventional procedures, appeared to benefit from oral GP IIb/IIIa antagonist therapy.

Another recently presented large scale trial, SYMPHONY-I[110] (with sibrafiban in AeS patients) showed no significant difference between aspirin alone and silvafiban alone in 9233 patients. The follow-up study, SYMPHONY-II, was recently halted by the sponsor.

Thus, despite initial high hopes, the oral IIb/IIIa antagonists will probably not have a clinical role in patients undergoing coronary intervention, at least in the forseeable future.

Conclusion

There is now a large body of evidence that the GPIIb/IIIa inhibitors reduce the risk of adverse ischemic events in both high-risk and low-risk patients undergoing percutaneous coronary intervention. The differences in efficacy between the clinically available agents remain controversial. The re-adjudication of the RESTORE trial end points demonstrates the difficulties and pitfalls of comparing different trials with similar but not identical endpoint definitions. In addition, the methodology used in determining the end points of MI is also extremely important.

A yet unresolved but important efficacy issue of GPIIb/IIIa blockade is the duration of treatment both before and after intervention. The CAPTURE and PRISM-PLUS trials demonstrated the potential for 'vessel wall passivation' by prolonged pre-treatment influencing the MI rate prior to intervention. The TACTICS study will, in part, shed some light on tirofiban's ability to pacify the vessel wall. The EPIC study suggested that the use of abciximab resulted in a reduction of target vessel revascularization beyond 6 months, however, this finding was not confirmed in subsequent abciximab interventional trials. Whether the use of longer infusions of GPIIb–IIIa inhibitors could result in a significant and clinically important reduction in target vessel revascularization remains to be determined.

Long-term therapy with oral IIb/IIIa blockers does not appear to convey significant clinical advantages. Oral IIb/IIIa antagonists may even (in low doses) be harmful for recovery that are as yet not well understood.

There are also important and unresolved pharmacological safety issues in the use of these newer antiplatelet agents in coronary intervention. For example, would a further decrease in the heparin dose (or indeed no heparin) further decrease the haemorrhagic risk without affecting the periprocedural thrombotic rates in patients undergoing PTCA with adjunctive GPIIb/IIIa inhibitors? When should ticlopidine or clopidogrel be started and for how long should it be continued to obtain optimal benefits?

The continued challenge to these agents also remains their cost-effectiveness in the setting of decreasing budgets and managed care. Should all interventions be covered with GPIIb/IIIa blockade? There appears compelling evidence from the EPIC, EPILOG, RESTORE and PRISM-PLUS trials, that patients presenting with both acute coronary syndromes as well as chronic stable angina benefit from this form of therapy. It should be acknowledged that the predominant influence of these agents is in reducing non-Q-wave MI and large (over twice normal) CK-MB leaks. The significance of the non-Q-wave infarction/CK-MB leaks is currently hotly debated. It is probably fair to say that myonecrosis cannot be considered to be a good outcome of intervention, but the reduction of asymptomatic non-Q-wave infarcts by the 'blanket' use of GPIIb/IIIa antagonists would prove to be prohibitively expensive and potentially crippling to an already cost-constrained health care system. Research is clearly needed to ascertain the significance of these CK findings, relate them to the other markers of myonecrosis, including the troponins, and define the medium and long-term outcome of patients who suffer such ischemic events. Once such data exists, it will be much easier to advocate the widespread use of these potent antiplatelet agents in all patient groups undergoing coronary intervention and therefore justify the expense.

References

1. Davies MJ, Thomas AC. Thrombosis and acute coronary artery lesions in sudden ischemic death. *N Engl J Med* 1984; **310**:1137–40.
2. Falk E. Unstable angina with fatal outcome: dynamic coronary thrombosis leading to infarction and/or sudden death: autopsy evidence of recurrent mural thrombosis with peripheral embolization culminating in total vascular occlusion. *Circulation* 1985;**71**: 699–708.
3. Pope CF, Ezekowitz MD, Smith EO, et al. Detection of platelet deposition at the site of peripheral balloon angioplasty using Indium-111 platelet scintigraphy. *Am J Cardiol* 1985;**55**:495–7.
4. Gasperetti CM, Gonias SL, Gimple LW, et al. Platelet activation during coronary angioplasty in humans. *Circulation* 1993;**88**: 2728–34.
5. ISIS-2 Second International Study of Infarct Survival Collaborative Group. Randomized trial of intravenous streptokinase, oral aspirin, both, or neither among 17 187 cases of suspected acute myocardial infarction: ISIS-2. *Lancet* 1988;**2**:349–60.
6. Theroux P, Ouimet H, McCans J, et al. Aspirin, heparin or both to treat acute unstable angina. *N Engl J Med* 1988;**318**: 1105–11.
7. The RISC Group. Risk of myocardial and death during treatment with low-dose aspirin and intravenous heparin, in men with unstable coronary artery disease. *Lancet* 1990; **336**:827–30.
8. Antiplatelet Trialists' Collaboration. Collaborative overview of randomised trials of antiplatelet therapy, 1: prevention of death, myocardial infarction, and stroke by prolonged antiplatelet therapy in various categories of patients. *Br Med J* 1994;**308**: 81–106.
9. Cohen M, Adams PC, Parry G, et al and the Antithrombotic Therapy in Acute Coronary Research Group. Combination antithrombotic therapy in unstable rest angina and non-Q-wave infarction in non-prior aspirin users: primary end points analysis from the ATACS trial. *Circulation* 1994;**89**:81–8.
10. Levine MN, Hirsh J, Landefeld S, Raskob G. Hemorrhagic complications of anticoagulant treatment. *Chest*1992;**102**(**4 Suppl**): 352S–363S.
11. Ridker PM, Manson JE, Gaziano JM, Buring JE, Hennekens CH. Low-dose aspirin therapy for chronic stable angina. A randomized, placebo-controlled clinical trial. *Annals Intern Med* 1991;**114**(**10**):835–9.
12. Chesebro JH, Webster MWI, Smith HC, et al. Antiplatelet therapy in coronary disease progression: Reduced infarction and new lesion formation. *Circulation* 1989;**80**(**Suppl II**): II–266.
13. Lewis HD Jr, Davis JW, Archibald DG, Steinke WE, Smitherman TC, Doherty JE, et al. Protective effects of aspirin against acute myocardial infarction and death in men with unstable angina. Results of a Veterans Administration Cooperative Study. *N Engl J Med* 1983;**309**(**7**):396–403.
14. Cairns JA, Gent M, Singer J, Finnie KJ, Froggatt GM, Holder DA, et al. Aspirin, sulfinpyrazone, or both in unstable angina. Results of a Canadian multicenter trial. *N Engl J Med* 1985;**313**(**22**):1369–75.
15. Theroux P, Ouimet H, McCans J, Latour JG, Joly P, Levy G, et al. Aspirin, heparin, or both to treat acute unstable angina. *N Engl J Med* 1988;**319**(**17**):1105–11.
16. Henderson WG, Goldman S, Copeland JG, Moritz TE, Harker LA. Antiplatelet or anticoagulant therapy after coronary artery bypass surgery. A meta-analysis of clinical trials. *Annals Intern Med* 1989;**111**(**9**):743–50.
17. Schwartz L, Bourassa MG, Lesperance J, Aldridge HE, Kazim F, Salvatori VA, et al. Aspirin and dipyridamole in the prevention of restenosis after percutaneous transluminal coronary angioplasty. *N Engl J Med* 1988;**318**(**26**):1714–19.

18. Mufson L, Black A, Roubin G, et al. A randomised trial of aspirin in PTCA. effect of high vs low dose aspirin on major complications and restenosis. *J Am Coll Cardiol* 1988;**11**:236A.

19. Burch JW, Stanford N, Majerus PW. Inhibition of platelet prostaglandin synthetase by oral aspirin. *J Clin Invest* 1978;**61**:314–19.

20. Patrignani P, Filabozzi P, Patrono C. Selective cumulative inhibition of platelet thromboxane production by low-dose aspirin in healthy subjects. *J Clin Invest* 1982;**69**:1366–72.

21. Dabaghi SF, Kamat SG, Payne J, et al. Effects of low-dose aspirin on platelet aggregation in the early minutes after ingestion in normal subjects. *Am J Cardiol* 1994;**74**:720.

22. Vu T-KH, Hung DT, Wheaton VI, et al. Molecular cloning of a functional thrombin receptor reveals a novel proteolytic mechanism of receptor activation. *Cell* 1991;**64**:1057.

23. Greco NJ, Tandon NN, Jackson BW, et al. Identification of a nucleotide binding site on glycoprotein IIb. *J Biol Chem* 1991;**266**:13 627.

24. Kobilka BK, Matsui H, Kobilka TS, et al. Cloning, sequencing and expression of the gene coding for the human platelet α_2-adrenergic receptor. *Science* 1987;**238**:650.

25. Jaffe EA, Wexler BB. Recovery of endothelial cell prostacyclin production after inhibition by low doses of aspirin. *J Clin Invest* 1979;**63**:532–5.

26. Coller BS. Platelets in cardiovascular thrombosis and thrombolysis. In: Fozzard HA, et al. (eds) The Heart and Cardiovascular System (New York, Raven Press, 1992) 219–73.

27. The EPIC Investigators. Use of a monoclonal antibody directed against the platelet glycoprotein IIb/IIIa receptor in high-risk coronary angioplasty. *N Engl J Med* 1994;**330**:956–61.

28. Topol EF, Ferguson JJ, Weisman HF, et al. Long-term protection from myocardial ischemic events in a randomized trial of brief integrin beta3 blockade with percutaneous coronary intervention. EPIC Investigator Group. Evaluation of Platelet IIb/IIIa Inhibition for Prevention of Ischemic Complication. *JAMA* 1997;**278**:479–84.

29. The EPILOG Investigators. Platelet glycoprotein IIb/IIIa receptor blockade and low-dose heparin during percutaneous coronary revascularization. *N Engl J Med* 1997;**336**:1689–96.

30. The CAPTURE Investigators. Randomised placebo-controlled trial of abciximab before and during coronary intervention in refractory unstable angina: the CAPTURE study. *Lancet* 1997;**349**:1429–35.

31. The EPISTENT investigators: Randomised placebo-controlled and balloon-angioplasty-controlled trial to assess safety of coronary stenting with use of platelet glycoprotein-IIb/IIIa blockade. *Lancet* 1998;**352**:87–91.

32. Brener SJ, Barr LA, Burchenal JE, Katz S, George BS, Jones AA, et al. Randomized, placebo-controlled trial of platelet glycoprotein IIb/IIIa blockade with primary angioplasty for acute myocardial infarction. ReoPro and Primary PTCA Organization and Randomized Trial (RAPPORT) Investigators. *Circulation* 1998;**98**(8):734–41.

33. The ERASER Investigators. Acute platelet inhibition with abciximab does not reduce in-stent restenosis (ERASER study). *Circulation* 1999;**100**:799–806.

34. IMPACT-II Investigators. A randomised placebo-controlled trial of effect of eptifibatide on complications of percutaneous coronary intervention: Integrilin to Minimise Platelet Aggregation and Coronary Thrombosis-II [see comments]. Clinical Trial, Phase III. *Lancet* 1997;**349**(9063):1422–8.

35. The RESTORE Investigators. Effects of platelet glycoprotein IIb/IIIa blockade with tirofiban on adverse cardiac events in patients with unstable angina or acute myocardial infarction undergoing coronary angioplasty. *Circulation* 1997;**96**:1445–53.

36. The PURSUIT Trial Investigators. Inhibition of platelet glycoprotein IIbIIIa with eptifibatide in patients with acute coronary syndromes. *N Engl J Med* 1998;**339**:436–43.

37. The Platelet Receptor Inhibition in Ischemic Syndrome Management in Patients Limited by Unstable Signs and Symptoms (PRISM-PLUS) Study Investigators. Inhibition of the platelet glycoprotein IIb/IIIa receptor with tirofiban in unstable angina and non-Q-wave myocardial infarction. *N Engl J Med*

1998;**338**:1488–97.

38. Coller BS, Peerschke EI, Scudder LE, et al. A murine monoclonal antibody that completely blocks the binding of fibrinogen to platelets produces a thrombasthenic-like state in normal platelets and binds to glycoproteins IIb and/or IIIa. *J Clin Invest* 1983;**72**:325–38.

39. Knight DM, Wagner C, Jordan R, et al. The immunogenicity of the 7E3 murine monoclonal Fab antibody fragment variable region is dramatically reduced in humans by substitution of human for murine constant regions. *Mol Immunol* 1995;**32**:1271–81.

40. Delebasse P, Maffrand JP. Pharmacology of ticlopidine: a review. *Semin Thromb Haemost* 1989;**15**:159–66.

41. Hass WK, Easton JD, Adams HP, et al for the Ticlopidine Aspirin Stroke Study Group. A randomised trial comparing ticlopidine hydrochloride with aspirin for the prevention of stroke in high-risk patients. *N Engl J Med* 1989;**321**:501–7.

42. CAPRIE Steering Committee. A randomised, blinded, trial of clopidogrel versus aspirin in patients at risk of ischaemic events (CAPRIE). *Lancet* 1996;**348**(9038):1329–39.

43. Miltenburg AJM van, Simoons ML, Veerhoek RJ, et al. Incidence and follow up of Braunwald subgroups in unstable angina pectoris. *J Am Coll Cardiol* 1995;**25**:1286–92.

44. Braunwald E. Unstable angina: a classification. *Circulation* 1989;**80**:410–14.

45. The TIMI IIIB Investigators. Effects of tissue plasminogen activator and a comparison of early invasive and conservative strategies in unstable angina and non-Q-wave myocardial infarction. Results of the TIMI IIIB Trial. *Circulation* 1994;**89**:1545–56.

46. VANQWISH Boden WE, Dai H, on behalf of the VANQWISH Trial Investigators. Long-term outcomes in non-Q-wave infarction patients randomised to an "invasive" versus "conservative" strategy: results of the multicentre VA Non-Q-Wave Infarction Strategies In-hospital (VANQWISH) trial (abstract). *Eur Heart J* 1997;**18**(Suppl):351.

47. Lefkovits J, Ivanhoe RJ, Califf RM, et al. For the EPIC investigators. Effect of platelet glycoprotein IIb/IIIa receptor blockade by a chimeric monoclonal antibody (abciximab) on acute and 6-month outcomes after percutaneous transluminal coronary angioplasty for acute myocardial infarction. *Am J Cardiol* 1996;**77**:1045–51.

48. Gibson CM, Goel M, Cohen D, et al. Six-month angiographic and clinical follow-up of patients prospectively randomizes to receive either tirofiban or placebo during angioplasty in the RESTORE trial. *J Am Coll Cardiol* 1998;**32**(1):28–34.

49. Tcheng J. Glycoprotein IIbIIIa receptor inhibitors: Putting EPIC, IMPACTII, RESTORE and EPILOG Trials into perspective. *Am J Cardiol* 1996;**78**(3A):35–40.

50. Adhesion of activated platelets to endothelial cells: evidence for a GPIIbIIIa-dependent bridging mechanism and novel roles for endothelial intercellular adhesion molecule 1 (ICAM-1), alphavbeta3 integrin, and GPIb-alpha. *J Exp Med* 1998;**187**(3):329–39.

51. Expression of integrins and examination of their adhesive function in normal and leukemic hematopoietic cells. *Blood* 1993;**81**(1):112–21.

52. Hanson S. Personal communication.

53. Fuster 1992. The pathogenesis of coronary artery disease and the acute coronary syndromes. *N Engl J Med* 1992;**326**(4):242–50.

54. The GUSTO Angiographic Investigators. The effects of tissue plasminogen activator, streptokinase, or both on coronary-artery patency, ventricular function, and survival after acute myocardial infarction. *N Engl J Med* 1993;**329**:1615–22.

55. Brodie BR, Grines CL, Ivanhoe R, et al. Six-month clinical and angiographic follow-up after direct angioplasty for acute myocardial infarction. *Circulation* 1994;**25**:156–62.

56. The Primary Angioplasty in Myocardial Infarction Study Group (PAMI). A comparison of immediate angioplasty with thrombolytic therapy for acute myocardial infarction. *N Engl J Med* 1993;**328**(10): 673–9.

57. Stone GW. Stenting in acute myocardial infarction: the promise and the proof. *Circulation* 1998;**97**(25):2482–5.

58. Myocardial Infarction Stent Pilot Trial Investigators. Prospective, multicenter study of the safety and feasibility of primary stenting in acute myocardial infarction: in-hospital and

30-day results of the PAMI stent pilot trial. *J Am Coll Cardiol* 1998;31(1):23–30.

59. Miller JM, Ohman EH, Schildcrout RW, et al. *J Am Coll Cardiol* 1998;31(Suppl A): 191A.

60. Abdelmeguid AE, Ellis SG, Sapp SK, Simpfendorfer C, Franco I, Whitlow PL. Directional coronary atherectomy in unstable angina. *J Am Coll Cardiol* 1994;24(1):46–54.

61. Mabin TA, Holmes DR, Smith HC. Intracoronary thrombus role in coronary occlusion complicating PTCA. *J Am Coll Cardiol* 1985;5:198–202.

62. Tenaglia A, Fortin D, Califf R. Predicting the risk of abrupt closure after angioplasty in an individual patient. *J Am Coll Cardiol* 1994;24(4):1004–11.

63. Rucco NA, Ring ME, Holubkov R, et al. Results of coronary angioplasty of chronic total occlusions (the NHLBI 1985–1986 PTCA registry). *Am J Cardiol* 1992;69: 69–76.

64. Tan K, Sulke N, Taub N, Sowton E. Clinical and lesion morphologic determinants of coronary angioplasty success and complications: Current experience. *J Am Coll Cardiol* 1995;25:855–65.

65. Serruys PW, de Jaegere P, Kiemeneij F, Macaya C, Rutsch W, Heyndrickx, G, et al. A comparison of balloon-expandable-stent implantation with balloon angioplasty in patients with coronary artery disease. Benestent Study Group [see comments]. *N Engl J Med* 1994;331(8):489–95.

66. Fischman DL, Leon MB, Baim DS, Schatz RA, Savage MP, Penn I, et al. A randomized comparison of coronary-stent placement and balloon angioplasty in the treatment of coronary artery disease. Stent Restenosis Study Investigators [see comments]. *N Engl J Med* 1994;331(8):496–501.

67. Roubin GS, Cannon AD, Agrawal SK, Macander PJ, Dean LS, Baxley WA, et al. Intracoronary stenting for acute and threatened closure complicating percutaneous transluminal coronary angioplasty. *Circulation* 1992;85(3):916–27.

68. Hearn JA, King SB, 3rd, Douglas JS, Jr, Carlin SF, Lembo NJ, Ghazzal ZM. Clinical and angiographic outcomes after coronary artery stenting for acute or threatened closure after

percutaneous transluminal coronary angioplasty. Initial results with a balloon-expandable, stainless steel design [see comments]. *Circulation* 1993;88(5):2086–96.

69. Schomig A, Kastrati A, Mudra H, Blasini R, Schuhlen H, Klauss V, et al. Four-year experience with Palmaz-Schatz stenting in coronary angioplasty complicated by dissection with threatened or present vessel closure. *Circulation* 1994;90(6):2716–24.

70. Mak KH, Belli G, Ellis SG, Moliterno DJ. Subacute stent thrombosis: evolving issues and current concepts. *J Am Coll Cardiol* 1996;27(2):494–503.

71. Eeckhout E, Kappenburger L, Goy JL. Stents for intracoronary placement: current status and future direction. *J Am Coll Cardiol* 1996;27:757–65.

72. Bailey SR, Kiesz RS. Intravascular stents: current applications. *Curr Probl Cardiol* 1995; 20(9):614–78.

73. Serruys PW, Strauss BH, Beatt KJ, Bertrand ME, Puel J, Rickards AF, et al. Angiographic follow-up after placement of a self-expanding coronary-artery stent. *N Engl J Med* 1991;324(1):13–17.

74. Bittl JA. Advances in coronary angioplasty. *N Engl J Med* 1996;335:1290–302.

75. Nath FC, Muller DW, Ellis SG, Rosenschein U, Chapekis A, Quain L, et al. Thrombosis of a flexible coil coronary stent: frequency, predictors and clinical outcome. *J Am Coll Cardiol* 1993;21(3):622–7.

76. Nakamura S, Colombo A, Gaglione A, Almagor Y, Goldberg SL, Maiello L, et al. Intracoronary ultrasound observations during stent implantation. *Circulation* 1994;89(5): 2026–34.

77. Goldberg SL, Colombo A, Nakamura S, Almagor Y, Maiello L, Tobis JM. Benefit of intracoronary ultrasound in the deployment of Palmaz-Schatz stents. *J Am Coll Cardiol* 1994;24(4):996–1003.

78. Schuhlen H, Hadamitzky M, Walter H, Ulm K, Schomig A. Major benefit from antiplatelet therapy for patients at high risk for adverse cardiac events after coronary Palmaz-Schatz stent placement: analysis of a prospective risk stratification protocol in the Intracoronary Stenting and Antithrombotic

Regimen (ISAR) trial. *Circulation* 1997; **95**(8):2015–21.

79. Leon MB, Baim DS, Popma JJ, Gordon PC, Cutlip DE, Ho KKL, et al for the Stent Anticoagulation Restenosis Study (STARS) investigators. *N Engl J Med* [In press].

80. Bertrand M, Legrand V, Boland J, et al. Randomized multicenter comparison of conventional anticoagulation versus antiplatelet therapy in unplanned and elective coronary stenting: the full anticoagulation versus ticlopidine plus aspirin after stent implantation. A randomized multicenter European study: the FANTASTIC trial. *Circulation* 1996;**94**:I–685 [Abstract].

81. Cutlip DE, Leon MB, Ho KK, et al. Acute and nine-month clinical outcomes after "suboptimal" coronary stenting: results from the Stent Anti-thrombotic Regimen Study (STARS) registry, *J Am Coll Cardiol* 1999; **34**:698–706.

82. Urban P, Macaya C, Rupprecht HJ, et al Randomized evaluation of anticoagulation versus antiplatelet therapy after coronary stent implantation in high-risk patients: the Multicenter aspirin and ticlopidine trial after intracoronary stenting in high risk patients. *J Am Coll Cardiol* 1998;**31**:397A [Abstract].

83. Kereiakes DJ, Miller DP, Tcheng JE, Weisman HF, Topol EJ. Abciximab reduces risk of unplanned coronary stent deployment; Epilog Trial Results. *Circulation* 1997;**96**:I–163 [Abstract].

84. Kereiakes DJ, Lincoff AM, Miller DP, Tcheng JE, Cabot CF, Anderson KM, et al. Abciximab therapy and unplanned coronary stent deployment: favorable effects on stent use, clinical outcomes, and bleeding complications. EPILOG Trial Investigators. *Circulation* 1998;**97**(9):857–64.

85. Barr LA, Brener SJ, Jones AA, et al. Abciximab reduces the need for bailout stenting during primary angioplasty: the RAPPORT trial. *J Am Coll Cardiol* 1998;**31**:237A [Abstract].

86. Zidar JP, Kruse KR, Thel MC, et al for the IMPACT-II Investigators: Integrilin for emergency coronary artery stenting. *J Am Coll Cardiol* 1996;**27**:138A [Abstract].

87. Kereiakes DJ, Lincoff AM, Simoons ML, et al. Complementarity of stenting and abciximab for percutaneous coronary intervention. *J Am Coll Cardiol* 1998;**31**:54A [Abstract].

88. Dehmer GJ, Nichols TC, Bode AP, et al. Assessment of platelet activation by coronary sinus blood sampling during balloon angioplasty and directional coronary atherectomy. *Circulation* 1996;**94**:I–198 [Abstract].

89. Topol EJ, Leya F, Pinkerton CA, Whitlow PL, Hofling B, Simonton CA, et al. A comparison of directional atherectomy with coronary angioplasty in patients with coronary artery disease. The CAVEAT Study Group. *N Engl J Med* 1993;**329**(4):221–7.

90. Holmes DR, Jr, Topol EJ, Califf RM, Berdan LG, Leya F, Berger PB, et al. A multicenter, randomized trial of coronary angioplasty versus directional atherectomy for patients with saphenous vein bypass graft lesions. CAVEAT-II Investigators. *Circulation* 1995; **91**(7):1966–74.

91. Ghaffari S, Kereiakes DJ, Kelly T, et al. Platelet GPIIb/IIIa receptor blockade reduces ischemic complications in patients undergoing directional coronary atherectomy. *Circulation* 1996;**94**:I–198 [Abstract].

92. Ghaffari S, Kereiakes DJ, Lincoff AM, Kelly T, et al for the EPILOG investigators: Platelet GPIIbIIIa receptor blockade with abciximab reduces ischemic complications in patients undergoing directional coronary atherectomy. *Am J Cardiol* [In press].

93. Reisman M, Shuman B, Fei R, et al. Analysis and comparison of platelet aggregation with high-speed rotational atherectomy. *J Am Coll Cardiol* 1997;**29**:186A [Abstract].

94. Williams MS, Coller BS, Vaananen HJ, et al. Activation of platelets in platelet rich plasma by rotation is speed dependant and can be inhibited by abciximab. *J Am Coll Cardiol* 1998;**31**:237A [Abstract].

95. Bier JD, Mukherjee S, Schubert P, et al. Predictors of no reflow during rotational atherectomy. *Circulation* 1996;**94**:I–249 [Abstract].

96. Sharma SK, Dangas G, Mehran R, et al. Risk factors for the development of slow flow during rotational coronary atherectomy. *Am J Cardiol* 1997;**80**:219–22.

97. Leon MB, Baim BS, Popma JJ et al. A clinical

trial comparing three antithrombotic-drug regimens after coronary-artery stenting. Stent Anticoagulation Restenosis Study Investigators. *N Engl J Med* 1998;**339**:1665–71.

98. Kastrati A, Schuhlen H, Hausleiter J et al. Restenosis after coronary stent placement and randomization to a 4-week combined antiplatelet or anticoagulant therapy: six-month angiographic follow-up of the Intracoronary Stenting and Antithrombotic Regimen (ISAR) Trial. *Circulation* 1997;**96**:462–7

99. Schuhlen H, Hadamitzky M, Walter H et al. Major benefit from antiplatelet therapy for patients at high risk for adverse cardiac events after coronary Palmaz-Schatz stent placement: analysis of a prospective risk stratification protocol in the Intracoronary Stenting and Antithrombotic Regimen (ISAR) trial. *Circulation* 1997;**95**:2015–21.

100. Albeiro R, Hall P, Itoh A et al. Results of a consecutive series of patients receiving only antiplatelet therapy after optimized stent implantation. Comparison of aspirin alone versus combined ticlopidine and aspirin therapy. *Circulation* 1997;**95**:1145–56.

101. Moussa I, Oetgen M, Roubin G et al. Effectiveness of clopidogrel and aspirin versus ticlopidine and aspirin in preventing stent thrombosis after coronary stent implantation. *Circulation* 1999;**99**:2364–6.

102. Bertrand M. Oral presentation. ACC (1999)

103. O'Neill. Oral presentation. ACC (1999).

104. Tierstein PS, Yakubov SJ, Thel MC, Wildermann N, Kereiakes DJ, Popma JJ, et al. Platelet IIbIIIa blockade with integrilin: atherectomy patients. *J Am Coll Cardiol* 1996;**27**:334A.

105. Altman D, Popma J, Hong M, et al. CPK-MB elevation after angioplasty of sephanous vein grafts. *J Am Coll Cardiol* 1993;**21**:232A.

106. Challapalli RM, Eisenberg MJ, Sigmon K, et al for the EPIC investigators: Platelet GPIIb/IIIa monoclonal antibody (c7E3) reduces distal embolization during percutaneous intervention of saphenous vein grafts. *Circulation* 1995;**92**:I–607 [Abstract].

107. Mak KH, Challapalli R, Eisenberg MJ, Anderson KM, Califf RM, Topol EJ. Effect of platelet glycoprotein IIb/IIIa receptor inhibition on distal embolization during percutaneous revascularization of aortocoronary saphenous vein grafts. EPIC Investigators: Evaluation of IIb/IIIa platelet receptor antagonist 7E3 in preventing ischemic complications. *Am J Cardiol* 1997;**80**(8):985–8.

108. Tcheng JE, Anderson K, Tardiff BE, et al. Reducing the risk of pecutaneous intervention after coronary bypass surgery: beneficial effects of abciximab treatment. *J Am Coll Cardiol* 1997;**29**:187A [Abstract].

109. Cannon. Oral presentation. ACC (1999).

110. Topol EJ. Oral presentation. ESC (1999).

111. Montalescot G. Oral presentation. ACC (1999).

16

Acute coronary syndromes

K Martijn Akkerhuis and Jaap W Deckers

Introduction

Acute coronary syndromes (ACS), which include unstable angina, non-Q-wave myocardial infarction (MI), Q-wave MI, sudden ischemic death and the acute complications resulting from interventional procedures, are the leading causes of morbidity and mortality in the Western world.

In Western European countries, 14% of all deaths (414 000 annually) have been attributed to acute MI and other ischemic heart diseases.[1] In the USA, more than 13 million people suffer from ischemic heart disease, and ACS yearly account for almost 500 000 deaths. Each year, an estimated 1.1 million Americans have a new or recurrent coronary attack, and about one-third of them die. At least 250 000 deaths attributed to MI occur within 1 hour of onset of symptoms and before treatment can be started.[2] More than 650 000 Americans are discharged each year with a primary diagnosis of unstable angina. This number approaches that of patients discharged with a primary diagnosis of MI (747 000).[3] Over 10% of patients admitted to the hospital with unstable angina develop an MI within 2 weeks of diagnosis, and 1-year mortality of these patients ranges from 5% to as much as 14%.[4] The ACS therefore have a considerable impact on public health and result in substantial medical expenditure.

Although current interventional and phar-macologic therapies have been effective in reducing the incidence of ischemic events, novel therapeutic targets and strategies are urgently needed to improve further the clinical outcome in patients presenting with ACS.

In the last decade, numerous studies have provided a more detailed understanding of the pathogenesis of ACS. From these insights, new therapeutic targets and pharmacologic approaches to the treatment of ACS have emerged. Additionally, the results of these studies have led to an appreciation of the reasons for the drawbacks and shortcomings, including the relatively limited effectiveness, of the conventional drugs used in the management of patients with ACS and the emerging role of antiplatelet therapy as an adjunct in clinical situations where conventional therapies may not be adequate.

Pathophysiology of ACS

ACS share the common pathophysiology of myocardiol ischemia caused by varying degrees of coronary artery occlusion by platelet-rich thrombi, initiated by the process of disruption or erosion of the covering endothelial layer of an atherosclerotic plaque.[5,6] The two critical events in the pathogenesis of ACS, therefore, are disruption or ulceration (erosion) of an atherosclerotic plaque and the subsequent superimposed formation of a partially or completely occlusive platelet-rich thrombus through the stages of platelet adhesion, activation and aggregation of individually activated platelets.[5,6] The clinical presentation of the ischemia resulting from the platelet-rich coronary thrombus depends on the extent and duration of obstruction of myocardial blood supply.

Disruption or erosion of atherosclerotic plaques

Early plaque development involves the proliferation of smooth muscle cells, the production of collagen and the accumulation of lipid within macrophages, as well as in the extracellular milieu within the lesion.[6] These initial plaques are often asymptomatic owing to the remodelling capacity of the affected coronary artery. An atherosclerotic plaque can become symptomatic, either because additional lipid acquisition leads to plaque growth, causing chronic stenosis which may clinically manifest as stable angina, or because the plaque undergoes erosion or disruption of the covering endothelium, resulting in coronary thrombosis which may present as an acute ischemic coronary syndrome.[5,6] Not all plaque disruptions followed by platelet thrombus formation, however, lead to an acute ischemic coronary event. Plaque ruptures with subclinical thrombosis result in the incorporation of thrombi into the lesion, stimulating plaque growth. In this way, plaque ruptures also contribute to the progression of the atherosclerotic process, which leads to the development of the chronic stenoses that cause stable angina.[5,6] The probability of plaque disruption is determined by several factors, including the shape of the plaque, its composition, some properties of the local circulation and external factors (e.g. blood pressure).

Most patients with coronary artery disease have both concentric plaques, resulting in a fixed degree of obstruction, and eccentric plaques, which may vary in the degree of stenosis owing to changes in coronary artery muscle tone.[5] Concentric plaques are more commonly associated with stable angina, while eccentric plaques carry an increased risk of disruption or erosion, resulting in an ACS.[5–7]

Susceptibility to disruption or fissuring is determined to a great extent by the relative content of the major constituents of the plaque—namely intracellular lipid, extracellular lipid, collagen and proteoglycans. Fibrous plaques are composed primarily of collagen and proteoglycans and are considered 'stable' plaques. In contrast, high lipid content predisposes atherosclerotic plaques to an increased risk of disruption. These plaques contain a lipid-rich core that is separated from the blood by a fibrous cap whose strength is proportional to its thickness. Therefore, the susceptibility of the lipid-rich plaques to rupture may vary depending on the thickness of the fibrous cap and the collagen content, which lends stability to the cap. Lipid-rich atherosclerotic lesions with a thin fibrous cap and a lack of collagen are more susceptible to disruption and are therefore considered 'vulnerable' plaques.[5,8]

High shear forces in the area of stenosis increase the probability of plaque rupture, especially if it concerns a vulnerable plaque that lacks a stable fibrous cap.[8] Changes in coronary tone and pressure can also affect plaque susceptibility to rupture or fissuring by altering the degree of stenosis and the related local shear forces.

Thrombotic response to plaque rupture and platelet thrombus formation

When an atherosclerotic plaque ruptures or

ulcerates, platelets in the circulation are exposed to the highly thrombogenic environment within the plaque or the subendothelium. Platelet adhesion is the first step in platelet-mediated thrombosis. Platelet adhesion is mediated primarily by the binding of the platelet glycoprotein (GP)Ib receptor to the subendothelial form of von Willebrand factor (vWF).[9] Adhesion of platelets is followed by platelet activation. Adherent platelets are activated via several potent platelet agonists. The plaque and the subendothelial layer both contain large amounts of collagen while lipid-laden macrophages in the plaque core produce large quantities of tissue factor. Tissue factor stimulates the generation of thrombin (factor IIa) by initiating the coagulation cascade.[10] Thrombin and collagen are two of the major inducers of platelet activation.[11] Another potent platelet agonist is the high shear force of the circulation in the stenotic region.[10,11] These agonists activate several signal transduction pathways within the platelet. The final outcome of platelet activation includes a change in platelet shape and the secretion of additional platelet agonists (adenosine diphosphate [ADP], serotonin and thromboxane A_2), adhesive glycoproteins (fibrinogen and vWF), clotting factors and other vasoconstrictors, thus promoting vasospasm and further platelet accumulation and activation.[6,10,11] Activation of platelets by any agonist results in the expression of more than 50 000–80 000 copies of the GPIIb/IIIa receptor on the surface of each and every platelet, and its conversion to a high-affinity binding site for its primary ligands, fibrinogen and vWF. Bivalent molecules of fibrinogen cross-link ligand-competent GPIIb/IIIa receptors on adjacent platelets. Eventually, bridging of platelets by their GPIIb/IIIa receptors on a large scale generates a platelet-rich thrombus at the site of plaque injury.[11] Additionally, the aggregate of activated platelets is the primary source of the negatively-charged phospholipid surface on which the coagulation cascade proceeds, further increasing thrombin generation and the conversion of fibrinogen to fibrin.[9] Local generation of thrombin and fibrin then further enhance both platelet activation and aggregation. Most important, regardless of the proaggregatory stimulus, the final common pathway to platelet aggregation and thus to the formation of the platelet-rich thrombus, a pivotal event in the development of ACS, involves aggregation of activated platelets via their GPIIb/IIIa receptors. Further details of coagulation and platelet function can be found in Chapters 1 and 2.

Clinical presentation

The clinical presentation of the myocardial ischemia resulting from the platelet-rich coronary thrombus depends on the extent and acuteness of myocardial blood flow obstruction, as well as on the duration of decreased myocardial perfusion.[6]

The magnitude of the plaque injury determines the strength of the subsequent thrombotic response and is therefore related to the clinical outcome. Minor plaque fissuring usually results in the formation of small intraintimal platelet thrombi, which are subsequently incorporated into the plaque. These thrombi usually remain asymptomatic but stimulate further plaque growth.[5,6] In lesions that have been more deeply disrupted, increasing platelet activation results in the formation of larger thrombi. These thrombi may grow intraluminally and can be either non-occlusive (mural) or occlusive.[5] The non-occlusive, intraluminal thrombi consist primarily of platelets and fibrin ('white' thrombi).[5,12,13] The outer surface of the white thrombus mass consists of a layer of activated platelets.[5] An occlusive coronary thrombus is composed of a platelet-rich or 'white' part located inside the disrupted athero-sclerotic plaque and an intraluminal, occlusive 'red' part. The occlusive part of the thrombus consists mainly of fibrin and red blood cells, while platelets are scarce.[5,12,13] The transitional zone between the intraplaque white thrombus part and the occlusive red thrombus is characterized by a layer of activated platelets, which provide a highly active surface on which the occluding red thrombus layer is generated.[5] Therefore, the aggregation of individual activated platelets by cross-linking of their GPIIb/IIIa receptors to form a white mural thrombus represents an essential step in the generation of the completely occlusive red thrombus.

The presence or absence of a well-developed collateral circulation to the affected vessel is also an important factor determining the clinical outcome of intracoronary thrombosis.[5,14] Disruption of highly stenotic plaques is less likely to interfere significantly with myocardial perfusion since the distal territory is usually supplied by collaterals.[15,16] In contrast, disruption of moderately stenotic plaques carries an increased risk of developing an ACS since the collateral circulation has usually been less well-developed.

The clinical manifestations of ACS depend primarily on the degree and acuteness of coronary blood flow obstruction and the duration of decreased myocardial perfusion.[6] At one end of the spectrum, patients presenting with the ACS of unstable angina usually have non-occlusive, intraluminal thrombi, which are composed primarily of platelets (Figures 16.1 and 16.2).[12,13] Additionally, platelet aggregates may embolize distally, causing foci of myocardial necrosis.[5] These patients usually present with ST-segment depression and elevated troponin T or troponin I levels on their electrocardiogram (ECG). In non-Q-wave infarction, the angiographic form of the responsible

lesions is very similar to that seen in unstable angina. In 25% of the non-Q-wave MI patients, however, the infarct-related artery is occluded but the distal myocardium remains perfused by the collateral vasculature. In the remaining 75% of subjects, the mural platelet-rich thrombus is non-occlusive.[6] The principal difference between unstable angina and non-Q-wave MI is the elevated level of cardiac enzymes (creatine kinase-MB) in the latter patient population, reflecting myocardial necrosis resulting from a longer duration of coronary blood flow obstruction. In Q-wave infarction, an occlusive thrombus on a deeply injured plaque leads to an abrupt, complete and prolonged cessation of myocardial perfusion.[6] This results in subsequent myocardial ischemia and necrosis of the myocardium supplied by the affected coronary artery. The intraluminal thrombi found in patients with Q-wave MI are occlusive and consist mainly of fibrin and trapped red blood cells (see Figures 16.1 and 16.2).[12,13] The ECG shows ST-segment elevation and subsequent development of abnormal Q-waves. As in non-Q-wave MI, elevated levels of cardiac enzymes reflect the myocardial necrosis. The pathophysiology of sudden ischemic death involves a rapidly progressing lesion with subsequent occlusive thrombosis.[6] The abrupt and complete obstruction of coronary blood flow results in severe ischemia and fatal ventricular arrhythmias.[6] The probability of sudden ischemic death in patients with acute thrombotic occlusion is increased in absence of a well-developed collateral circulation.

Goals in the management of acute coronary syndromes

In the majority of patients presenting with the ACS of unstable angina and non-Q-wave MI,

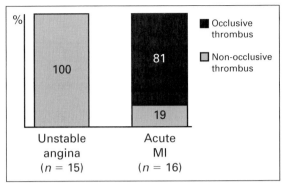

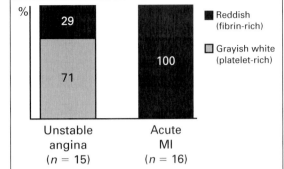

Figure 16.1
Occlusive and non-occlusive thrombi in acute coronary syndromes. Adapted from White 1997[12] and Mizuno et al 1992.[13]

Figure 16.2
Thrombus composition in acute coronary syndromes. Adapted from White 1997[12] and Mizuno et al 1992.[13]

the platelet-rich thrombus is only partially occlusive. Antithrombotic (anticoagulant in combination with antiplatelet) agents aim to maintain vessel patency by preventing the progression of a non-occlusive thrombus to an occlusive thrombus, and to inhibit the generation of new thrombi by preventing further platelet aggregation. In patients with acute MI, characterized by ST-segment elevation, the affected coronary artery is completely occluded. Therefore, the first goal is to achieve rapid reperfusion by the administration of thrombolytic therapy. Secondly, it is of utmost importance to maintain patency of the infarct-related artery, and to prevent recurrent thrombosis leading to reocclusion and recurrent ischemia. For this reason, thrombolytic therapy is commonly used in combination with antithrombotic drugs.[17]

Angioplasty has been used successfully in patients with all ACS. Although effective in establishing adequate myocardial reperfusion, angioplasty does not affect the underlying pathophysiologic processes, platelet aggregation and thrombus formation. Drawbacks of angioplasty include a significant incidence of both acute (abrupt vessel closure) and long-term (restenosis) ischemic complications, which may result in MI or death.[18,19] These have been managed by intracoronary stent implantation, but stenting is also accompanied by adverse effects, most notably stent thrombosis.[20]

Although current interventional and pharmacological therapies have been effective in the treatment of patients with ACS, none of the current management strategies effectively prevents platelet thrombus formation, and the more thorough understanding of the pathophysiology of ACS has pointed to their drawbacks and limited effectiveness. Additionally, studies have identified the pivotal role of the GPIIb/IIIa receptor in platelet aggregation and coronary thrombosis. This receptor has emerged as a new therapeutic target and several inhibitors of its function have been developed and studied in large clinical trials.[11] Based on the results of these trials, the GPIIb/IIIa receptor inhibitors have shown promising results in improving the outcomes of patients with ACS and those experiencing the ischemic complications of the invasive therapies of these diseases.

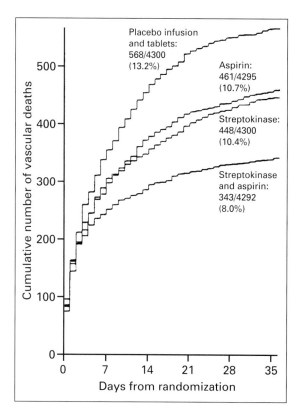

Figure 16.3
Cumulative vascular mortality in the ISIS-2 trial in Days 0–35 among patients allocated: (a) active streptokinase only; (b) active aspirin only; (c) both active treatments; and (d) neither. Reprinted from ISIS-2 Collaborative Group 1988,[22] with permission from The Lancet.

Antithrombotic therapy

Antithrombotic therapy consisting of the intravenous infusion of unfractionated heparin plus the oral administration of aspirin is used routinely in the treatment of the various ACS.

Aspirin

In patients with a broad spectrum of cardio-vascular diseases, antiplatelet therapy offers protection against recurrent adverse ischemic events.[21] The most widely used antiplatelet drug today is acetylsalicylic acid (aspirin). Aspirin reduces the incidence of death, recurrent MI and stroke in patients presenting with acute MI (Figure 16.3).[21,22] Aspirin also reduces mortality and MI when used in the acute management of unstable angina.[23–26] The principal side-effects of aspirin include dose-dependent gastrointestinal symptoms and renal toxicity. Aspirin inhibits the synthesis of the potent platelet activator thromboxane A_2 by blocking the cyclo-oxygenase pathway.[27] However, like many other platelet activation antagonists, aspirin inhibits only one of the pathways to platelet activation, leaving the others intact. Most of the platelet agonists can stimulate platelet aggregation by activating the GPIIb/IIIa receptor via numerous alternate platelet activation pathways.[10] Although safe and very cost-effective, aspirin is therefore not a potent platelet antagonist.

Unfractionated heparin

Unfractionated heparin is a heterogeneous mixture of polysaccharides with a molecular weight of 5000–30 000 Da. The mechanism of action of heparin involves binding to antithrombin III (AT III), thereby greatly increasing its anticoagulant activities.[28] AT III is a protein capable of inhibiting multiple steps in the intrinsic and common coagulation pathways, and of blocking the actions of free thrombin. Thrombin is thought to play an important role in the pathophysiology of coronary artery thrombosis. It promotes platelet activation and aggregation, cleaves fibrinogen to form fibrin, and catalyses the cross-linkage of the fibrin clot. Additionally, thrombin can self-amplify by means of a positive feedback loop. By binding to AT III, heparin increases the affinity of AT III for thrombin 1000-fold. In this way, the heparin-AT III complex is capable of blocking a higher level of thrombin activity and increasing the time to clot formation.[28] Heparin fragments with a lower molecular weight bound to AT III are more capable of inhibiting factor Xa activity than blocking the actions of thrombin.[28]

Heparin is the most widely used antithrombin therapy for patients with ACS. In clinical trials, heparin, alone and in combination with aspirin, has been effective in reducing the adverse ischemic outcomes, including death and non-fatal MI among patients with unstable angina and non-Q-wave MI.[25,26,29] A meta-analysis of multiple studies has shown a 33% reduction in MI or death during heparin therapy in patients with unstable angina treated with aspirin plus heparin compared with those treated with aspirin alone.[4] The usefulness of unfractionated heparin in the management of patients presenting with acute ST-elevation MI is not unequivocal. ACC/AHA guidelines recommend the use of intravenous heparin in patients treated with tPA and in patients who do not receive thrombolytics, while in those who are treated with streptokinase and are not at high risk for systemic emboli the addition of heparin is not recommended.[30,31]

The use of unfractionated heparin is associated with several potential drawbacks. The effectiveness of heparin is limited by several factors, including its inability to inhibit clot-bound thrombin, its dependence on AT III, its neutralization by protein binding and platelet factor 4, which is secreted by activated platelets and blocks the interaction between heparin and AT III, and the rebound clinical events that follow the discontinuation of unfractionated heparin. Unfractionated heparin is therefore inconsistent in its effect within and between patients. Furthermore, it leads to thrombocytopenia in about 5% of patients, and requires hospitalization for frequent monitoring of the activated partial thromboplastin

time (aPTT) and careful titration to achieve aPTT of 50–70 sec.[32–35] In the GUSTO-I trial, aPTT values exceeding 70 sec were related to a progressively increased rate in moderate-to-severe bleeding and were also associated with higher mortality and reinfarction rate.[36] In the GUSTO-IIa trial, a more intensive heparin regimen was accompanied by a 2-fold risk of haemorrhagic stroke in patients receiving thrombolytic therapy.[37] In patients with acute MI, fibrinolytic therapy exposes thrombin, which results not only in the autocatalytic formation of more thrombin but also in enhanced platelet activation. The thrombin activity, but not the increasing formation of more thrombin, may be inhibited by concomitant heparin during thrombolytic therapy. Furthermore, activated platelets create an environment that is potentially resistant to the effects of heparin. When complexed with activated platelets, factor Xa is also relatively resistant to inactivation by the heparin-AT III complex.[38]

The need for increased efficacy and the limitations of unfractionated heparin have led to the development of alternative and more potent antithrombotic drugs, including low-molecular-weight (LMW) heparins and direct thrombin inhibitors.

Low-molecular-weight heparin

LMW heparins are produced by depolymerization of standard heparin, resulting in shorter polysaccharide fragments with a molecular weight of 4000–8000 Da. LMW heparins have several potential advantages over unfractionated heparin. Owing to a higher resistance to inactivation by platelet factor 4 and a lower affinity for heparin-binding proteins, LMW heparins have a more predictable pharmacokinetic profile, greater bioavailability and longer plasma half-life, all of which result in more predictable and reliable levels of anticoagulant effect.[34,39] LMW heparins can therefore be administered once or twice daily as subcutaneous injections at fixed or weight-adjusted doses, thus simplifying treatment in the acute phase without the need for laboratory monitoring. The lower-molecular-weight distribution not only decreases the variability of the anticoagulant effect, but also modifies the anticoagulant mechanism. LMW heparins have a higher Xa/IIa inhibition ratio, but a lesser platelet inhibitory effect.[40]

Several clinical trials have evaluated the efficacy and safety of LMW heparins in patients presenting with ACS.

In the FRISC (Fragmin During Instability in Coronary Artery Disease) study, 1506 patients with unstable angina or non-Q-wave infarction were randomized to receive subcutaneous dalteparin (Fragmin; 120 U/kg twice daily for 6 days, followed by 7500 IU once daily for 35–45 days) or placebo in addition to aspirin.[41] The primary endpoint (death or new MI at 6 days) was significantly lower in the group taking dalteparin (1.8% versus 4.8%). The composite endpoint of death, new MI, revascularization or need for intravenous heparin also showed a significant difference in favour of dalteparin (5.4% versus 10.3%). These differences persisted at 40 days but were no longer significant at 4–5 months after the end of treatment. However, survival analysis showed a risk of reactivation and reinfarction when the dose was decreased. The treatment regimen was safe and compliance was adequate. Of note, this study did not compare dalteparin with unfractionated heparin, but with placebo.

In the ESSENCE (Efficacy and Safety of Subcutaneous Enoxaparin in Non-Q-wave Coronary Events) trial the effect of the LMW heparin enoxaparin (1 mg/kg every 12 h) was compared with unfractionated heparin (adjusted to achieve an aPTT of 55–85 s) in

3171 patients with unstable angina or non-Q-wave MI.[42] All patients received aspirin. The median duration of treatment for both trial therapies was 2.6 days. At 14 days, the risk of death, MI or recurrent angina was significantly lower in patients assigned to enoxaparin than in those randomized to unfractionated heparin (16.6% versus 19.8%). The risk of this composite endpoint remained significantly lower at 30 days (19.8% versus 23.3%). Although the significance of the treatment effect was driven by the differences in the rates of recurrent angina, the risks of both death and MI at 30 days were reduced as well by 20% and 25%, respectively. Treatment with enoxaparin did not increase the incidence of major bleeding complications, although there were slightly more minor bleedings, primarily because of ecchymoses at injection sites.

In the ESSENCE trial, the theoretical advantages of LMW heparin over unfractionated heparin have been translated into a clinical benefit. The more consistent anticoagulant effect together with the higher Xa/IIa inhibition ratio may, in part, account for the better therapeutic index that LMW heparin has over unfractionated heparin. A major advantage of LMW heparin is, however, that it can be used in fixed doses without the necessity of monitoring, thus simplifying therapy and allowing its continuation beyond hospital discharge. More studies are, however, needed to assess the optimal length of treatment and the long-term outcome. Future clinical trials will investigate the efficacy and safety of LMW heparins in new therapeutic settings and in combination with thrombolytic and other new potent antithrombotic and antiplatelet therapy. A substudy in the GUSTO-IV trial will investigate the simultaneous treatment of unstable angina patients with a GPIIb/IIIa inhibitor (abciximab) and LMW heparin.

Direct thrombin inhibitors

Direct thrombin inhibitors, such as hirudin and hirulog, have some potential advantages over heparin. They do not require AT III as a cofactor, are capable of inhibiting both free circulating as well as clot-bound thrombin and are not inactivated by plasma proteins or platelet factor 4.[43]

The TIMI 9B trial compared the efficacy and safety of hirudin with intravenous heparin in 3002 patients with acute MI presenting within 12 h from onset and treated with streptokinase or tissue-type plasminogen activator.[44,45] Comparison of the primary endpoint of death, MI, congestive heart failure or shock at 30 days between treatment groups did not show a significant difference (heparin 11.8% versus hirudin 12.8%). The incidence of major bleeding events including intracranial bleeding was also similar between groups.

The HERO (Hirulog Early Reperfusion/ Occlusion) trial compared the efficacy of two doses of hirulog with heparin in achieving TIMI grade 3 flow at 90 min among 412 patients with acute ST-elevation MI who were treated with aspirin and streptokinase.[46] TIMI grade 3 flow at 90 min was 35% with heparin, 46% with low-dose, and 48% with - high-dose hirulog. At 2–4 days after treatment, similar rates of TIMI grade 3 flow were present in the three groups. Hirulog was more effective in producing early patency without increasing the risk of major bleeding.

In the large GUSTO-IIB (Global Use of Strategies to Open Occluded Coronary Arteries) trial, 12 142 patients with ACS were randomized to receive 72 h of therapy with either intravenous heparin or hirudin.[47] At 24 h, the risk of death or MI was significantly lower in the hirudin group than in the group assigned to heparin (1.3% versus 2.1%). This dif-

ference was still significant 48 h after the initiation of treatment (2.3% versus 3.1%). Although hirudin demonstrated an important effect in reducing early events, the extent of the benefit at 30 days was small and of marginal statistical significance (incidence of death or MI at 30 days: 8.9% versus 9.8% in heparin group, representing an 11% risk reduction, $p = 0.058$). The benefit was similar in patients with ST-segment elevation and in those without. Although there was no significant difference in the incidence of severe bleeding complications, treatment with hirudin was associated with a significantly higher incidence of moderate bleeding (8.8% versus 7.7%, $p = 0.03$).

Results from trials with direct thrombin inhibitors have questioned the hypothesis that potent direct inhibition of thrombin results in a clinically meaningful long-term benefit in clinical outcome. Although thrombin is one of the most potent platelet activators, inhibition of thrombin only targets a single platelet activation pathway, leaving numerous alternate routes for platelet activation available. Further, it was demonstrated that, while capable of inhibiting thrombin activity, hirudin, like heparin, was incapable of blocking thrombin generation resulting in an accumulation of thrombin exceeding the ability of hirudin to block its activity.[48,49] Therefore, antagonism higher in the coagulation cascade, as achieved using LMW heparin, may appear to be more effective. The lack of long-term benefit may also reflect the lack of passivation of the vessel surface or the rebound hypercoagulability after the discontinuation of treatment.[50] Higher doses of hirudin, however, resulted in excessive bleeding (including intracerebral haemorrhage) in the prematurely discontinued TIMI 9A and GUSTO-IIA trials without indication of improved efficacy.[37,51] Therefore, like heparin, hirudin also requires careful titration to achieve aPTT of 50–70 s. The GUSTO-IIB trial showed that patients treated with hirudin required significantly fewer dose adjustments to maintain therapeutic levels of anticoagulation than those treated with heparin.[47] Most important, future trials will have to find ways to improve the durability over time of the therapeutic effect as observed in the early phase, and to assess the additional benefit of a combination of direct thrombin inhibiting agents and platelet GPIIb/IIIa receptor blockers.

Thrombolysis

Thrombolytic therapy has been effective in reducing mortality in patients presenting with acute MI with ST-segment elevation (Figure 16.3).[22,52] Although primary angioplasty is being used to an increasing extent, thrombolysis is still the most widely used modality of reperfusion therapy. Nevertheless, thrombolytic therapy has significant and relevant efficacy as well as safety limitations.

In patients with acute MI, achievement of rapid, complete and sustained restoration of coronary flow through the infarct-related artery (TIMI—Thrombolysis In Myocardial Infarction—grade 3 flow) results in lower mortality, irrespective of the thrombolytic regimen.[53,54] In the angiographic substudy of the landmark GUSTO-I trial, death occurred in 4.4% of patients with normal coronary flow at 90 min, whereas mortality was as high as 8.9% among patients with no flow.[53,54] The most potent currently available thrombolytic therapy, a combination of accelerated alteplase, aspirin and intravenous heparin, produces complete myocardial reperfusion in only 53% of patients, however.[53]

Treatment with thrombolytics is associated with an increased risk of intracerebral bleeding, particularly in older patients and in those with hypertension.[55] In the recently completed GUSTO-III trial, the incidence of haemorrhagic stroke was 0.9%, or approximately 1 in 100 patients.[56]

Furthermore, primary angioplasty for the treatment of acute MI is capable of achieving higher rates of infarct vessel patency (TIMI grade 3 flow approximately 90%) and is associated with a significant reduction in mortality and recurrent MI as compared with pharmacological reperfusion.[57–60]

The primary reason for the lack of efficacy and the relatively high failure rate of thrombolytic therapy is related to the prothrombotic effects of fibrinolytics and the lack of a potent antiplatelet approach in the treatment of acute MI. When fibrinolysis occurs, there is exposure of free thrombin, which not only increases its own production but also leads to platelet activation, thereby strongly promoting further platelet aggregation. The platelet-rich part at the core of the thrombus is, however, fully resistant to fibrinolytic therapy. In addition, activated platelets inhibit fibrinolysis by releasing large amounts of plasminogen activator inhibitor-1, the most potent endogenous inhibitor of fibrinolysis, and by secreting rapid-acting α_2 antiplasmin. Release of coagulation factor XIII further increases resistance to thrombolytics by cross-linking fibrin.[61–63]

These interactions in response to fibrinolytic therapy stimulate the formation of platelet-rich thrombi and contribute to the ongoing and recurrent thrombosis observed in the infarct-related coronary artery. Together with the inability of fibrinolytics to interfere with the formation of the platelet-rich (white) thrombi and the lack of a potent antiplatelet approach, they may contribute to the failure of reperfusion and to the reocclusion that are present in many patients treated with thrombolytic therapy.[64]

The prothrombotic state following fibrinolytic therapy may not only account for the lack of benefit of fibrinolysis in patients with unstable angina and non-Q-wave MI, in whom the thrombus is composed primarily of platelets,[65] but also explain the adverse clinical effects of angioplasty after preceding thrombolysis in patients with acute MI.[66–68]

The importance of a potent antiplatelet approach is endorsed by the results of the ISIS-2 trial. Despite the fact that aspirin is a relatively weak antiplatelet agent and its anti-aggregatory effect in the acute phase is only modest, this study showed that early administration of aspirin resulted in a 23% risk reduction in mortality in patients with acute MI. This benefit was as large as the mortality reduction achieved with the use of streptokinase alone (see Figure 16.3).[22]

A more potent antiplatelet therapy can be achieved with the use of GPIIb/IIIa receptor antagonists. The addition of GPIIb/IIIa receptor blockade to thrombolytic therapy in patients presenting with acute MI has the potential to counteract the prothrombotic tendencies of fibrinolytic agents, and to result in more rapid, complete and sustained reperfusion, and improved survival.

Platelet glycoprotein IIb/IIIa receptor inhibitors

Based on a more thorough understanding of the pathogenesis of ACS and the identification of the platelet GPIIb/IIIa receptor as the final common pathway to platelet aggregation, a new class of therapeutic agents has emerged, the GPIIb/IIIa receptor antagonists.[11] Several inhibitors of the GPIIb/IIIa receptor have been developed. They act either as irreversible, non-competitive GPIIb/IIIa receptor blockers (monoclonal antibodies) or as reversible, competitive GPIIb/IIIa receptor antagonists (fibrinogen analogs). However, while the common limitation of all antiplatelet agents that target the platelet activation stage of thrombus formation is the existence of numerous alternate platelet activation pathways, all of the GPIIb/IIIa receptor antagonists are potent inhibitors of platelet–platelet interaction and capable of fully blocking platelet aggregation, which represents the final common pathway to coronary thrombosis and ACS.[69] Several of these agents have been evaluated in large-scale, randomized, placebo-controlled clinical trials, and they have been shown to be effective in reducing recurrent adverse ischemic events in the treatment of patients undergoing percutaneous intervention and in patients with unstable angina or non-Q-wave infarction.

Abciximab, the Fab fragment of a chimeric human-mouse antibody (c7E3) directed against the GPIIb/IIIa receptor, was the first to undergo clinical evaluation in the EPIC trial,[70] and was approved for use in percutaneous coronary intervention in 1995. In the EPIC (Evaluation of c7E3 for the Prevention of Ischemic Complications) trial, 2099 patients scheduled to undergo angioplasty who were at high risk of ischaemic complications (severe unstable angina, evolving acute MI, or high-risk coronary morphologic characteristics) were randomized to placebo, a bolus of abciximab, or a bolus and 12-hour infusion of abciximab.[70] The composite endpoint of death, non-fatal MI or urgent revascularization at 30 days was reduced by 35% using bolus/infusion abciximab compared with placebo.[70] This benefit was sustained at 6 months, mainly due to lesser need for repeat revascularization,[71] and also at 3 years, most notably among patients with unstable angina or evolving acute MI.[72] Abciximab treatment resulted in particular and incremental benefit for patients enrolled with the ACS severe unstable angina or evolving acute MI; in the subset of 64 patients enrolled with acute MI, the composite endpoint was reduced by 83% (26.1% with placebo versus 4.5% with abciximab bolus/infusion). At 6 months, ischemic events were significantly reduced from 47.8% with placebo to 4.5% with abciximab bolus/infusion, with a significant reduction in reinfarction and a significantly lessened need for repeat revascularization.[73] Patients with severe unstable angina experienced particularly marked reductions in the risk of death and MI with abciximab treatment during coronary intervention (62% reduction in the rate of the 30-day endpoint, mainly owing to reduction in the incidences of death and MI); by 6 months, cumulative death and MI were further reduced using abciximab.[74] Among patients who presented with ACS, the incidence of mortality at 3 years with abciximab was less than half that in the placebo group.[72] The long-term results in the EPIC trial extended the benefits of abciximab from reducing the acute-phase ischemic complications from abrupt vessel closure to a diminished need for subsequent revascularization.[71,75] These sustained and, in some respects, incremental long-term benefits might be a result of the phenomenon of culprit vessel wall passivation, whereby the injured vessel wall is transformed from a platelet-reactive surface into one that does not support platelet thrombus formation and deposition.[76]

The particular benefit of a potent antiplatelet therapy in patients with ACS undergoing percutaneous intervention was further endorsed by the CAPTURE (c7E3 Antiplatelet Therapy in Unstable Refractory Angina) trial.[77] In 1265 patients with refractory unstable angina for whom percutaneous coronary intervention was planned, but not immediately performed, there was a significant 30% reduction in the primary endpoint of death, MI or urgent intervention at 30 days in

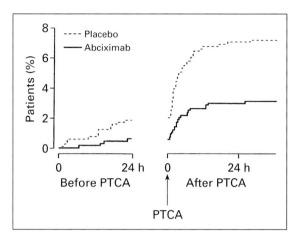

Figure 16.4
Development of myocardial infarction during treatment with abciximab or placebo, before and in association with PTCA. Results from the CAPTURE study. Reprinted from the CAPTURE Investigators 1997[77] with permission from The Lancet.

the abciximab group (11.3% versus 15.9% in the placebo group). In contrast to the EPIC trial, the CAPTURE trial involved the administration of placebo or abciximab starting 18–24 hours prior to percutaneous coronary intervention and continuing until 1 h after completion of the intervention. A unique observation in the CAPTURE trial was the significant reduction of MI occurring before PTCA in patients receiving abciximab during the 24 h preceding coronary intervention (Figure 16.4).[77] This finding also lends support to the hypothesis that GPIIb/IIIa receptor blockers can stimulate culprit vessel passivation and stabilize patients with ACS, such that subsequent coronary intervention may even be avoided.[77] Treatment with abciximab also showed to reduce significantly procedure-related infarctions. In fact, most infarcts occurred during or within 24 h following

PTCA (see Figure 16.4). This suggests that longer treatment with potent GPIIb/IIIa receptor blockers without subsequent coronary intervention might be an alternative or perhaps even the preferred option for patients with ACS, who are at particular high-risk of procedure-related thrombotic complications such as MI, with early coronary revascularization recommended only for patients with recurrent ischaemia despite intensive medical therapy. This new concept of potent antiplatelet therapy with GPIIb/IIIa blockade being effective in achieving culprit vessel wall passivation and stabilizing patients with non-ST-segment elevation ACS on a durable basis, without systematic early coronary revascularization, will be tested in the forthcoming large GUSTO-IV trial.

The effectiveness of platelet GPIIb/IIIa blockade on adverse cardiac events in patients with ACS undergoing coronary angioplasty was further supported by the results of several large clinical trials using several other GPIIb/IIIa receptor inhibitors: eptifibatide (Integrilin™), a cyclic heptapeptide that mimics fibrinogen structure and acts as a reversible, competitive GPIIb/IIIa receptor antagonist, reduced the rates of early ischaemic events at 30 days in the IMPACT-II (Integrilin to Minimise Platelet Aggregation and Coronary Thrombosis-II) trial.[78] Analysis of the treated patient population at 6 months showed a sustained reduction in the composite incidence of death and MI in patients who received eptifibatide.

Tirofiban, another GPIIb/IIIa blocker, was studied in the RESTORE (Randomized Efficacy Study of Tirofiban for Outcomes and REstenosis) trial and provided protection against early cardiac events related to thrombotic closure.[79] At 30 days, the relative reduction was sustained, although to a lesser extent.

The efficacy of platelet GPIIb/IIIa inhibitors as primary therapy in patients with ACS without ST-segment elevation has also been investigated in clinical trials without protocol-mandated revascularization strategies.

In the PURSUIT (Platelet glycoprotein IIb/IIIa in Unstable angina: Receptor Suppression Using Integrilin Therapy) trial, more than 10 000 patients with unstable angina or non-Q-wave infarction were studied.[80] Treatment with eptifibatide resulted in a significant 1.5% absolute reduction in the primary endpoint (death/non-fatal MI at 30 days) compared with placebo (14.2% versus 15.7%). This reduction was reached by 96 h and maintained for 30 days.[80] Using investigator-determined infarctions, the 30-day incidence of the primary endpoint was 8.1% in the eptifibatide group versus 10% in the placebo group. This almost 2.0% absolute reduction was highly significant. In conformity with the results from the CAPTURE study, eptifibatide reduced the event rate in patients treated medically, with an added benefit if they underwent coronary intervention while receiving study drug.[77,80] As with other antithrombotic therapies, eptifibatide was associated with increased bleeding and need for transfusion but not with an increased risk of haemorrhagic stroke.[80] The PURSUIT trial represented the largest phase III study of a GPIIb/IIIa receptor inhibitor used as primary ACS therapy in a setting that closely resembled clinical practice. The results from PURSUIT confirm that early treatment using GPIIb/IIIa inhibitors improves outcomes in abroad spectrum of ACS patients presenting without persistent ST-segment elevation.[80]

Three other large studies have evaluated two other small-molecule GPIIb/IIIa inhibitors as primary treatment in patients presenting with unstable angina or non-Q-wave MI. Tirofiban was studied in the PRISM (Platelet Receptor Inhibition in Ischemic Syndrome Management) and PRISM-PLUS

(Platelet Receptor Inhibition in Ischemic Syndrome Management in Patients Limited by Unstable Signs and Symptoms) trials.[81,82] In both trials, treatment with tirofiban was associated with a significant reduction in adverse ischemic events including death and non-fatal MI in the acute setting. At 30 days, the benefits had been eroded somewhat but the treatment effect still favoured tirofiban, with a significant reduction in mortality in the PRISM study and a significant reduction in death or MI in the PRISM-PLUS study.

In the PARAGON-A study of 2282 patients with unstable angina or non-Q-wave MI lamifiban, a nonpeptide platelet GPIIb/IIIa inhibitor, showed no significant benefit for reduced death or MI in the overall study cohort at 30 days (10% relative reduction).[83] At 6 months, however, there was a highly statistically significant 40% reduction in death or MI for the low-dose lamifiban/heparin group as compared with heparin alone. At 1 year, mortality was reduced from 8.7% to 7.0% in the same low-dose lamifiban/heparin group. These findings of incremental late benefit support the arterial passivation hypothesis. In agreement with other trials evaluating the efficacy of GPIIb/IIIa inhibitors in patients with ACS undergoing PTCA, lamifiban reduced the incidence of death and MI at 30 days in the subset of patients undergoing angioplasty (6.8% versus 15.8% with placebo).[84]

Platelet glycoprotein IIb/IIIa receptor inhibition has now been evaluated in large randomized clinical trials enrolling more than 30 000 patients. In trials, GPIIb/IIIa receptor antagonists were compared with standard therapy in patients undergoing coronary revascularization,[70,77–79,85] and in four trials GPIIb/IIIa receptor inhibition was evaluated as primary therapy in patients with unstable angina or non-Q-wave infarction.[80–83] While the magnitude of benefit has varied, the results of these trials have all demonstrated a consistent benefit in the reduction of death and non-fatal MI for different GPIIb/IIIa receptor blockers (Figure 16.5). Four studies have demonstrated that GP IIb/IIIa inhibition therapy, added to heparin and aspirin in the acute-phase treatment of patients with unstable angina or non-Q-wave MI, improves outcomes in these patients beyond the benefit offered by heparin and aspirin.[80–83] A meta-analysis of the trials shows a very strong and highly significant 20% reduction in death or MI at 30 days (see Figure 16.5).[63] Although in the first trial with GPIIb/IIIa blockers a doubling of significant bleeding complications occurred,[70] recent trials have only shown a slightly higher bleeding event rate in the

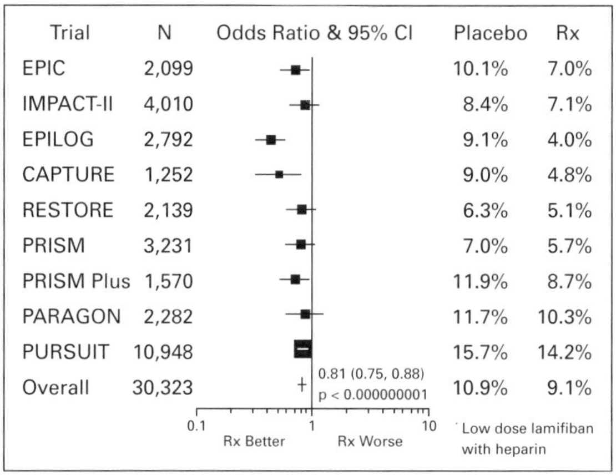

Trial	N	Odds Ratio & 95% CI	Placebo	Rx
EPIC	2,099		10.1%	7.0%
IMPACT-II	4,010		8.4%	7.1%
EPILOG	2,792		9.1%	4.0%
CAPTURE	1,252		9.0%	4.8%
RESTORE	2,139		6.3%	5.1%
PRISM	3,231		7.0%	5.7%
PRISM Plus	1,570		11.9%	8.7%
PARAGON	2,282		11.7%	10.3%
PURSUIT	10,948		15.7%	14.2%
Overall	30,323	0.81 (0.75, 0.88) $p < 0.000000001$	10.9%	9.1%

0.1   1   10
Rx Better   Rx Worse

Low dose lamifiban with heparin

Figure 16.5
Odds ratios and 95% confidence intervals for the nine large-scale (over 1000 patients), randomized, placebo-controlled trials of platelet GPIIb/IIIa inhibitors for percutaneous coronary intervention or unstable angina/non-Q-wave MI. Overall, in 30 323 patients, there is a highly statistically significant 20% reduction in death or MI at 30 days. Reprinted from Topol 1998[63] with permission from Circulation.

GPIIb/IIIa inhibitor group, mainly because of bleeding at the femoral access site in patients undergoing angioplasty. It has been demonstrated that risk can be reduced using reduced heparin dosing on a weight-adjusted basis along with more attention to the catheter-access site bleeding.[85,86] Most importantly, GPIIb/IIIa inhibition therapy has not been associated with an excess of intracerebral bleedings in patients enrolled in the large intervention trials.[63] Of note, all trials used aspirin in the placebo group. The effect of the GPIIb/IIIa receptor inhibitors is therefore additional and of a magnitude (25%) that is comparable with that achieved with aspirin more than a decade ago. In addition, at least two trials with different GPIIb/IIIa inhibiting agents have shown evidence for durability or incremental late benefit of the treatment effect achieved in the early phase.[72,83]

GPIIb/IIIa inhibitors in the treatment of acute MI

As discussed, platelet thrombus formation is a major contributor to both the failure of thrombolysis and the pathogenesis of reocclusion in patients with acute MI. Therefore, GPIIb/IIIa receptor blockade therapy added to thrombolytics or used as an adjunct to direct angioplasty may significantly improve treatment outcomes in patients with acute ST-segment elevation MI.

Thrombolytic therapy combined with GPIIb/IIIa receptor blockade

Experimental, preclinical studies have shown that combining GPIIb/IIIa inhibitors with thrombolytic therapy results in more rapid, complete and sustained reperfusion, and that the dosage of fibrinolytics can be decreased with concomitant use of GPIIb/IIIa receptor blockers.[63] In the first clinical study, TAMI 8,

60 patients receiving full-dose alteplase, aspirin and heparin for acute MI received bolus injections of the murine 7E3 monoclonal antibody Fab at varying time points after initiation of the thrombolytic therapy.[87] Ten control patients were treated with alteplase but not with m7E3 Fab. The infarct-related artery was patent (TIMI grade 2 or 3 flow) in 92% of patients receiving m7E3 Fab compared with 56% of patients in the control group. There was no excess of major bleeding complications among patients treated with the combination of alteplase and m7E3 Fab. The IMPACT-AMI (Integrilin to Manage Platelet Aggregation to Combat Thrombus in Acute Myocardial Infarction) trial investigated the preliminary efficacy and safety of a combination of full-dose, accelerated alteplase, aspirin and heparin with variable dosing of the GP IIb/IIIa inhibitor eptifibatide in a pilot study of 180 patients with acute MI.[88] Patients treated with the highest eptifibatide dose had a 69% higher rate of TIMI grade 3 flow than placebo-treated patients (66% versus 39%) at 90 min, and a shorter median time to ST-segment recovery on continuous 12-lead ST-segment monitoring. The combined use of alteplase and eptifibatide was not associated with an excess of significant bleeding complications. In the PARADIGM (Platelet Aggregation Receptor Antagonist Dose Investigation and Reperfusion Gain in Myocardial Infarction) trial, 345 patients with acute MI treated with either alteplase or streptokinase were randomly assigned intravenous lamifiban at three different doses or placebo. While there was no trend in reducing clinical endpoints between groups, the continuous 12-lead ECG monitoring showed more rapid and stable resolution of the ST-segment elevation among patients treated with the combination of lamifiban and thrombolytics, suggesting improved early and complete reperfusion.[63,64]

Furthermore, concomitant use of potent antiplatelet therapy facilitating fibrinolysis may allow for lower doses of fibrinolytics needed to achieve reperfusion. Lower doses of fibrinolytic therapy minimize the adverse pro-thrombotic effects and could reduce the risk of significant bleeding complications including intracerebral haemorrhage.[63] The SPEED (Strategies for Patency Enhancement in the Emergency Department) trial was a dose-finding, Phase II study that compared abciximab alone with abciximab plus reduced-dose reteplase in patients with acute ST-elevation MI. The dose of reteplase was escalated to establish the optimal dose of r-PA in combination with full-dose abciximab. Preliminary 60-min angiographic results showed a dose-response with increasing doses reteplase with a higher TIMI 3 flow rate.[89] TIMI 3 flow at 60 min was achieved in 52% of patients receiving abciximab plus 10 units r-PA versus 45% in the t-PA meta-analysis.[89] The ongoing TIMI 14A trial evaluates the additional benefit of abciximab when used as adjunct to several fibrinolytic regimens in the management of patients with acute MI. Preliminary data showed that treatment with abciximab alone was capable of achieving TIMI 3 flow rates similar to those seen with a full-dose of strep-tokinase in the GUSTO-I trial. When added to streptokinase and t-PA, abciximab increased the rate and extent of reperfusion with reduced doses of the fibrinolytics.[90] The high-est TIMI 3 flow rate (79%) was achieved with a 60-min infusion of 50 mg t-PA in combination with abciximab.[90] Although the angio-graphic results and/or ST-monitoring data from these studies suggest that the rate and speed of reperfusion can be enhanced by com-bining GPIIb/IIIa receptor inhibitors with thrombolytic therapy, larger, Phase III trials are needed to assess further the ability of GPIIb/IIIa inhibitors, alone or in combination with full- or reduced-dose fibrinolytics, to improve clinical outcomes with fewer signifi-cant bleeding complications in patients with acute ST-segment elevation MI.

Combining direct angioplasty and GP IIb/IIIa blockade

Initial data pointing to the beneficial effects of adding GP IIb/IIIa receptor blockade to direct angioplasty for acute MI were provided by the subgroup analysis of patients from the EPIC trial enrolled with acute MI and undergoing primary or rescue angioplasty. These have already been discussed in this chapter. In the recent RAPPORT (Reopro and Primary PTCA Organization and Randomized Trial) trial, abciximab was compared with placebo in patients undergoing primary angioplasty for acute MI. Abciximab significantly reduced the incidence of death, reinfarction or urgent tar-get vessel revascularization at 30 days (5.8% versus 11.2%).[91] Furthermore, the need for unplanned, 'bail-out' stenting was reduced by 42% in the abciximab group. Treatment with abciximab was, however, associated with an increased risk of major bleeding (16.6% ver-sus 9.5%). Larger trials will have to confirm the beneficial effects of GPIIb/IIIa inhibition in patients undergoing direct angioplasty for acute ST-segment elevation MI.

In the next few years, it is likely that GP IIb/IIIa inhibitors will come to play an impor-tant role in the treatment of patients with acute ST-segment elevation MI. They have the potential to achieve high rates of reperfusion without an increased risk of significant bleed-ing complications when used combined with low-dose fibrinolytics, and are capable of enhancing the safety of primary or (subse-quent) rescue angioplasty.

Oral GPIIb/IIIa receptor antagonists

Where intravenous GP IIb/IIIa receptor inhibitors have shown significant effect in reducing acute ischemic complications in patients undergoing angioplasty and in those with ACS, additional and, potentially, incremental long-term benefit might be obtained by subsequent, continuing longer-term treatment with oral platelet GP IIb/IIIa antagonists. However, whether prolonged administration of oral GP IIb/IIIa blockers is capable of preventing subsequent events in at-risk patients and providing secondary prevention awaits the results of large-scale trials.

References

1. *World Health Statistics Annual 1994* (Geneva, Switzerland, World Health Organisation, 1995).
2. American Heart Association, *Heart and Stroke Facts* (Dallas, Tex, American Heart Association National Center, 1996).
3. Brunelli C, Spallarossa P, Rossettin P, Caponnetto S. Recognition and treatment of unstable angina. *Drugs* 1996;**52**:196–208.
4. Oler A, Whooley MA, Oler J, Grady D. Adding heparin to aspirin reduces the incidence of myocardial infarction and death in patients with unstable angina. A meta-analysis. *J Am Med Assoc* 1996;**276**:811–15.
5. Davies MJ. A macro and micro view of coronary vascular insult in ischemic heart disease. *Circulation* 1990;**82(Suppl. II)**:II-38–II-46.
6. Fuster V, Badimon L, Badimon JJ, Chesebro JH. The pathogenesis of coronary artery disease and the acute coronary syndromes. *N Engl J Med* 1992;**326**:242–50, 310–18.
7. Hangartner JRW, Charleston AJ, Davies MJ, Thomas AC. Morphological characteristics of clinically significant coronary artery stenosis in stable angina. *Br Heart J* 1986;**56**:501–8.
8. Richardson PD, Davies MJ, Born GVR. Influence of plaque configuration and stress distribution on fissuring of coronary atherosclerotic plaques. *Lancet* 1989;**2**:941–4.
9. Ware JA, Coller BS. Platelet morphology, biochemistry, and function. In: Beutler E, Lichtman MA, Coller BS (eds), *Williams Hematology*, 5th edn (New York, McGraw-Hill, 1995) 1161–201.
10. Coller BS. Platelets in cardiovascular thrombosis and thrombolysis. In: Fozzard HA, Haber Jennings RB, Katz AM, Morgan HE (eds) *The Heart and Cardiovascular System: Scientific Foundations*, 2nd edn (New York, Raven Press, 1992) Vol.1, 219–73.
11. Lefkovits J, Plow EF, Topol EJ. Platelet glycoprotein IIb/IIIa receptors in cardiovascular medicine. *N Engl J Med* 1995;**332**:1553–9.
12. White HD. Unmet therapeutic needs in the management of acute ischemia. *Am J Cardiol* 1997;**80(4A)**:2B–10B.
13. Mizuno K, Satomura K, Miyamoto A et al. Angioscopic evaluation of coronary artery thrombi in acute coronary syndromes. *N Engl J Med* 1992;**326**:287–91.
14. Davies MJ. The role of plaque pathology in coronary thrombosis, *Clin Cardiol* 1997;**20 (Suppl. I)**:I-2–I-7.
15. Cohen M, Sherman W, Rentrop KP, Gorlin R. Determinants of collateral filling observed during sudden controlled coronary artery occlusion in human subjects. *J Am Coll Cardiol* 1989;**13**:297–303.
16. Habib GB, Heibig J, Forman SA et al, and the TIMI Investigators. Influence of coronary collateral vessels on myocardial infarct size in humans. Results of phase I Thrombolysis in Myocardial Infarction (TIMI) trial. *Circulation* 1991;**83**:739–46.
17. Neuhaus KL. Coronary thrombosis-defining the goals, improving the outcome. *Clin Cardiol* 1997;**20(Suppl I)**:I-8–I-13.
18. Landau C, Lange RA, Hillis LD. Percutaneous transluminal coronary angioplasty. *N Engl J Med* 1994;**330**:981–93.
19. Ferguson JJ, Wilson JM. Early and late ischemic complications of PTCA. *J Invas Cardiol* 1994;**6(Suppl A)**:3A–12A.
20. Bittl JA. Coronary stent occlusion: Thrombus horribilis. [Editorial]. *J Am Coll Cardiol* 1996;**28**:368–70.
21. Antiplatelet Trialists' Collaboration. Collaborative overview of randomised trials of antiplatelet therapy I: prevention of death, myocardial infarction, and stroke by prolonged antiplatelet therapy in various categories of patients, *Br Med J* 1994;**308**:81–106.
22. ISIS-2 (Second International Study of Infarct Survival) Collaborative Group. Randomised trial of intravenous streptokinase, oral aspirin, both, or neither among 17 187 cases of suspected myocardial infarction, *Lancet* 1988;**2**:349–60.

23. Lewis HDJ, Davies JW, Archibald DG et al. Protective effects of aspirin against acute myocardial infarction and death in men with unstable angina. Results of a Veterans Administration Cooperative Study. *N Engl J Med* 1983;**309**:396–403.

24. Cairns JA, Gent M, Singer J et al. Aspirin, sulfinpyrazone, or both in unstable angina. Results of a Canadian multicenter trial. *N Engl J Med* 1985;**313**:1369–75.

25. Théroux P, Ouimet H, McCans J et al. Aspirin, heparin, or both to treat acute unstable angina. *N Engl J Med* 1988;**319**:1105–11.

26. The RISC Group. Risk of myocardial infarction and death during treatment with low-dose aspirin and intravenous heparin in men with unstable coronary artery disease. *Lancet* 1990;**336**:827–30.

27. Almony GT, Lefkovits J, Topol EJ. Antiplatelet and anticoagulant use after myocardial infarction. *Clin Cardiol* 1996;**19**:357–65.

28. Fiore L, Deykin D. Anticoagulant therapy. In: Beutler E, Lichtman MA, Coller BS (eds) *Williams Hematology*, 5th edn (New York, McGraw-Hill, 1995) 1562–84.

29. Cohen M, Adams PC, Parry G, et al, and the Antithrombotic Therapy in Acute Coronary Syndromes Research Group. Combination antithrombotic therapy in unstable rest angina and non-Q-wave infarction in nonprior aspirin users. Primary end points analysis from the ATACS trial. *Circulation* 1994;**89**:81–8.

30. The GUSTO Investigators. An international randomized trial comparing four thrombolytic strategies for acute myocardial infarction. *N Engl J Med* 1993;**329**:673–82.

31. Ryan TJ, Anderson JL, Antman EM et al. ACC/AHA guidelines for the management of patients with acute myocardial infarction: executive summary: a report of the American College of Cardiology/American Heart Association Task Force on Practice Guidelines (Committee on Management of Acute Myocardial Infarction). *Circulation* 1996;**94**:2341–50.

32. Weitz JI, Hudoba M, Massel D, Maraganore J, Hirsh J. Clot-bound thrombin is protected from inhibition by heparin-antithrombin III but is susceptible to inactivation by antithrombin III-independent inhibitors. *J Clin Invest* 1990;**86**:385–91.

33. Hirsh J. Heparin. *N Engl J Med* 1991;**324**: 1565–74.

34. Melandri G, Semprini F, Cervi V, et al. Comparison of efficacy of low molecular weight heparin (parnaparin) with that of unfractionated heparin in the presence of activated platelets in healthy subjects. *Am J Cardiol* 1993;**72**:450–54.

35. Théroux P, Waters D, Lam J, Juneau M, McCans J. Reactivation of unstable angina after the discontinuation of heparin. *N Engl J Med* 1992;**327**:141–5.

36. Granger CB, Hirsh J, Califf RM, et al. Activated partial thromboplastin time and outcome after thrombolytic therapy for acute myocardial infarction. Results from the GUSTO I trial. *Circulation* 1996;**93**:870–78.

37. The Global Use of Strategies to Open Occluded Coronary Arteries (GUSTO) IIa Investigators. Randomized trial of intravenous heparin versus recombinant hirudin for acute coronary syndromes, *Circulation* 1994;**90**:1631–7.

38. Jesty J, Nemerson Y. The pathways of blood coagulation. In: Beutler E, Lichtman MA, Coller BS (eds), *Williams Hematology*, 5th edn (New York, McGraw-Hill, 1995)1227–38.

39. Hirsh J, Levine MN. Low molecular weight heparin. *Blood* 1992;**79**:1–17.

40. Nurmohamed MT, ten Cate H, ten Cate JW. Low molecular weight heparin(oids)s—clinical investigations and practical recommendations. *Drugs* 1997;**53**:736–51.

41. Fragmin During Instability in Coronary Artery Disease (FRISC) Study Group. Low-molecular-weight heparin during instability in coronary artery disease. *Lancet* 1996;**347**:561–8.

42. Cohen M, Demers C, Gurfinkel EP et al. for the Efficacy and Safety of Subcutaneous Enoxaparin in Non-Q-Wave Coronary Events Study Group: A comparison of low-molecular-weight heparin with unfractionated heparin for unstable coronary artery disease. *N Engl J Med* 1997;**337**:447–52.

43. Lefkovits J, Topol EJ. Direct thrombin inhibitors in cardiovascular medicine. *Circulation* 1994;**90**:1522–36.

44. Ferguson JJ. Meeting highlights American Heart Association 68th Scientific Sessions, Anaheim, California, November 3–15, 1995. *Circulation* 1996;**93**:843–6.

45. Ferguson JJ, Lau TK. Newer antithrombotic and antiplatelet agents for acute coronary syndromes. *Acute Coronary Syndromes* 1997; 1:9–18.

46. White HD, Aylward PE, Frey MJ, et al, on behalf of the Hirulog Early Reperfusion/Occlusion (HERO) Trial Investigators. Randomized, double-blind comparison of hirulog versus heparin in patients receiving streptokinase and aspirin for acute myocardial infarction (HERO). *Circulation* 1997;**96**:2155–61.

47. The Global Use of Strategies to Open Occluded Coronary Arteries (GUSTO) IIb Investigators. A comparison of recombinant hirudin with heparin for the treatment of acute coronary syndromes. *N Engl J Med* 1996;**335**:775–82.

48. Zoldhelyi P, Janssens S, Lefèvre G, Collen D, Van de Werf F, for the GUSTO IIa Investigators. Effects of heparin and hirudin (CGP 39393) on thrombin generation during thrombolysis for acute myocardial infarction. *Circulation* 1995;**92** (Suppl. I):I-740 [Abstract].

49. Merlini PA, Ardissino D, Bauer KA, et al. Persistent thrombin generation during heparin treatment in patients with acute coronary syndromes. *Circulation* 1995;**92**(Suppl. I):I-623 [Abstract].

50. Flather M, Weitz J, Campeau J, et al. Evidence for rebound activation of the coagulation system after cessation of intravenous anticoagulant therapy for acute myocardial ischemia: *Circulation* 1995;**92**(Suppl. I):I-485 [Abstract].

51. Antman EM, for the TIMI 9A Investigators. Hirudin in acute myocardial infarction. Safety report from the Thrombolysis and Thrombin Inhibition in Myocardial Infarction (TIMI) 9A trial. *Circulation* 1994;**90**:1624–30.

52. Fibrinolytic Therapy Trialists' (FTT) Collaborative Group. Indications for fibrinolytic therapy in suspected acute myocardial infarction: collaborative overview of early mortality and major morbidity results from all randomised trials of more than 1000 patients. *Lancet* 1994;**343**:311–22.

53. The GUSTO Angiographic Investigators. The effects of tissue plasminogen activator, streptokinase, or both on coronary-artery patency, ventricular function, and survival after acute myocardial infarction. *N Engl J Med* 1993;**329**:1615–22.

54. Simes RJ, Topol EJ, Holmes DR, et al, for the GUSTO-I Investigators. Link between the angiographic substudy and mortality outcomes in a large randomized trial of myocardial infarction. Importance of early and complete infarct artery reperfusion. *Circulation* 1995;**91**:1923–8.

55. Gore JM, Granger CB, Simoons ML, et al. Stroke after thrombolysis: mortality and functional outcomes in the GUSTO-I trial. *Circulation* 1995;**92**:2811–18.

56. The GUSTO-III Investigators. An international, randomized comparison of reteplase with alteplase for acute myocardial infarction. *N Engl J Med* 1997; **337**:1118–23.

57. Stone GW, O'Neill WW, Jones D, Grines CL. The central unifying concept of TIMI-3 flow after primary PTCA and thrombolysis therapy in acute myocardial infarction. *Circulation* 1996;**94**(Suppl.):I-515 [Abstract].

58. Grines CL, Browne KF, Marco J, et al. A comparison of immediate angioplasty with thrombolytic therapy for acute myocardial infarction. *N Engl J Med* 1993;**328**:673–9.

59. Zijlstra F, de Boer MJ, Hoorntje JCA, Reiffers S, Reiber JHC, Suryapranata H. A comparison of immediate coronary angioplasty with intravenous streptokinase in acute myocardial infarction. *N Engl J Med* 1993;**328**:680–84.

60. The GUSTO-II Angioplasty Substudy Investigators. A clinical trial comparing primary coronary angioplasty with tissue plasminogen activator and recombinant hirudin with heparin for acute myocardial infarction. *N Engl J Med* 1997;**336**:1621–8.

61. Coller BS. Platelets and thrombolytic therapy. *N Engl J Med* 1990;**322**:33–42.

62. Coller BS. Augmentation of thrombolysis with antiplatelet drugs. *Cor Artery Dis* 1995;**6**: 911–14.

63. Topol EJ. Toward a new frontier in myocardial reperfusion therapy. Emerging platelet preeminence. *Circulation* 1998;**97**:211–18.

64. Alexander JH, Ohman EM, Harrington RA. Platelet GPIIb/IIIa inhibitors in acute MI: pathophysiology and clinical effects. *Acute Coronary Syndromes* 1998;**1**:46–51.

65. The TIMI IIIB Investigators. Effects of tissue plasminogen activator and a comparison of

early invasive and conservative strategies in unstable angina and non-Q-wave myocardial infarction. Results of the TIMI IIIB trial. *Circulation* 1994;**89**:1545–56.

66. Topol EJ, Califf RM, George BS, for the Thrombolysis and Angioplasty in Myocardial Infarction Study Group. A randomized trial of immediate versus delayed elective angioplasty after intravenous tissue plasminogen activator in acute myocardial infarction. *N Engl J Med* 1987;**317**:581–8.

67. Simoons ML, Arnold AER, Betriu A, et al. Thrombolysis with tissue plasminogen activator in acute myocardial infarction: no additional benefit from immediate percutaneous transluminal coronary angioplasty. *Lancet* 1988;**1**:197–203.

68. TIMI Research Group. Immediate versus delayed catheterization and angioplasty following thrombolytic therapy for acute myocardial infarction. TIMI IIA results, *J Am Med Assoc* 1988;**260**:2849–58.

69. Topol EJ. Targeted approaches to thrombus inhibition – an end to the shotgun approach. *Clin Cardiol* 1997;**20(Suppl. I)**:I-22–I-26.

70. The EPIC Investigators. Use of a monoclonal antibody directed against the platelet glycoprotein IIb/IIIa receptor in high-risk coronary angioplasty. *N Engl J Med* 1994;**330**:956–61.

71. Topol EJ, Califf RM, Weisman HF, et al, on behalf of the EPIC Investigators. Randomised trial of coronary intervention with antibody against platelet IIb/IIIa integrin for reduction of clinical stenosis: results at six months. *Lancet* 1994;**343**:881–6.

72. Topol EJ, Ferguson JJ, Weisman HF, et al for the EPIC Investigator Group. Long-term protection from myocardial ischemic events in a randomized trial of brief integrin β_3 blockade with percutaneous coronary intervention, *J Am Med Assoc* 1997;**278**:479–84.

73. Lefkovits J, Ivanhoe RJ, Califf RM et al, for the EPIC Investigators. Effects of platelet glycoprotein IIb/IIIa receptor blockade by a chimeric monoclonal antibody (abciximab) on acute and six-month outcomes after percutaneous transluminal coronary angioplasty for acute myocardial infarction. *Am J Cardiol* 1996;**77**:1045–51.

74. Lincoff AM, Califf RM, Anderson KM et al, for the EPIC Investigators. Evidence for prevention of death and myocardial infarction with platelet membrane glycoprotein IIb/IIIa receptor blockade by abciximab (c7E3 Fab) among patients with unstable angina undergoing percutaneous coronary revascularization. *J Am Coll Cardiol* 1997;**30**:149–56.

75. Ip JH, Fuster V, Israel D, Badimon L, Badimon J, Chesebro JH. The role of platelets, thrombin and hyperplasia in restenosis after coronary angioplasty. *J Am Coll Cardiol* 1991;**17**:77B–88B.

76. Bates ER, Walsh DG, Mu DX, Abams GD, Luchessi BR. Sustained inhibition of the vessel wall-platelet interaction after deep coronary artery injury by temporary inhibition of the platelet glycoprotein IIb/IIIa receptor. *Cor Art Dis* 1993;**3**:67–76.

77. The CAPTURE Investigators. Randomised placebo-controlled trial of abciximab before and during coronary intervention in refractory unstable angina: the CAPTURE study. *Lancet* 1997;**349**:1429–35.

78. The IMPACT-II Investigators. Randomised placebo-controlled trial of effect of eptifibatide on complications of percutaneous coronary intervention: IMPACT-II, *Lancet* 1997;**349**:1422–8.

79. The RESTORE Investigators. Effects of platelet glycoprotein IIb/IIIa blockade with tirofiban on adverse cardiac events in patients with unstable angina or acute myocardial infarction undergoing coronary angioplasty. *Circulation* 1997;**96**:1445–53.

80. The PURSUIT Investigators. Inhibition of platelet glycoprotein IIb/IIIa with eptifibatide in patients with acute coronary syndromes without persistent ST-segment elevation. *N Engl J Med* 1998;**339**:436–43.

81. The PRISM Study Investigators. A comparison of aspirin plus tirofiban with aspirin plus heparin for unstable angina. *N Engl J Med* 1998;**338(21)**:1498–505.

82. The PRISM-PLUS Study Investigators. Inhibition of the platelet glycoprotein IIb/IIIa receptor with tirofiban in unstable angina and non-Q-wave myocardial infarction. *N Engl J Med* 1998;**338(21)**:1488–97.

83. The PARAGON Investigators. An international, randomized, controlled trial of lami-

fiban, a platelet glycoprotein IIb/IIIa inhibitor, heparin or both in unstable angina. *Circulation* 1998;**97**:2386–95.

84. Alexander JH, Newby NK, Moliterno DJ et al, for the PARAGON A Investigators. Relationship of outcomes to treatment with lamifiban in patients undergoing PTCA: analysis of PARAGON A. *J Am Coll Cardiol* 1997; **29(Suppl. A)**:409A [Abstract].

85. The EPILOG Investigators. Platelet glycoprotein IIb/IIIa receptor blockade and low-dose heparin during percutaneous coronary revascularization. *N Engl J Med* 1997;**336**:1689–96.

86. Lincoff AM, Tcheng JE, Califf RM, et al, for the PROLOG Investigators. Standard versus low-dose weight-adjusted heparin in patients treated with the platelet glycoprotein IIb/IIIa receptor antibody fragment abciximab (c7E3 Fab) during percutaneous coronary revascularization. *Am J Cardiol* 1997;**79**:286–91.

87. Kleiman NS, Ohman EM, Califf RM, et al. Profound inhibition of platelet aggregation with monoclonal antibody 7E3 Fab after thrombolytic therapy. Results of the Thrombolysis and Angioplasty in Myocardial Infarction (TAMI) 8 pilot study. *J Am Coll Cardiol* 1993;**22**:381–9.

88. Ohman EM, Kleiman NS, Gacioch G, et al, for the IMPACT-AMI Investigators. Combined accelerated tissue-plasminogen activator and platelet glycoprotein IIb/IIIa integrin receptor blockade with integrilin in acute myocardial infarction. Results of a randomized, placebo-controlled, dose-ranging trial. *Circulation* 1997;**95**:846–54.

89. Ohman EM. Dose-escalation evaluation of full dose abciximab in conjunction with low dose r-PA. The SPEED trial, Highlight report from the American College of Cardiology 47th Annual Scientific Session, March 29–April 1, 1998, Atlanta Georgia, USA.

90. Braunwald E. Dose-finding study assessing the value of abciximab as an adjunct to fibrinolytic therapy in acute myocardial infarction. The TIMI 14A study, Highlight report from the American College of Cardiology 47th Annual Scientific Session, March 29–April 1, 1998, Atlanta Georgia, USA.

91. Topol EJ. RAPPORT: outcomes in patients with acute myocardial infarction with abciximab and primary PTCA, Presented at the XIX Congress of the European Society of Cardiology, Stockholm, Sweden, August 24–28, 1997.

Section IV:

Directions for the future

17

Platelet GPIIb/IIIa inhibitor—device synergy during percutaneous coronary intervention

Dean J Kereiakes

Introduction

Recent data have suggested that platelet glyco-protein (GP)IIb/III blockade using abciximab improves clinical outcomes similarly when administered adjunctively for various interventional techniques[1,2] and for patients in both low- and high-risk clinical stratifications using the American Heart Association (AHA) criteria[3] (Figures 17.1 and 17. 2). The observation of appreciable and similar benefit across interventions and risk categories has prompted consideration for adjunctive GPIIb/IIIa therapy for *all* patients undergoing percutaneous coronary intervention. Nevertheless, close evaluation of data from both randomized trials and clinical series in the context of current knowledge of pathophysiologic mechanisms suggests that adjunct platelet GPIIb/IIIa blockade may offer preferential benefit for certain subgroups of patients undergoing percutaneous coronary intervention. The benefits of platelet GPIIb/IIIa blockade may be most evident in patients having coronary stents or undergoing revascularization using an atheroablative technique. Likewise, patients having saphenous vein grafts or those with an acute coronary syndrome requiring percutaneous coronary intervention may also benefit from GPIIb/IIIa inhibition.

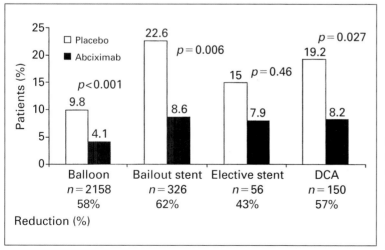

Figure 17.1
Primary endpoint (death, MI, urgent intervention at 30 days) following multiple intervention in the EPILOG trial. DCA, directional coronary atherectomy. Reproduced from Kereiakes et al,[1] 1997, with permission.

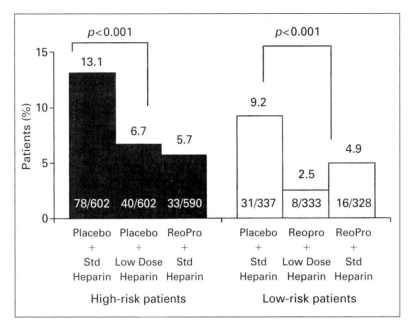

Figure 17.2
Incidence occurrence of primary endpoint (death, MI, urgent intervention) at 30 days by treatment strategy and American Heart Association (AHA) risk stratification in the EPILOG trial. Improvement in outcomes associated with abciximab therapy was similar in both risk groups as defined by AHA criteria. Std, standard weight-adjusted heparin.

Platelet GPIIb/IIIa blockade and coronary stenting
Unplanned or provisional coronary stenting

Elective or planned coronary stent deployment was discouraged by protocol in the EPILOG trial and coronary stenting was reserved for patients who had abrupt or threatened coronary closure; over 40% residual stenosis following balloon angioplasty or Types C–F coronary dissection.[3–5] A multivariate analysis of baseline angiographic morphology from patients who subsequently required unplanned stent deployment in the EPILOG trial identified several characteristics, including complex lesion morphology (AHA/ACC Class B2 or C; $p = 0.003$), lesion length over 10 mm ($p = 0.002$), lesion eccentricity ($p = 0.027$), irregular lesion contour ($p = 0.001$), and bifurcation involvement ($p = 0.019$) to be more common.[5] Despite the fact that these complex descriptors were distributed equally across the three randomized pharmacologic treatment arms in the EPILOG trial; the requirement for unplanned coronary stent deployment was significantly reduced in patients who received prophylactic abciximab and low-dose weight-adjusted heparin compared with patients who received placebo and standard-dose heparin (9.0% versus 13.7% respectively; $p < 0.001$).[4,5] Similarly, the requirement for bailout or unplanned coronary stent deployment was reduced by 41% ($p = 0.022$) in patients in the RAPPORT (Reopro and Primary PTCA Organization Randomization) trial who were randomized to receive abciximab therapy and who also had balloon angioplasty performed.[6] These observations have been extended by a meta-analysis of multiple trials in which 10 691 patients were randomized to receive platelet GPIIb/IIIa blockade or placebo (Figure 17.3). In these trials, platelet GPIIb/IIIa blockade was associated with a significant (27%) reduction in the requirement for unplanned coronary stent deployment ($p < 0.0005$).[7] These data suggest that prophylactic platelet GPIIb/IIIa blockade reduces the requirement for 'bailout' or unplanned coronary stent deployment and improves the outcomes of balloon angioplasty in complex lesions subsets.

A substantial foundation of data supports the premise that once a bailout or unplanned coronary stent is deployed, concomitant platelet GPIIb/IIIa blockade is associated with improvement in clinical outcomes. In the IMPACT II randomized trial of integrelin versus placebo, which were administered during percutaneous coronary intervention, the prophylactic administration of integrelin to patients who subsequently required an emergency/unplanned stent deployment was associated with a reduction in periprocedural myocardial infarction (MI) ($p = 0.017$) and in the composite occurrence of death, myocardial infarction and urgent revascularization ($p = 0.002$).[8] Likewise in the EPILOG trial, patients who required unplanned stent deployment derived considerable benefit from the prophylactic administration of abciximab (Figure 17.4).[4,5] Multiple ischemic outcomes, particularly periprocedural infarction and the need for urgent/emergent revascularization were reduced using abciximab therapy. A subsequent meta-analysis of 529 patients with coronary stent deployment (9.9%) from 5364 patients enrolled in the EPIC, EPILOG and CAPTURE placebo-controlled randomized trials of abciximab administration during percutaneous coronary intervention confirmed the benefit of prophylactic abciximab administration.[9] The prophylactic administration of abciximab was associated with enhanced survival at 30 days and marked reductions in the requirements for emergency bypass surgery and urgent revascularization (reductions of over 90% and 75% respectively; Figure 17.5a). The benefit of abciximab therapy was maintained at 6 months follow-up, with a

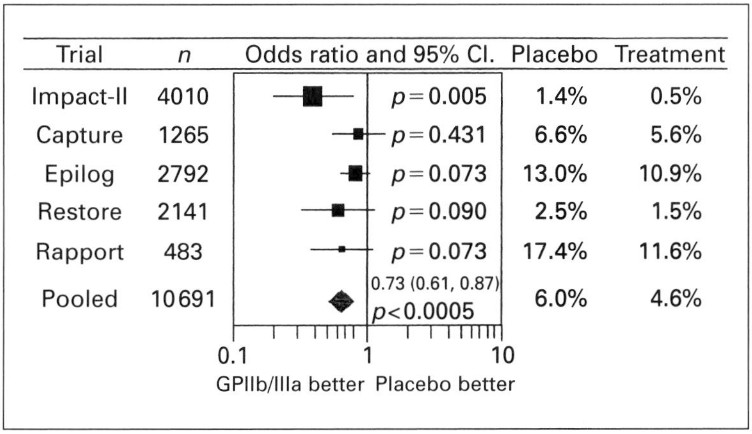

Trial	n	Odds ratio and 95% C.I.	Placebo	Treatment
Impact-II	4010	$p = 0.005$	1.4%	0.5%
Capture	1265	$p = 0.431$	6.6%	5.6%
Epilog	2792	$p = 0.073$	13.0%	10.9%
Restore	2141	$p = 0.090$	2.5%	1.5%
Rapport	483	$p = 0.073$	17.4%	11.6%
Pooled	10691	0.73 (0.61, 0.87) $p < 0.0005$	6.0%	4.6%

0.1   1   10
GPIIb/IIIa better   Placebo better

Figure 17.3
Unplanned stent deployment in randomized, placebo controlled trials of parenteral platelet GPIIb/IIIa blockade. Platelet GPIIb/IIIa blockade reduces the requirement for unplanned stent deployment. Reproduced from Bhatt et al,[7] with permission.

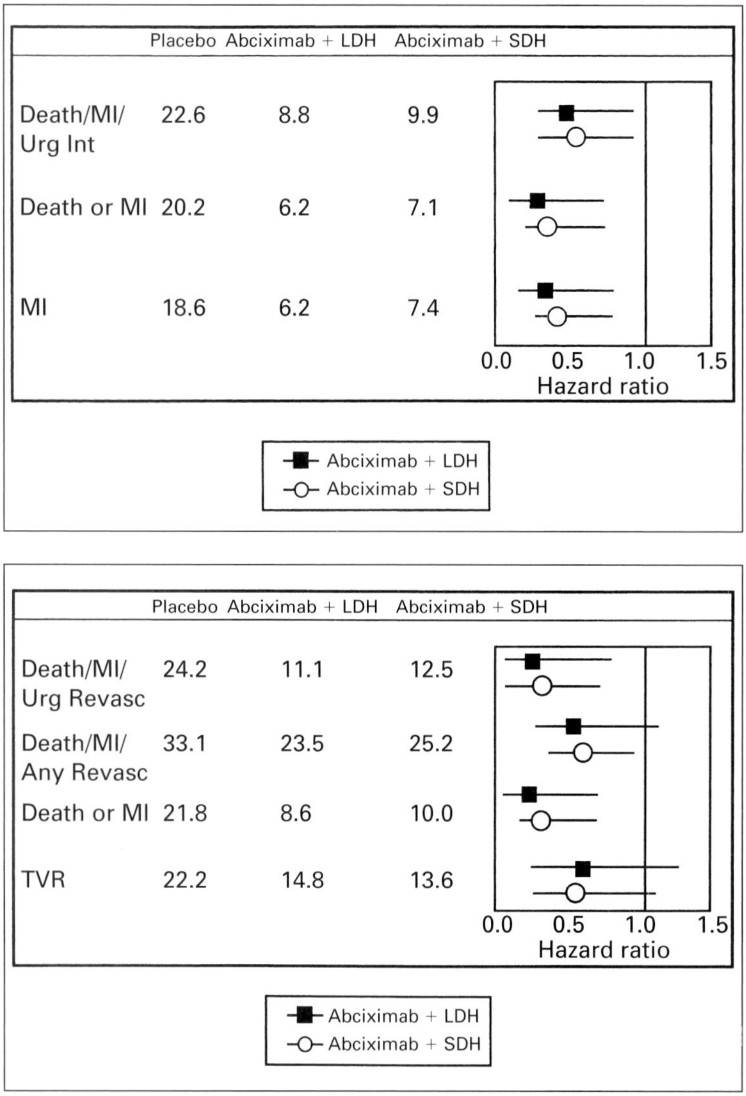

	Placebo	Abciximab + LDH	Abciximab + SDH
Death/MI/ Urg Int	22.6	8.8	9.9
Death or MI	20.2	6.2	7.1
MI	18.6	6.2	7.4

Hazard ratio

- ■- Abciximab + LDH
- ○- Abciximab + SDH

	Placebo	Abciximab + LDH	Abciximab + SDH
Death/MI/ Urg Revasc	24.2	11.1	12.5
Death/MI/ Any Revasc	33.1	23.5	25.2
Death or MI	21.8	8.6	10.0
TVR	22.2	14.8	13.6

Hazard ratio

- ■- Abciximab + LDH
- ○- Abciximab + SDH

Figure 17.4
Clinical outcomes at (a) 30 days and (b) 6 months following unplanned stent deployment in the EPILOG trial stratified by treatment regimen. Hazard ratios with 95% confidence intervals and event rates are shown. LDH, low-dose heparin; MI, myocardial infarction; SDH, standard-dose heparin; TVR, target vessel revascularization; Urg Int, urgent intervention). Adapted from Kereiakes et al, 1998.[5]

reduction in the composite occurrence of death, MI or urgent intervention; a 53% reduction in the composite of death and MI and a 30% reduction in target vessel revascularization (Figure 17.5b). These data suggest that prophylactic platelet GPIIb/IIIa blockade will significantly improve the outcomes of patients who subsequently require unplanned stent deployment.

Complex coronary stenting

In the era of optimal stent deployment strategies and adjunct antiplatelet therapy, subacute stent thrombosis has been associated with the

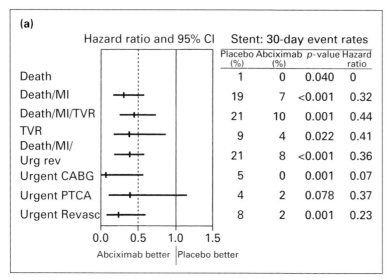

(a)

Hazard ratio and 95% CI   Stent: 30-day event rates

	Placebo (%)	Abciximab (%)	p-value	Hazard ratio
Death	1	0	0.040	0
Death/MI	19	7	<0.001	0.32
Death/MI/TVR	21	10	0.001	0.44
TVR	9	4	0.022	0.41
Death/MI/ Urg rev	21	8	<0.001	0.36
Urgent CABG	5	0	0.001	0.07
Urgent PTCA	4	2	0.078	0.37
Urgent Revasc	8	2	0.001	0.23

0.0   0.5   1.0   1.5

Abciximab better | Placebo better

(b)

Hazard ratio and 95% CI   Stent: 6-month event rates

	Placebo (%)	Abciximab (%)	p-value	Hazard ratio
Death	2	1	0.231	0.39
Death/MI	20	9	<0.001	0.38
Death/MI/TVR	30	22	0.026	0.67
TVR	19	15	0.11	0.7
Death/MI/ Urg rev	23	11	0.002	0.46
Urgent CABG	5	0.4	0.003	0.08
Urgent PTCA	5	2	0.125	0.42
Urgent Revasc	9	3	0.004	0.27

0.0   0.5   1.0   1.5   2.0

Abciximab better | Placebo better

Figure 17.5
*Clinical outcomes at **(a)** 30 days and **(b)** 6 months in patients taking abciximab in 529 patients having unplanned coronary stent deployment in EPIC, EPILOG and CAPTURE trials. Hazard ratios with 95% confidence intervals and event rates are shown. MI, myocardial infarction; TVR, target vessel revascularization; Urg Int urgent intervention; CABG, coronary artery bypass surgery; PTCA, percutaneous transluminal coronary angioplasty.*

use of combination stent designs as well as the number of stents deployed per coronary lesion.[10] Similarly, when two or more contiguous stents are deployed in a single coronary vessel, the need for target vessel revascularization at 6 months is increased.[11–14] In a series of 45 patients in whom multiple (three or more)

contiguous coronary stents were deployed for largely 'high-risk' indications (i.e. 13.3% abrupt closure, 57.8% coronary dissection, 13.3% suboptimal balloon angioplasty result) adverse events in hospital included stent occlusion (9%), death (4.4%), urgent bypass surgery (4.4%), urgent repeat angioplasty

(4.4%), the incidence of any in-hospital adverse event being 15.6%.[15] At 6 months follow-up of hospital survivals from this series, ischemic outcomes were observed in 23.3%. Interestingly, only 2 of these 45 patients received abciximab therapy at the time of their initial complex coronary stenting procedure. Recent data have also supported the concept of increased risk for patients in whom coronary stents are placed for coronary dissection or suboptimal balloon angioplasty results, as well as threatened or abrupt coronary closure.[5,16–18] Similarly, patients requiring contiguous stents or those in whom 'optimal' deployment cannot be obtained have increased risk for both in-hospital and late (6-month) ischemic outcomes. Although randomized trials (ISAR, STARS, FANTASTIC)[18–20] have demonstrated the superiority of antiplatelet therapy using ticlopidine and aspirin compared with anticoagulation with coumadin and aspirin for stented patients, these trials have enrolled largely low-risk, elective patients who have had 'optimal' stent deployment. Thus, the low incidence occurrence of ischemic outcomes observed following ticlopidine and aspirin therapy, which was initiated at the time of stent deployment (0.5% stent thrombosis to 30 days in STARS randomized patients), may not be extrapolated to other higher-risk groups of stented patients. Indeed, patients followed in the STARS registry because of less-than-optimal stent deployment had a 7-fold increase (3.5%) in the occurrence of subacute stent thrombosis.[18] In addition, although antiplatelet therapy using aspirin and ticlopidine proved superior to anticoagulation with coumadin and aspirin for 'high-risk' stented patients enrolled in the MATTIS trial, the composite occurrence of death, MI and urgent revascularization in this population was still 5.6% at 30 days.[16] Likewise, treatment with aspirin and ticlopidine may not

adequately suppress recurrent ischemic events following stent deployment in patients with unstable angina pectoris.[20] In this population, major ischemic complications (death, Q-wave and non-Q-wave) were observed in proportion to the severity of unstable angina using the Braunwald classification and were most frequent in Class III (14.1%, $p < 0.04$) and Class C (27%, $p < 0.01$) angina, despite therapy with aspirin and ticlopidine initiated at the time of the procedure.[21] Similarly, multivariable analysis of the ISAR database identified unstable angina to be a significant hazard for cardiac events following successful coronary stenting.[22] These observations are consistent with data demonstrating an increase in platelet surface expression of GPIIb/IIIa receptors (as reflected by CD41 immunofluorescence)[23] as well as increased platelet volume[24] in patients with unstable angina pectoris. These findings suggest that platelet activation is a dynamic process and that patients with acute coronary syndromes have an activated platelet population.

Also pertinent to this issue are data presented by Gregorini et al[25] that demonstrate both free thrombin generation and platelet activation in patients undergoing coronary stent deployment who had received up to 24 h of ticlopidine therapy before the procedure. Evidence of both thrombin generation (prothrombin fragment 1,2 and thrombin–antithrombin complexes) and platelet activation (serotonin release; CD62-membrane p-selection expression) during the procedure were suppressed to normal levels only in those patients who had received 72 h or more preprocedural therapy with ticlopidine.[25] Recent clinical data in support of this observation show that the incidence of non-Q-wave MI following coronary stenting is greatest in those patients who receive ticlopidine for the first time on the day of the procedure and is less frequent ($p = 0.024$) in patients pretreated with ticlopidine for 3 days or more.[26] Similarly, patients allocated to the stent-placebo treatment strategy, show a significant (13.4 versus 8.9%; $p = 0.03$) reduction in death, myocardial infarction or urgent revascularization to 30 days compared with patients who had not received ticlopidine prior to stent deployment.[27] Thus, a 'window of vulnerability' created by procoagulant activity may exist, and antiplatelet therapy with aspirin and ticlopidine initiated at the time of the stent procedure may not suppress adequately subsequent ischemic events. This premise is supported by examining the time course for occurrence of ischemic outcomes in stented patients and the benefit afforded by adjunct GPIIb/IIIa blockade in this population. For example, the follow-up of 529 patients receiving unplanned stent deployment in the EPIC, EPILOG and

CAPTURE trials demonstrates that the benefit attributed to prophylactic abciximab therapy for reducing death, MI, urgent revascularization and target vessel revascularization occurs within the first week following therapy and is then sustained to 6 months follow-up[9] (Figure 17.6).

Elective stent deployment

Elevation in the post-procedural creatine phosphokinase (CPK) levels above baseline preprocedural levels was observed in 22% of patients having planned, elective Palmaz-Schatz stent deployment in the STARS trial.[28] This finding suggests the potential for platelet GPIIb/IIIa blockade to reduce ischemic outcomes following elective stenting as well. For example, following 'optimal' elective stent deployment in the ERASER trial, abciximab bolus and 12-h infusion reduced the composite

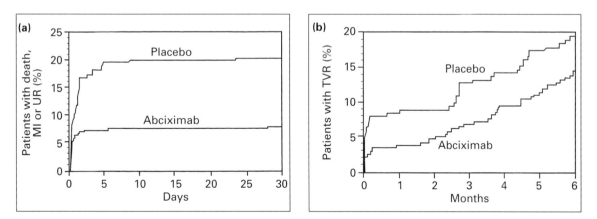

Figure 17.6
*Kaplan-Meier curves from the combined EPIC, EPILOG and CAPTURE trial datasets. **(a)** Percentage of patients out to 30 days with the composite occurrence of death, myocardial infarction (MI) or urgent revascularization (UR) and **(b)** Percentage of patients with target vessel revascularization (TVR) to 6 months following unplanned coronary stent deployment. The benefit associated with abciximab therapy is accrued within 1 week of treatment and sustained at 6 months.*

occurrence of death, MI and target vessel revascularization by 53% compared with placebo (aspirin and ticlopidine placebo) at 1 week follow-up[29]. More conclusive data concerning the benefit provided by adjunctive GPIIb/IIIa blockade comes from the EPISTENT trial.[30] In this trial, patients were randomized to one of three percutaneous revascularization strategies:

(1) Balloon angioplasty with adjunctive abciximab administration;
(2) Planned stent deployment with abciximab administration; or,
(3) planned stent deployment without concomitant abciximab.

All patients having stent deployment received aspirin and ticlopidine (250 mg twice daily) orally following the procedure. In stented patients who received adjunctive abciximab, the primary composite endpoint of death, MI, and urgent revascularization, to 30 days was significantly reduced (10.8 versus 5.3%; $p < 0.001$) compared with stented patients who did not receive adjunctive abciximab therapy (Figure 17.7). Interestingly, the magnitude of reduction in periprocedural MI was most marked for larger (over 5-fold CPK levels) non-Q-wave infarctions and the requirement for urgent revascularization was reduced by 38%.[30]

The benefit of abciximab in stented patients has been durable to 1 year follow-up as well. At 1 year, the composite occurrence of death, large MI (Q wave or 5-fold increase CK MB) and any revascularization was reduced by 16% ($p = 0.002$) in abciximab-treated stent patients compared with placebo-treated stent patients (Eric J Topol, personal communication). Remarkably, a survival advantage was observed in favor of abciximab treatment (1.0 versus 2.4% mortality at 1 year; $p = 0.037$). Overall, an 18% reduction in late (6 months)

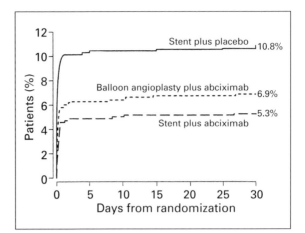

Figure 17.7
Primary endpoint events (death, MI or urgent revascularization) over time to 30 days by treatment strategy in the EPISTENT trial. A 51% reduction in primary endpoint events was observed in stented patients who received abciximab (5.3%) versus placebo (10.8%; p < 0.001).

target vessel revascularization, largely due to a 51% ($p = 0.02$) reduction in diabetic patients was observed in favor of abciximab in stented patients.[31] The angiographic substudy of EPISTENT documents the mechanism of abciximab benefit in stented diabetic patients to be a reduction in late loss (in stent) and 'normalization' of net gain to that of non-diabetic stent patients administered abciximab (Figure 17.8). The preferential benefit for reduction in angiographic restenosis and late target vessel revascularization in diabetic patients may reflect the greater propensity for neointimal proliferation in this population.[31] These observations have fueled speculation regarding the affinity of abciximab for the avϑ3 (vitronectin) receptor and the role of this adjunctive receptor in mediating smooth muscle cell migration and proliferation.

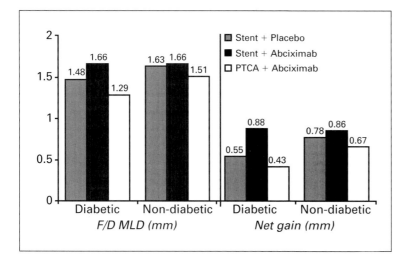

Figure 17.8
Minimum Lumen Diameter (MLD) and net gain in diabetics and non-diabetics by quantitative coronary angiography performed at 6 months in the EPISTENT trial. The adjunctive administration of abciximab to diabetic patients who had stent deployment 'normalized' net gain at late follow-up to that observed in non-diabetic patients.

The early benefit of abciximab conferred to stented patients is mediated by the antiplatelet, antithrombotic effects of this agent and appears to complement the more delayed antiplatelet action of ticlopidine. In this context, synergy for inhibition of platelet aggregation has been demonstrated for abciximab and ticlopidine administration following coronary stenting[32] (Figure 17.9). At least 1 week is required for ticlopidine alone (in combination with aspirin) to reach the levels of platelet inhibition achieved by administering abciximab at the time of the procedure followed by ticlopidine and aspirin.[32] Together, these data provide an explanation for the mechanism and time course of clinical benefit from GPIIb/IIIa blockade following coronary stent deployment and support the usefulness of GPIIb/IIIa blockade in coro-

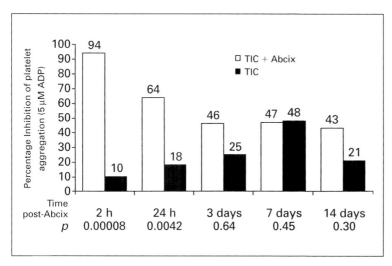

Figure 17.9
Inhibition of ex vivo platelet aggregation in response to agonist (5 μM ADP) following therapy with abciximab (Abcix), ticlopidine (TIC) and aspirin or ticlopidine and aspirin alone in patients undergoing coronary stent deployment. Abstracted from Kleiman et al, 1998.[32]

nary stenting. Although our current recommendations for abciximab administration during coronary stenting include stent deployment for abrupt or threatened coronary closure, multiple (two or more) contiguous stents, use of combination stent designs, suboptimal stent deployment, provisional/ unplanned deployment and deployment in patients with unstable and/or post-infarction angina pectoris, and patients undergoing coronary stent deployment who have not received preprocedural therapy for 72 h or more with ticlopidine. As previously noted, diabetic patients undergoing stent deployment appear to derive particular early and late (reduced target vessel revascularization) benefit from adjunctive abciximab administration and thus may represent another indication for its administration.[31]

Atheroablation

Directional coronary atherectomy

Multiple, randomized trials have demonstrated an increased incidence of non-Q-wave MI in patients undergoing directional coronary atherectomy compared with balloon angioplasty.[33–36] Direct activation of platelets by the directional atherectomy device or from exposure of deep arterial wall components has been demonstrated and significantly exceeds the degree of platelet activation observed during standard balloon angioplasty.[37] A meta-analysis of all patients undergoing directional coronary atherectomy in the EPIC and EPILOG trials demonstrated that prophylactic abciximab administration was associated with a reduction in both the combined occurrence of death, MI and urgent revascularization ($p = 0.008$) and also in the occurrence of MI ($p = 0.003$) up to 30 days following the procedure. Similarly, the occurrence of death, MI and target vessel revascularization ($p = 0.02$) as well as MI ($p = 0.002$) at 6 months follow-up was reduced[38,39] (Figure 17.10). These data suggest that adjunct platelet GPIIb/IIa blockade should be considered for patients undergoing directional coronary atherectomy procedures.

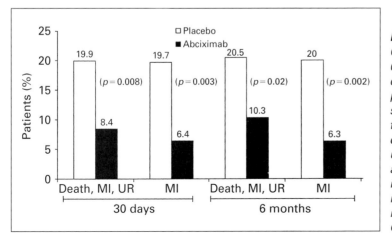

Figure 17.10
Clinical outcomes at 30 days and 6 months following directional coronary atherectomy by pharmacologic treatment strategy in the EPIC and EPILOG trials. Abciximab improved clinical outcomes in patients undergoing directional coronary atherectomy. MI, myocardial infarction; TVR, target vessel revascularization; UR, urgent revascularization. Adapted from Ghaffari et al, 1998.[39]

Rotational atherectomy

The incidence of non-Q-wave periprocedural MI may be as high as 19% following the use of rotational atherectomy[40] and can be influenced by both patient related[41,42] and technical factors.[41] Elevation of post procedural CPK-MB enzyme has been related to frequent burr decelerations (over 5000 rpm) and to prolonged ablation times (over 90 s).[43] In addition, stenosis length over 20 mm and ulcerative coronary lesion morphology have been associated with the occurrence of slow flow and periprocedural CPK-MB elevation.[41,42] Recent data also suggest that burr rotational speed may influence directly the degree of platelet activation that occurs with this device.[44,45] The formation of large platelet aggregates, the rate of platelet aggregate generation and the release of platelet granules are all significantly greater at a burr speed of 180 000 rpm compared with 14 000 rpm.[44,45] Rotablation-induced platelet aggregation can be inhibited by platelet GPIIb/IIIa receptor

blockade with abciximab and the degree of inhibition is not enhanced by the addition of 6D1, a specific antagonist of the GPIb/IX (von Willebrand) receptor[46] (Figure 17.11). In the IMPACT II trial, patients undergoing rotational atherectomy who were randomized to receive integrilin had a reduced incidence of abrupt coronary occlusion and in the composite endpoint of death, MI and urgent revascularization.[47] Similarly, in a small randomized trial of abciximab versus placebo administered during rotational atherectomy, significant reductions in both the incidence and magnitude of postprocedural CPK-MB elevation were observed following abciximab therapy.[48] Other evidence incriminating the platelet in the pathophysiology of slow flow and periprocedural infarction following rotational atherectomy comes from multivariate analyses of clinical variables that have identified unstable angina pectoris as a powerful correlate to these ischemic outcomes.[41,42] Indeed, angina pectoris at rest within 12 h of the interventional procedure closely correlated with the

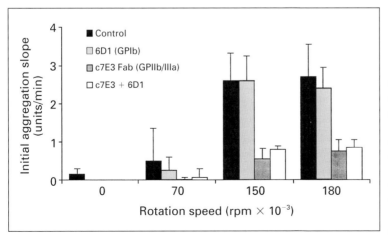

Figure 17.11
Inhibition of rotoblation induced platelet aggregation by platelet GPIIb/IIIa receptor blockade with abciximab. The addition of 6D1, a specific antagonist of the GPIb-IX (von Willebrand) receptor did not contribute to the effect of abciximab. Reproduced from Williams et al, 1998,[45] with permission.

occurrence of slow flow with an odds ratio of 15.8 ($p < 0.0001$).[42]

In general, these data suggest a pathophysiologic role for the platelet in mediating ischemic outcomes following both directional and rotational atherectomy. These atheroablative techniques appear to activate platelets directly. Adjunctive therapy with platelet GPIIb/IIIa blockade during directional or rotational atherectomy can effectively block platelet activation associated with these procedures and can significantly reduce the occurrence of ischemic outcomes. Recent data suggest that the currently recommended, labeled and approved dose regimen for tirofiban (PRISM PLUS) achieves only 60% inhibition of shear-induced platelet aggregation by rotational atherectomy in an *in vitro* artery model and that higher doses of tirofiban may be required to obtain maximal levels of platelet inhibition.[49]

Future directions

The specific benefit of adjunct platelet GPIIb/IIIa blockade in patients undergoing percutaneous intervention with extraction atherectomy or rheolytic thrombectomy has not been evaluated systematically. In addition, the potential for incremental benefit to accompany more prolonged preprocedural administration of a platelet GPIIb/IIIa inhibitor in clinical situations where thrombus is likely to be present (post-MI; aged saphenous vein grafts) has not been evaluated. For example, a reduction in angiographic thrombus was observed following abciximab administration (compared with unfractionated heparin administration) for 18–24 h to patients with medically refractory unstable angina pectoris in the CAPTURE trial.[50] Prolonged abciximab infusion has also been associated with a reduction in thrombus burden documented by angioscopy in patients with native vessel or saphenous vein graft disease (R. Guagliumi, personal communication). In contrast, however, the prolonged intravenous infusion of unfractionated heparin was not associated with an improvement in the angiographic appearance of the thrombus in patients with unstable angina.[51]

The potential for more prolonged postprocedural administration of platelet GPIIb/IIIa receptor blockade as may be achieved by sequencing a parenteral and an orally active GPIIb/IIIa inhibitor to influence late (6 months or more) post-procedural outcomes has not been evaluated. Likewise, the role of prolonged concomitant β_3-integrin blockade (aVβ_3 or vitronectin receptor) to reduce neointimal proliferation and thus, the restenotic process has not been addressed. Recent observations that upregulation of β_3-intregrins on vascular smooth muscle follows balloon injury[52] and that β_3-integrin blockade by abciximab or other β_3-integrin specific monoclonal antibodies (LM 609) can inhibit smooth muscle cell migration and proliferation[53,54] has spurred interest in administering agents with β_3-integrin-blocking capabilities in an attempt to interrupt the vascular response to injury and thus, restenosis. For example, prolonged intravenous administration of abciximab to baboons following both femoral balloon angioplasty and carotid stenting significantly reduced the degree of subsequent neointimal vascular hyperplasia measured at 30 days. These experimental observations are consistent with the EPISTENT trial clinical observations of a marked reduction in late loss (in-stent) on 6-month angiographic follow-up of diabetic patients who received abciximab therapy during coronary stent deployment. Recent data have suggested that blockade of specific epitope binding sites on the β_3-integrin receptor may influence smooth muscle cell proliferation in response to specific stimuli such as thrombin, thrombospondin or platelet derived growth factors.[55] For example, β_3-integrin binding by abciximab inhibited smooth muscle cell proliferation in response to thrombospondin and thrombin but not platelet derived growth factors.[55] Thus, further understanding of the β_3-integrin receptor physiology may allow for more effective, specific antagonists to be developed.

Another mechanism that may in part influence the benefit attributable to abciximab is via the CD11B/18 or MAC1 receptor. This receptor is present on neutrophils and monocytes and modulates white cell adhesion, white cell–platelet interactions and the inflammatory response to vessel injury.[56] The MAC1 receptor is upregulated following balloon angioplasty and is inhibited by abciximab.[57] Thus, the potential exists for abciximab to influence multiple steps over the time course of the vascular response to injury including thrombosis (GP IIb/IIIa), inflammation (MAC1) and neointimal proliferation ($\alpha V\beta 3$). Whether similar degrees of clinical benefit following percutaneous coronary intervention can also be provided by agents having only GP IIb/IIIa receptor blocking activity (small molecule antagonists) awaits evaluation.

References

1. Kereiakes DJ, Cabot C, Melsheimer RM, Lincoff AM, Califf RM, Topol EJ. Abciximab-mediated platelet GPIIb/IIIa blockade improves outcomes following multiple interventional technologies: Results of the EPILOG trial. *Am J Cardiol* 1997;**80**:9S [Abstract].

2. Bhatt DL, Topol EJ. The benefit of abciximab in interventional cardiology is not device specific. *Circulation* 1998;**98**:I-17 [Abstract].

3. The EPILOG Investigators. Platelet glycoprotein IIb/IIIa receptor blockade and low-dose heparin during percutaneous coronary revascularization. *N Engl J Med* 1997;**336**:1689–96.

4. Kereiakes DJ, Lincoff AM, Miller DP, Tcheng JE, Weisman HF, Topol EJ. Abciximab reduces risk of unplanned coronary stent deployment: EPILOG trial results. *Circulation* 1997;**96**:I-163 [Abstract].

5. Kereiakes DJ, Lincoff AM, Miller DP, Tcheng JE, Cabot CF, Anderson KM, et al for the EPILOG Trial Investigators. Abciximab therapy and unplanned coronary stent deployment: favorable effects on stent utilization, clinical outcomes and bleeding complications. *Circulation* 1998;**97**:857–64.

6. Barr LA, Brener SJ, Jones AA, Moliterno DJ, Effron MB, Topol EJ. Abciximab reduces the need for bail-out stenting during primary angioplasty: the RAPPORT Trial. *J Am Coll Cardiol* 1998;**31**:237A [Abstract].

7. Bhatt DL, Lincoff AM, Kereiakes DJ, Tcheng JE, Godfrey N, Califf RM, et al. Reduction in need for unplanned stenting with the use of platelet glycoprotein IIb/IIIa blockade in percutaneous coronary intervention. *Am J Cardiol* (In press).

8. Zidar JP, Kruse KR, Thel MC, Kereiakes DJ, Muhlestein JB, Davidson CJ, et al for the IMPACT II Investigators. Integrilin for emergency coronary artery stenting. *J Am Coll Cardiol* 1996;**27**:138A [Abstract].

9. Kereiakes DJ, Lincoff AM, Simoons ML, deBoer MJ, Tcheng JE, Vahanian A, et al. Complementarity of stenting and abciximab for percutaneous coronary intervention. *J Am Coll Cardiol* 1998;**31**:54A [Abstract].

10. Moussa I, DiMario C, Reimers B, Akiyama T, Tobis J, Colombo A. Subacute stent thrombosis in the era of intravascular ultrasound-guided coronary stenting without anticoagulation: frequency, predictors and clinical outcome. *J Am Coll Cardiol* 1997;**29**:6–12.

11. Allabadi D, Bowers TR, Tilli FV, Spybrook M, Breenberg HL, Goldstein JA, et al. Multiple stents increases target vessel revascularization rates. *J Am Coll Cardiol* 1997;**29**:276A [Abstract].

12. Gaxiola E, Vlietstra RE, Browne KF, Ebersole DG, Brenner AS, Weeks TT, et al. Six-month follow-up of patients with multiple stents in a single coronary artery. *J Am Coll Cardiol* 1997;**29**:276A [Abstract].

13. Moussa I, DiMario C, Moses J, Reimers B, Blengino S, Colombo A. Single versus multiple Palmaz-Schatz stent implantation: immediate and follow-up results. *J Am Coll Cardiol* 1997;**29**:276A [Abstract].

14. Kornowski R, Mintz GS, Mehran R, Pichard AD, Kent KM, Satler LF, et al. The 'full metal jacket': procedural results and late clinical outcomes after placement of three or more coronary stents. *J Am Coll Cardiol* 1997;**29**:188A [Abstract].

15. Mathew V, Hasdai D, Holmes DR, Garratt KN, Bell MR, Lerman A, et al. Clinical outcome of patients undergoing endoluminal coronary artery reconstruction with three or more stents. *Am Coll Cardiol* 1977;**30**:676–81.

16. Urban P, Macaya C, Rupprecht HJ, Kiemeneij F, Emanuelsson H, Fontanelli P, et al for the MATTIS Investigators. Multicenter aspirin and ticlopidine trial after intracoronary stenting in high-risk patients. *J Am Coll Cardiol* 1998;**31**:397A [Abstract].

17. Leon MB, Baim DS, Popma JJ, Gordon PC, Cutlip DE, Ho KKL, et al for the Stent Anti-

coagulation Restenosis Study Investigators. A clinical trial comparing three antithrombotic-drug regimens after coronary-artery stenting. *New Engl J Med* 1999;**339**:1665–71.

18. Leon MB, Baim DS, Popma JJ, Gordon PC, Cutlip DE, Ho KKL et al for the Stent Anticoagulation Restenosis Study (STARS) Investigators. *New Engl J Med* 1998;**339**:1665–71.

19. Schomig A, Neumann FJ, Kastrati A, Schuhlen H, Blasini R, Hadamitzky M, et al. A randomized comparison of antiplatelet and anticoagulant therapy after the placement of coronary artery stents. *New Engl J Med* 1996;**334**:1084–9.

20. Bertrand M, Legrand V, Boland J, et al. Full anticoagulation versus ticlopidine plus aspirin after stent implantation. A randomized multicenter European study: the FANTASTIC trial. *Circulation* 1996;**94**:I-685 [Abstract].

21. Angioi M, Danchin N, Gangloff C, Gretzinger A, Jacquemin L, Berder V, et al. Ticlopidine-aspirin as anti-thrombotic regimen for intracoronary stenting for unstable angina: is there a need for further antiplatelet therapy? *J Am Coll Cardiol* 1998;**31**:100A [Abstract].

22. Kastrati A, Neumann FJ, Schöemig A. Operator volume and outcome of patients undergoing coronary stent placement. *J Am Coll Cardiol* 1998;**32**:970–6.

23. Lu Y, Therous P, Xiao Z, Ghitescu M. Increased expression of GPIIb/IIIa platelet membrane receptor in acute ischemic syndromes. *Circulation* 1996;**94**:I-515 [Abstract].

24. Pizzulli L, Yang A, Martin JF, Luderitz B. Changes in platelet size and count in unstable angina compared to stable angina or non-cardiac chest pain. *Eur Heart J* 1998;**19**:80–84.

25. Gregorini L, Marko J, Fajadet J, Cassagneau B, Brunel II P, Gapiache Y, et al. Ticlopidine attenuates post stent implantation thrombin generation. *J Am Coll Cardiol* 1996;**27**:334A [Abstract].

26. Steinhubl SR, Lauer MS, Mukerjee DP, Moliterno DJ, Ellis SG. Pre-treatment with ticlopidine reduces non-Q-wave myocardial infarctions following intra-coronary stenting. *J Am Coll Cardiol* 1998;**31**:100A [Abstract].

27. Steinhubl SR, Balog C, Topol EJ. Pretreatment with ticlopidine prior to stenting is associated with a substantial decrease in complications: data from the EPISTENT trial. *Circulation* 1998;**98**:I-573. [Abstract].

28. Cutlip DE, Chauhan M, Lasorda A, Bailey S, Davidson C, Ito S, et al. Influence of post-procedural myocardial infarction on late clinical outcome in the stent anti-thrombotic regimen study (STARS). *Circulation* 1997;**96**: I-31 [Abstract].

29. Ellis SG, Serruys PW, Popma JJ, Teirstein PS, Ricci DR, Gold HK, et al. Can abciximab prevent neointimal proliferation in Palmaz-Schatz Stents? The final ERASER results. *Circulation* 1997;**96**:I-87 [Abstract].

30. The EPISTENT investigators. Randomised placebo-controlled and balloon-angioplasty-controlled trial to assess safety of coronary stenting with use of platelet glycoprotein IIb/IIIa blockade. *Lancet* 1998;**352**:87–92.

31. Lincoff AM, Moliterno DJ, Ellis SG, Debowey D, Cabot CF, Booth JE, et al. Six month angiographic outcome with abciximab and stents: the EPISTENT angiographic substudy. *Circulation* 1998;**98**:I:768.

32. Kleiman NS, Graziadei N, Lance E, et al. Synergy of abciximab and ticlopidine in patients undergoing coronary stenting. *J Am Coll Cardiol* 1998;**31**:238A [Abstract].

33. Topol EJ, Leya F, Pinkerton CA, Whitlow PL, Hofling B, Simonton CA et al for the CAVEAT study group. A comparison of directional atherectomy with coronary angioplasty in patients with coronary artery disease. *New Engl J Med* 1993;**329**:221–7.

34. Holmes DR, Topol EJ, Califf RM, Berdan LG, Leya F, Berger PB, et al. A multicenter randomized trial of coronary angioplasty versus directional atherectomy for patients with saphenous vein bypass graft lesions. *Circulation* 1995;**91**:1966–74.

35. The EPIC Investigators. Use of a monoclonal antibody directed against the platelet glycoprotein IIb/IIIa receptor in 'high-risk' coronary angioplasty. *N Engl J Med* 1994;**330**:956–61.

36. Baim DS, Cutlip DE, Sharma SK, Ho KKL, Fortuna R, Schreiber TL et al for the BOAT investigators. Final results of the balloon vs. optimal atherectomy trial (BOAT). *Circulation* 1998;**97**:322–31.

37. Dehmer GJ, Nichols TC, Bode AP, Liles D,

Sigman J, Li S, et al. Assessment of platelet activation by coronary sinus blood sampling during balloon angioplasty and directional coronary atherectomy. *Am J Cardiol* 1997;80:871–7.

38. Ghaffari S, Kereiakes DJ, Kelly T, Tcheng JE, Timmis GC, Miller DP, et al. Platelet GPIIb/IIIa receptor blockade reduces ischemic complications in patients undergoing directional coronary atherectomy. *Circulation* 1996;94:I-198 [Abstract].

39. Ghaffari S, Kereiakes DJ, Lincoff AM, Kelly TA, Timmis GC, Kleiman NF, et al for the EPILOG Investigators. Platelet glycoprotein IIb/IIIa receptor blockade with abciximab reduces ischemic complications in patients undergoing directional coronary atherectomy. *Am J Cardiol* 1998;82:7–12.

40. Teirstein PS, Warth DC, Haq N, Jenkins NS, McCowan LC, Aubanel-Reidel P, et al. High-speed rotational coronary atherectomy for patients with diffuse coronary artery disease. *J Am Coll Cardiol* 1991;18:1694–701.

41. Bier JD, Mukherjee SN, Schubert P, Cohen JS, Cupples LA, Jacobs AK. Predictors of no reflow during rotational atherectomy. *Circulation* 1996;94:I-249 [Abstract].

42. Sharma SK, Dangas G, Mehran R, Duvvuri S, Kini A, Cooke TP, et al. Risk factors for the development of slow flow during rotational coronary atherectomy. *Am J Cardiol* 1997;80:219–22.

43. Horrigan MC, Eccleston DS, Williams DO, Lasorda DM, Moses JW, Whitlow PL. Technique dependence of CKMB elevation after rotational atherectomy. *Circulation* 1996;94:I-560 [Abstract].

44. Reisman M, Shuman B, Fei R, Dillard D, Nguyen S, Gordon L. Analysis and comparison of platelet aggregation with high-speed rotational atherectomy. *J Am Coll Cardiol* 1997;29:186A [Abstract].

45. Williams MS, Coller BS, Vaananen HJ, Scudder LE, Marmur JD. Activation of platelets in platelet rich plasma by rotablation is speed dependent and can be inhibited by abciximab. *J Am Coll Cardiol* 1998;31:237A [Abstract].

46. Williams MA, Coller BS, Väänänen HJ, Scudder LE, Sharma SK, Marmur JD. Activation of platelets in platelet-rich plasma by rotablation is speed-dependent and can be inhibited by abciximab (c7E3); ReoPro). *Circulation* 1998;98:742–8.

47. Teirstein PS, Yakubov SJ, Thel MC, Wildermann N, Kereiakes DJ, Popma JJ, et al. Platelet IIb/IIIa blockade with integrelin: atherectomy patients. *J Am Coll Cardiol* 1996;27:334A [Abstract].

48. Braden GA, Applegate RJ, Young TM, Love WW, Sane DC. Abciximab decreases both the incidence and magnitude of creatine kinase elevation during rotational atherectomy. *J Am Coll Cardiol* 1977;29:499A [Abstract].

49. Reisman M, Fei R, Dillard D, Bogosian S, Harms V. Tirofiban prevents platelet aggregation induced by rotational atherectomy in an invitro model. *J Am Coll Cardiol* 1999;33: 71A.

50. van den Brand M, de Scheerder I, Heyndrickx G, Laarman GJ, Beatt K, Steg PG, et al. Assessment of coronary angiograms prior and after treatment with abciximab in patients with refractory unstable angina. *Eur Heart J* 1997;18:243 [Abstract].

51. Cura F, Piraino R, Guzman L, Padilla L, Fernandez J, Marchetti G, et al. Does pretreatment with intravenous heparin produce any angiographic improvement in patients admitted with unstable angina? *J Am Coll Cardiol* 1998;31:457A [Abstract].

52. Stouffer GA, Hu Z, Sajid M, Li H, Jin G, Nakada MT, et al. β_3 integrins are upregulated after vascular injury and modulate thrombospondin- and thrombin-induced proliferation of cultured smooth muscle cells. *Circulation* 1998;97:907–15.

53. Liaw L, Skinner MP, Raines EW, Ross R, Cheresh DA, Schwartz SM, et al. The adhesive and migratory effects of osteopontin are mediated via distinct cell surface integrins. *J Clin Invest* 1995;95:713–24.

54. Brown SL, Lundgren CH, Nordt T, Fujii S. Stimulation of migration of human aortic smooth muscle cells by vitronectin: implications for atherosclerosis. *Cardiovasc Res* 1994;28:1815–20.

55. Marijanowski MM, Nakada M. Sundell BI, Kelly AB, Jordan RE, Jakubowski JA, et al. Abciximab reduces vascular lesion formation in non-human primates. *J Am Coll Cardiol* 1999;33:69A.

56. Hughes BJ, Hollers JC, Crockett-Torabi E, Smith CW. Recruitment of CD11b/CD18 to the neutrophil surface and adherence-dependent cell locomotion. *J Clin Invest* 1992;**90**:1687–96.

57. Mickelson JK, Ali MN, Kleiman NS, Lakkis NM, Chow TW, Hughes BJ, et al. Chimeric 7E3 Fab (ReoPro) decreases detectable CD11b on neutrophils from patients undergoing coronary angioplasty. *J Am Coll Cardiol* 1999;**33**:97–106.

18

Drug–drug synergy
Pierre Theroux and Richard Gallo

Introduction

There exists a strong rationale for using a combination of antithrombotic agents in many clinical situations, more specifically in coronary artery disease. Clot formation involves close interactions between platelets, the coagulation system and the fibrinolytic system. The role of these components is of critical importance in the different thromboembolic manifestations of coronary disease.

The difference between venous thrombosis and arterial thrombosis is particularly striking; the coagulation system primarily involved in the former and platelets in the latter. The pathophysiology of arterial thrombosis may also vary from one vascular area to another; for example the cerebrovascular versus the coronary circulation, or the peripheral circulation versus the intracardiac cavities, or variations within the same arterial area may be caused by disease.

The triggers of clot formation are also different in a stable plaque compared with those in an acute injury induced by a balloon, or in an inflammatory plaque that spontaneously ruptures, or in a profoundly injured plaque. Figure 18.1 illustrates how plaque constitution, triggers of coagulation, and shear rate influence formation of the thrombus. Coronary angioplasty of a stable plaque induces acute vessel injury at high shear rates from

inside the lumen through the wall. The thrombogenic material released from the plaque rupture may largely be normal constituents of the arterial wall, for example, von Willebrand factor abundant in the Webel-Palade bodies in the subendothelium, and collagen more deeply embedded in the arterial wall. Glycoprotein (GP)1b/IX on the platelet surface recognizes the former and glycoprotein GPIa/IIa recognizes collagen. The unstable plaque, on the other hand, has a different structure and is rich in inflammatory cells and in tissue factor. Shear rates may be high in moderate-to-severe obstruction and low in very severe obstruction; high shear rates facilitate the binding of von Willebrand factor to the GPIIb/IIIa receptor. Tissue factor that is present in these plaques readily forms a complex with factor VIIa in the circulation to stimulate the coagulation cascade, generation of thrombin, and fibrin deposition (Figure 18.2).[1] Completely occlusive thrombi that occur in myocardial infarction (MI) are associated with no flow, blood stasis and deposition of large amount of fibrin. Antiplatelet therapy is highly effective in preventing platelet aggregation in angioplasty, and thrombolytic agents are highly effective in lysing the fibrin clot. Unstable angina (implicating platelets and tissue factor) may require antiplatelet and anticoagulant therapy for optimum efficacy.

The distinction between the role of platelet

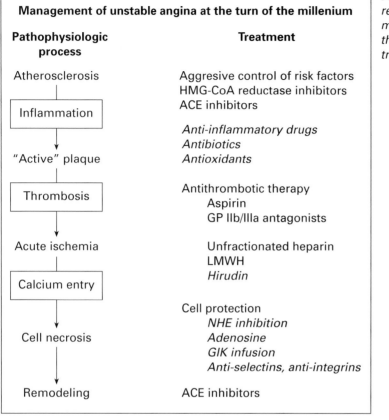

Management of unstable angina at the turn of the millenium

Pathophysiologic process	Treatment
Atherosclerosis	Aggresive control of risk factors HMG-CoA reductase inhibitors ACE inhibitors
Inflammation	*Anti-inflammatory drugs* *Antibiotics* *Antioxidants*
"Active" plaque	

Thrombosis	Antithrombotic therapy
	    Aspirin
	    GP IIb/IIIa antagonists

Acute ischemia	Unfractionated heparin LMWH *Hirudin*

Calcium entry	Cell protection
	    NHE inhibition
	    Adenosine
	    GIK infusion
	    Anti-selectins, anti-integrins

Cell necrosis	
Remodeling	ACE inhibitors

Figure 18.1 *Schematic representation of various mechanisms for intracoronary thrombosis, and implications for treatment selection.*

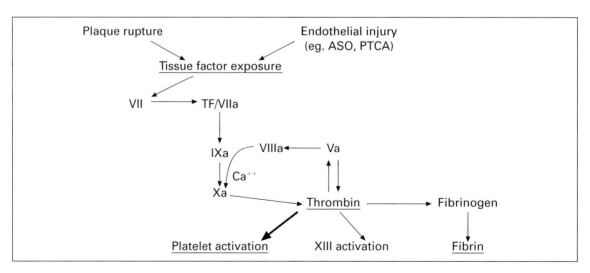

Figure 18.2
Tissue factor is the physiologic indicator of coagulation.

and of intravascular coagulation is obscured by the close interaction between these two components of thrombus formation, namely platelets and thrombin. Whereas thrombin may be the most important platelet agonist in vivo, platelets act as a surface where blood coagulation occurs. Efficient inhibition of thrombus formation will therefore often require concomitant inhibition of both platelets and thrombin.

The need for combination therapy is further emphasized by stimuli to thrombus formation that persist beyond the acute phase; the clot itself is thrombogenic by releasing entrapped thrombin, thus amplifying its own generation, and at times the treatment may be directly or indirectly partly thrombogenic. This is true for heparin, which is a platelet agonist at therapeutic concentrations, and for thrombolytic agents, which stimulate platelet and coagulation when administered during an acute coronary syndrome.

Since the various antithrombotic agents have relatively specific targets, a combination of agents is often needed. This chapter reviews the clinical situations in which a combination of therapies may be advantageous, and discusses common forms of combination therapy.

The rationale for using combined antithrombotic therapy may be listed as follows:

(1) Distinct role of platelets, thrombin, and the fibrinolytic system in various thrombogenic states;
(2) Close interactions between platelets, coagulation, and fibrinolysis;
(3) Relatively specific targets of various drugs;
(4) Pro-thrombotic effects of certain drugs;
(5) Persisting thrombogenic state.

Anticoagulant plus antiplatelet therapy
Aspirin and heparin

Aspirin and heparin have been shown individually to be effective in the acute coronary syndromes. The Antiplatelet Trialists' Collaboration meta-analysis of more than 100 000 patients documented a 18% reduction in the odds of vascular death in high-risk patients, a 35% reduction in the odds of non-fatal MI and a 31% reduction in non-fatal strokes using antiplatelet therapy.[2] In another overview of 26 randomized studies of anticoagulant therapy in suspected acute MI, anticoagulant therapy reduced mortality by 23%, stroke by 46%, pulmonary emboli by 48% ($p < 0.001$), and reinfarction by 13% (NS); whereas the risk of major bleeds was increased 2.3-fold ($p = 0.01$).[3] In the presence of aspirin, however, heparin reduced mortality by only 5% ($p = 0.03$), reduced reinfarction by 8% ($p = 0.04$), reduced pulmonary emboli by 30% ($p = 0.01$), but increased the rate of stroke by 6% (NS) and major bleeds by 46% ($p < 0.0001$). The authors concluded that the clinical evidence from randomized trials did not justify the routine addition of either intravenous or subcutaneous heparin to aspirin in the treatment of acute MI.

In unstable angina, moderately powered trials with unfractionated heparin and with low-molecular-weight heparins have shown the benefits of heparin to be additive to those of aspirin. In the Montreal trial, the combination of aspirin and heparin prevented recurrence of ischemic events following the discontinuation of heparin.[4] In the RISC study, the combination resulted in a significant risk reduction in death and MI at 5 days.[5] In the ATACS trial, heparin followed by coumadin to an INR 2–2.5, reduced at 14 days the combined endpoint of death and MI. A meta-analysis in this report showed a 56% reduction in the incidence of the hard endpoints of fatal and non-fatal MI with the combination therapy of unfractionated heparin compared with aspirin alone.[6] Another more recent meta-analysis demonstrated a significant risk reduction of 33% in the rate of death or MI with a combination of aspirin plus heparin compared with aspirin alone.[7]

The trials using the low-molecular-weight heparins also document a benefit in combination with aspirin.[8–12] In the Fragmin during Instability in Coronary Artery Disease (FRISC) study of 1506 patients with unstable angina or non-Q-wave MI, patients were randomized to subcutaneous dalteparin twice daily or placebo in addition to aspirin. Dalteparin reduced by 63% the risk of death or MI during the first 6 days.[8] After 6 days, the dose was reduced to a once daily administration for 35–45 days. Although an excess of events followed the dose reduction, the benefits were still statistically significant after 40 days. Four large trials have compared directly a low-molecular-weight heparin to unfractionated heparin. The two trials with enoxaparin have shown a moderate but statistically significant advantage of the low-molecular-weight heparin.[9,10] One trial using dalteparin and one using nadroparin have not documented such a benefit.[11,12] The combination therapy of aspirin and unfractionated heparin (or low-molecular-weight heparin) is now used routinely in patients with acute coronary syndromes. Recent study results have suggested that hirudin combined with aspirin may be superior to the combination of unfractionated heparin with aspirin, at least during the acute phase.[13,14]

Aspirin and coumadin

The addition of coumadin to aspirin holds the promise of prolonging the benefit observed during the acute phase by combining antiplatelet and anticoagulant. The APRICOT (Antithrombotics in the Prevention of Reocclusion in Coronary Thrombolysis) trial examined the angiographic and clinical outcomes of 248 patients randomized to one of three antithrombotic regimens (aspirin, 325 mg, versus coumadin, INR 2.8–4.0, versus placebo) after successful thrombolysis with streptokinase or APSAC.[15] After 3 months, aspirin appeared slightly better than coumadin in reducing angiographic reocclusion, reinfarction, and mortality (25% versus 30% versus 32% respectively, $p > 0.05$). An event-free clinical course was observed in 93% of patients treated with aspirin ($p < 0.001$), 82% of those treated with warfarin ($p < 0.05$) and 76% of those given placebo. These data suggest that oral anticoagulation with warfarin has little benefit to offer over aspirin.

The ATACS (Antithrombotic Therapy in Acute Coronary Syndromes Research Group) trial compared combined therapy with aspirin (162.5 mg/day) and anticoagulation (intravenous heparin, then warfarin, INR 2–3) versus aspirin alone in patients with unstable angina and non-Q-wave MI.[6] This study showed a significant reduction in recurrent ischemic events in the combination group versus aspirin alone (10.5% versus 27%, $p = 0.004$). However, bleeding complications were slightly more frequent, using the combination therapy. The CARS study, showed no benefit using a low-dose coumadin. In this trial, 8803 patients were randomized 3–21 days following MI to asprin (160 mg), warfarin (1 mg) plus aspirin (80 mg), or warfarin (3 mg) plus aspirin (80 mg).[16] During a median follow-up of 14 months, the primary outcome composite of reinfarction, non-fatal ischemic stroke or cardiovascular death occurred at rates of 8.6%, 8.8%, and 8.4%

respectively; major hemorrhage was observed in 0.74% of the aspirin patients and in 1.4% of the 3 mg warfarin/80 mg aspirin patients. The INRs were 1.51 at Week 1, 1.27 at Week 4, and 1.19 at 6 months using the 3 mg warfarin/80 mg aspirin combination. Similar negative results were observed in the OASIS pilot study in 309 patients randomized to a fixed-dose regimen of 3 mg of coumadin plus aspirin.[17] A moderate dose of coumadin titrated to an INR of 2–2.5, however, in 197 patients reduced the risk of death, MI, or refractory angina by 58% ($p = 0.08$), and the need for rehospitalization for unstable angina by 58% ($p = 0.03$). The results are consistent with a large body of literature, suggesting that warfarin is effective only at INR ranges of 2–3.5. A small, randomized double-blind study of 57 patients allocated to warfarin (INR 2–2.5), or placebo, in addition to aspirin and using repeated coronary angiography, reported less progression after 10 weeks in the culprit lesion using coumadin (4% of patients versus 33%) and more regression (19% versus 9%).[18]

The WARIS (Warfarin Re-Infarction Study) trial involved 1214 patients randomized to placebo or warfarin and followed for 37 months after an acute MI.[19] Warfarin, compared with placebo, significantly reduced mortality from 20% to 15%, reinfarction rates from 20% to 14%, and cerebrovascular accidents from 7% to 3%. The reduction in reinfarction from 5.1% in the placebo to 2.3% in the warfarin group over 37 months was confirmed by the ASPECT Study[20] in post-infarction patients at lower risk.

The Thrombosis Prevention Trial suggests that warfarin at lower INR of approximately 1.5 may be beneficial in primary prevention, in men aged between 45 and 69 years in the top 20% of a risk score distribution.[21] The design was factorial, the four treatment groups being

(1) Active warfarin (to an INR of about 1.5) and active aspirin (75 mg controlled-release);
(2) Active warfarin and placebo aspirin;
(3) Placebo warfarin and active aspirin; and
(4) Placebo warfarin and placebo aspirin.

The mean warfarin dose required was 4.1 mg daily (range 0.5–12.5 mg). Warfarin vs no warfarin reduced events by 21% ($p = 0.02$) chiefly by a 39% reduction in fatal events ($p = 0.003$) so that warfarin reduced the death rate from all causes by 17% ($p = 0.04$). Aspirin vs no aspirin reduced cardiac events by 20%, almost entirely by a 32% reduction ($p = 0.004$) in non-fatal events. In the individual treatment groups, the absolute reductions in cardiac events compared with placebo, were warfarin 2.6, aspirin 2.3, and warfarin/aspirin 4 per 1000 person years. Neither warfarin nor aspirin alone affected the incidence of all stroke, although the combination increased haemorrhagic strokes ($p = 0.009$). Major non-cerebral bleeding episodes were about twice as frequent in the active treatment groups as in the double placebos (NS) and there was no significant difference in frequency among the three active treatment groups.

Thrombolytic and antithrombotic therapy

The success of thrombolysis is only partial; resistance to recanalization is observed in 19% of patients with optimal flow restoration (TIMI grade 3 flow) in only 54% of patients with accelerated rt-PA.[22] Reocclusion occurs in at least 5–7%, and substantial bleeding in 0.8–1.5%, including rates of intracerebral bleeding in the order of 0.5–0.9%.[23] The success of thrombolysis is limited by an ongoing thrombotic process, and possibly also by a thrombogenic stimulation induced by these agents. Attempts to improve the success rates include development of newer lytic agents and use of various anticoagulant and antiplatelet agents as adjuvant therapy.

Anticoagulants

Heparin

Several studies have documented the importance of conjunctive heparin therapy when using fibrin-specific thrombolytic agents. The Heparin Aspirin Reinfarction Trial (HART) randomized 205 patients to either heparin or low-dose aspirin (100 mg/day) given as conjunctive therapy to standard-dose rt-PA.[24] Patency at 7–24 h was observed in 82% in the heparin group and 52% in the aspirin group ($p < 0.0001$). In a small, randomized pilot study by Bleich et al, patency of the infarct related artery was 71% with heparin group and tPA, and 44% with placebo and tPA ($p < 0.02$).[25,26] The GUSTO trial has compared a regimen of accelerated tPA administration with intravenous heparin to steptokinase with subcutaneous or intravenous administration to show the superiority of tPA with heparin. Heparin is administered routinely with tPA following this trial, although there was no group of patients with tPA and no heparin.[22] The role of conjunctive therapy with heparin in addition to non-fibrin specific agents is more controversial. In an ISIS-2 pilot study, patients treated with intravenous heparin 12 h after streptokinase had lower reinfarction rates than those patients who did not receive heparin (2.2% versus 4.9%; $p < 0.05$).[27] Furthermore, a subgroup analysis of those patients who received heparin demonstrated that mortality was 8.3% in those patients receiving intravenous heparin, and 10.1% in those patients who did not receive heparin ($p < 0.05$) and vascular mortality was also reduced by 19%.[28] Lastly, data from Eisenberg et al[29] and Owen et al,[30] documenting that

therapy with streptokinase significantly increased levels of fibrinopeptide A, and that the levels decreased with heparin therapy, provides compelling evidence for the efficacy of heparin with streptokinase.

Conversely, the argument against using heparin as conjunctive therapy with streptokinase is that streptokinase therapy accentuates the systemic lytic effect. The large ISIS-3[31] and GISSI-2[32] trials showed that subcutaneous heparin after thrombolytic therapy either with rt-PA or streptokinase (4 h in ISIS-3, 12 h in GISSI-2) did not decrease mortality or reinfarction. Since therapeutic levels of heparin may not be reached before 24–48 hours with subcutaneous administration, the GUSTO trial compared subcutaneous heparin administration to intravenous administration, but failed to show any mortality reduction (7.9% and 8.2%).[22] Heparin is therefore not recommended routinely with streptokinase, rather it is recommended in patients at high risk of systemic or venous thromboembolism.

An overview by Collins et al of trials involving heparin with and without aspirin and a thrombolytic agent showed that rates of death, reinfarction, stroke, and pulmonary embolus were markedly less compared with the pre-aspirin/fibrinolysis era.[33,34] Although the addition of heparin led to a reduction of death (5/1000, $p = 0.03$), reinfarction (3/1000, $p = 0.04$), and pulmonary embolus (1/1000, $p = 0.01$), the benefits were small, and the statistical significance was marginal. The small mortality benefits observed at 7 days in the ISIS-3 and GISSI-2 trials (which contributed most of the patients) became less and were no longer statistically significant at 35 days and 6 months of follow-up. Interestingly, the rate of major bleeding with heparin was also less than in the pre-aspirin/fibrinolysis era (3/1000, $p = 0.0001$). Hence the physician is faced with a modest early benefit of heparin of about 5 fewer deaths, 3 fewer reinfarctions, and 1 fewer pulmonary embolus, balanced against 3 more major bleeds.

Low-molecular-weight heparins have not been tested in combination with thrombolytic therapy in large trials. Among patients with a recently diagnosed acute MI treated with streptokinase, treatment with low-molecular-weight heparin for an additional 25 days prevented recurrent ischemic events in the month and up to 6 months following initiation of therapy.[35]

Hirudin

More reproducible thrombin inhibition is achieved with hirudin, a direct thrombin inhibitor. The TIMI-5 trial randomized 246 patients to standard-dose heparin versus one of four escalating doses of hirudin in combination with front-loaded rt-PA.[35] A trend to better TIMI grade 3 flow at 90 min was observed with hirudin compared with heparin (61.8% versus 49.4% $p = 0.07$); the trend became highly significant at 18–36 h (98% patency versus 89%, $p = 0.01$). Reocclusion was also slightly less frequent (1.6% versus 6.7%). The incidence of in-hospital death or reinfarction was 6.8% for hirudin and 16.7% for heparin ($p = 0.02$), and of death, MI, severe coronary heart failure (CHF) or cardiogenic shock 19.0% versus 9.3%, $p = 0.03$. The incidence of major spontaneous hemorrhage was more common with heparin group (4.7% versus 1.2%).

The HIT-I trial randomized 143 patients to heparin or two doses of hirudin (bolus 0.1–0.15 mg/kg, infusion 0.07–0.15 mg/kg/h) in combination with front-loaded rt-PA. TIMI grade 3 flow at 60 min was present in 50%, 57% and 61% of patients, and at 36–48 h 72%, 76% and 92% respectively.[37] Reocclusion and reinfarction rates were also less frequent, but bleeding more frequent.

The TIMI-6 study was a dose-ranging clinical study of hirudin versus heparin with streptokinase in 193 patients; no safety issues were raised.[38] However, three large-scale trials comparing hirudin to heparin (TIMI 9A, GUSTO IIa, and HIT III) were discontinued prematurely because of increased incidences of major bleeding with hirudin, including intracerebral hemorrhage.[39–41] The TIMI 9A and GUSTO IIa trials evaluated hirudin as a bolus of 0.6 mg/kg followed by 0.2 mg/kg/h for 96 h with no monitoring of the aPTT (activated prothrombin time); the HIT-III study used hirudin as a bolus of 0.4 mg/kg followed by 0.15 mg/kg/h for 48 h. Bleeding complications in heparin-treated patients tended to occur in older patients, and in those with higher aPTTs (especially within 12 h). In the hirudin group, it was noted that there was an increased risk of bleeding in patients with elevated creatinine levels. The TIMI and GUSTO investigations were resumed with lower levels of anticoagulation (heparin regimen 1000 U/h, titrated to an aPTT of 55–85 s) and the dose of hirudin was reduced to a bolus of 0.1 mg/kg followed by an infusion of 0.1 mg/kg/h. Neither trials documented clearly a benefit of hirudin. In the GUSTO IIb study, the primary endpoint of death or non-fatal MI or reinfarction at 30 days was non-significantly reduced in the hirudin-treated patients (8.9% versus 9.8% $p = 0.06$); in the TIMI 9B study, the composite endpoint of death, MI, congestive heart failure, and shock, occurred in 11.9% of the heparin-treated patients and 12.9% of the hirudin-treated patients ($p > 0.05$).[42,43] Although, serious bleeding complications were not more frequent with hirudin, more frequent intracranial bleeding occurred. The GUSTO IIB trial yielded some positive findings for hirudin in secondary analyses: firstly, a significant reduction in the rate of death and of nonfatal MI was present early at 24 h (1.3%

versus 2.1%, $p = 0.001$); secondly, patients receiving streptokinase appeared to benefit more than patients administered tPA.

Other direct thrombin inhibitors

Bivilarudin (Hirulog)

In two angiographic pilot studies from the Montreal Heart Institute, hirulog, in combination with streptokinase, improved the 90-min patency of the infarct-related artery.[44,45] A higher dose of hirulog was not better than a moderate dose to prolong the aPTT.[45] This dose was also found to be the best in the HERO trial with a TIMI grade 3 flow at 90 min in 48% of patients compared with 46% with a lower dose and 35% with heparin.[46] These pilot studies have led to the launch of a large trial, HERO-2, with the combination of bivaluridin and streptokinase, looking at the rate of death and MI.

Argatroban

Argatroban, an arginine derivative, was evaluated in the Argatroban in Myocardial Infarction (AMI) study, which enrolled 910 patients treated with one of two doses of argatroban or placebo in conjunction with streptokinase. At 30 days, there was no difference in clinical events, but a positive trend in favor of argatroban in patients treated within 3 h of symptom onset. Similar negative results, but favorable trend, were observed in an angiographic substudy in this trial. Another study of combination of argatroban with t-PA, however, failed to show a benefit.

Inogatran

The Thrombin Inhibition in Myocardial Infarction (TRIM) trial compared inogatran to heparin in patients presenting with unstable angina or non-Q-wave MI. No benefits of the direct thrombin inhibitor on any endpoints were observed.[47]

Antiplatelet agents

Aspirin

The landmark ISIS-2 study of more than 17 000 patients with suspected MI has definitively established the clinical efficacy of aspirin in acute MI, used alone or with steptokinase.[28] The major endpoint was 5-week vascular mortality, which was reduced 25% by streptokinase alone, 23% by aspirin alone, and 42% by both agents compared with placebo ($p < 0.0001$). The benefit on mortality, which was evident at 35 days, persisted throughout a median follow-up of 15 months. The beneficial effect of aspirin was independent of the time of administration within the first 24 h and probably related to a reduction of early reinfarction. The in-hospital reinfarction rate was 3.7% in patients receiving streptokinase alone, to 2.9% in those given placebo, and 1.8% in those allocated to streptokinase plus aspirin. Major bleeding complications (requiring blood transfusions) occurred in 0.6% of those receiving streptokinase plus aspirin, compared with 0.5% with streptokinase alone and 0.3% in the placebo group. Streptokinase plus aspirin was associated with a reduced incidence of stroke (including fatal and disabling strokes) during the in-hospital period. The stroke incidence was 0.6% with streptokinase plus aspirin, 0.7% with streptokinase alone and 1.0% with placebo.

A meta-analysis by Roux et al of 32 trials including 4930 patients treated with either rt-PA or streptokinase demonstrated that aspirin reduces recurrent ischemia from 41% to 25%; angiographic reocclusion in a subgroup of patients who had an early and late hospital angiograms taken was reduced from 25% to 11%.[48]

Platelet membrane GPIIb/IIIa antagonists

The pilot studies of the GPIIb/IIIa antagonists in acute MI has not shown that these drugs alone would obviate the need for a thrombolytic agent. As suggested by recent pilot studies, they could have allowed the use of a lesser amount of thrombolytic agent to possibly reduce the risk of bleeding without compromising efficacy. A previous study of escalating bolus injections of c7E3 given after administration of rt-PA had shown a patent infarct-related artery in 92% of patients compared with 56% of control patients, while recurrent ischemia occurred in only 13% of patients compared with 20% of controls. This benefit was accompanied by with a 25% risk of major bleeding.[49,50] Further details of the TIMI 14 and SPEED studies combining abciximab and thrombolytic stenting are found in Chapter 8.

The RAPPORT trial involved 483 patients randomized to primary PTCA with or without adjunctive c7E3.[51] A TIMI 3 grade flow was present at the first dye injection in 14% of patients administered abciximab versus 7.7% of control patients. The composite endpoint of death, reinfarction, and emergency PTCA was also reduced by 74%. While no intracranial bleeding occurred, major bleeding was increased with the use of abciximab (16.6% versus 9.5%, $p = 0.02$) as well as the need for transfusion (13.7% versus 7.9%, $p < 0.05$).

Eptifibatide[52] and lamifiban[53] were also studied in conjunction with thrombolysis. With eptifibatide and tPA, a TIMI grade 3 flow was observed in 66% versus 39% of patients and the median time to ST-segment recovery was shorter, 65 min versus 116 min ($p = 0.05$) with no increase in the frequency of bleeding. The PARADIGM trial with lamifiban studied patients administered streptokinase or rt-PA. ST segments returned towards baseline more frequently in the lamifiban group (77% versus 56%, $p = 0.019$). Angiography performed in a subset of patients showed a similar patency rate. The frequency of major bleeds or need for transfusions was not increased. Large trials are now ongoing or planned with abciximab, eptifibatide, and lamifiban.

Thromboxane synthase inhibitors and thromboxane receptor antagonists, prostacyclin, and related compounds

Ridogrel, a thromboxane synthase inhibitor and thromboxane receptor antagonist demonstrated an efficacy similar to aspirin to restore patency of the infarct-related artery 7–14 days after administration of streptokinase, and significantly reduced the risk of recurrent ischemia (19% versus 13%).[54] Therapy with prostacyclin either alone or in conjunction with rt-PA had limited success owing to the high incidence of unacceptable side-effects of prostacycline.[53] A small trial with prostaglandin E_1 suggested a decreased time to reperfusion with streptokinase, but not with rt-PA.[56] Another prostacyclin analog, taprostene, demonstrated no increase in infarct-related artery patency when given in addition to single chain urokinase.[57]

Other combinations with antiplatelet therapy

GPIIb/IIIa antagonists and aspirin

GPIIb/IIIa antagonists occupy the obligatory receptor for platelet aggregation and inhibit aggregation to virtually all agonists. Assuming the mechanism for the benefit of antiplatelet therapy is prevention of platelet aggregation and that the effective level of inhibition required is well tolerated, no other concomitant antiplatelet therapy would theoretically be needed. When administered intravenously in the hospital setting, doses of GPIIb/IIIa antagonists have been shown to be effective in coronary angioplasty, in unstable angina and non-Q-wave MI they inhibited platelet aggregation to ADP by 85%; this level of inhibition was well tolerated. The effective doses for secondary prevention and tolerance in outpatients are not yet determined. Addition of aspirin may complement therapy, especially at low levels of blood concentration, and allow use of lower and safer doses of the inhibitors. Although GPIIb/IIIa antagonists are potent inhibitors of platelet aggregation, other platelet functions, including adhesion, activation and the release reaction of active procoagulants, vasoactive agents and growth factors, are not directly affected by these drugs. The mechanism for the benefit of aspirin and of ticlopidine and clopidogrel may be related partly to effects on platelet function other than aggregation. Thus, prevention of thromboxane A_2 vasoconstriction by aspirin may be beneficial; similarly, blockage of the effects of adenosine diphosphate (ADP) by the thienopyridines may afford benefit. Given its safety, documented efficacy and low cost, aspirin has been administered in all trials that have evaluated a GPIIb/IIIa antagonist intravenously in an acute setting. It is also administered in most trials with oral agents. The ongoing SYMPHONY trials of sibrafiban, an oral inhibitor of the GPIIb/IIIa antagonist, are testing the drug with and without aspirin, and also at a high dose without aspirin and at a low dose with aspirin.

GPIIb/IIIa antagonists and heparin

GPIIb/IIIa antagonists are potent inhibitors of platelet aggregation and may obviate the need of concomitant heparin administration. This may be particularly true in acute injury of a stable plaque such as during coronary angioplasty. The EPILOG trial has shown that reduced doses of heparin are associated with less bleeding in angioplasty without compromising on the protective effects of abcix-

imab.[58] In contrast, the inflammatory plaque in unstable angina and MI is rich in tissue factor, which triggers thrombin generation and intravascular coagulation; such plaques may require the combination of an antiplatelet therapy and of an anticoagulant for maximal benefit. The pivotal trials that have documented the benefits of intravenous GPIIb/IIIa antagonists have used concomitant heparin, providing compulsive, but not definitive, evidence that this combination is better. Pilot studies have been performed using lamifiban and with tirofiban without heparin. The Canadian Lamifiban study was a dose-ranging study in patients with unstable angina; heparin use was left optional to the treating physician and was used in 20% of patients only.[59] The combination was associated with an increase in the risk of bleeding. The larger PARAGON trial compared the effects of high- and a low-dose lamifiban with placebo; heparin was used with placebo, and heparin or placebo heparin with lamifiban.[60] The bleeding rate with heparin alone was 0.8%, with lamifiban and no heparin it was 1.0%, and with lamifiban with heparin it was 1.5%. The high dose of lamifiban resulted in an excess bleeding with and without heparin. A larger trial of 3232 patients, the Platelet Receptor Inhibition in Ischemic Syndrome Management (PRISM), has compared directly tirofiban with heparin.[61] The primary endpoint of death, MI or refractory ischemia was assessed at the end of a 48 h infusion period of the study drugs. A statistically significant 33% risk reduction was observed in favor of tirofiban, mainly by a reduction in the incidence of refractory ischemia. The benefit, however, was not sustained and not statistically significant after 1 week. The Platelet Receptor Inhibition in Ischemic Syndrome Management in Patients Limited by Unstable Signs and Symptoms (PRISM-PLUS) Study compared tirofiban with heparin to the combination in patients with documented unstable angina or non-Q-wave MI.[62] Treatment was applied for a mean duration of 71 h, including a 48 h medical management followed by coronary angiography and coronary angioplasty, if deemed clinically useful on study drug infusion. The primary endpoint was measured 1 week after randomization. The treatment arm with tirofiban alone was prematurely discontinued because of an excess mortality rate at 1 week, whereas the group that received the combination of tirofiban plus heparin fared significantly better at 1 week, 4 weeks, and 6 months. Although underpowered because of premature discontinuation, the results with tirofiban suggest that an anticoagulant is needed with platelet inhibition in these syndromes characterized by an active inflammatory ulcerated plaque. Indeed, the survival curves for the endpoint of MI up to 6 months were very similar in the groups administered tirofiban alone and heparin, and significantly reduced with the combination. The combination therapy was associated to a risk reduction in the rate of death or MI of 66% at 48 h, 43% at 1 week, and 30% at 1 month. The composite endpoint was also reduced significantly at all timepoints. The large PURSUIT trial involving 9461 patients with unstable angina and non-Q-wave MI documented a benefit of eptifibatide over placebo on a background of aspirin and of heparin with a risk reduction in the primary endpoint of death or MI at 1 month of 9% ($p = 0.04$).[63]

Ticlopidine plus aspirin or clopidogrel plus aspirin

Ticlopidine blocks the platelet effect of adenosine diphosphate (ADP) and aspirin block the thromboxane A_2 effects. The combination has therefore high potential for very effective and additive antiplatelet therapy since they inhibit two independent pathways to platelet aggregation. Many trials have now documented that ticlopidine used with aspirin in the setting of stent implantation affords significantly more protection than the combination of coumadin and aspirin. A trial in unstable angina compared ticlopidine with no ticlopidine and no aspirin and showed a significant long-term benefit but not in the first week, in complince with the known delay of the thienopyridines to reach full antiplatelet effects.[64] Clopidogrel has not yet been tested in acute situations; the favorable results observed in secondary prevention of stroke and MI in the CAPRIE trial with a 9% risk reduction over the benefit of aspirin suggest that the drug will be equally effective as ticlopidine and safer.[65]

The ideal drug–drug combination

The optimal antithrombotic therapy should be effective and safe. It will probably consist of a combination of drugs acting selectively on various steps of the process of platelet function and/or the coagulation system. The ideal therapy may vary in specific disease states. Triple antithrombotic therapy adding a GPIIb/IIIa receptor antagonist to aspirin and to heparin is now recommended in high-risk patients. Oral GPIIb/IIIa antagonists hold the promise of prolonging and accentuating the benefit observed in the acute phase for better plaque passivation and prevention of the recurrence of events. Other interventions tested are the combination of clopidogrel and aspirin, of aspirin and coumadin, and the subcutaneous administration of a low-molecular-weight heparin and of a long-acting hirudin on an outpatient basis.

References

1. Theroux P and Fuster V. Acute coronary syndromes: unstable angina and non-Q-wave myocardial infarction. *Circulation* 1998;**97**: 1195–206.

2. Antiplatelet Trialists' Collaboration. Collaborative overview of randomized trials of antiplatelet therapy: I. Prevention of death, myocardial infarction, and stroke by prolonged antiplatelet therapy in various categories of patients. *Br Med J* 1994;**308**:81–106.

3. Collins R, MacMahon S, Flather M, Baigent C, Remvig L, Mortensen S, et al. Clinical effects of anticoagulant therapy in suspected acute myocardial infarction: systematic overview of randomised trials. *Br Med J* 1996;**313**(7058): 652–9.

4. Theroux P, Waters D, Lam J, Juneau M, and McCans J. Reactivation of unstable angina after the discontinuation of heparin. *N Eng J Med* 1992;**327**:141–5.

5. The RISC Group. Risk of myocardial infarction and death during treatment with low-dose aspirin and intravenous heparin in men with unstable coronary artery disease. *Lancet* 1990;**336**:827–30.

6. Cohen M, Adams PC, Parry G, et al. Combination antithrombotic therapy in unstable rest angina and non-Q-wave infarction in nonprior aspirin users: primary endpoint analysis from the ATACS trial. *Circulation* 1994;**89**:81–8.

7. Oler A, Whooley MA, Oler J, Grady D. Adding heparin to aspirin reduces the incidence of myocardial infarction and death in patients with unstable angina. *J Am Med Assoc* 1996;**276**:811–15.

8. The FRISC Investigators. Low-molecular-weight heparin during instability in coronary artery disease, Fragmin during Instability in Coronary Artery disease (FRISC) Study. *Lancet* 1996;**347**:561–8.

9. Klein W, Buchwald A, Hillis SE, Monrad S, Sanz G, Turpie GG, et al. Comparison of low-molecular-weight heparin with unfractionated heparin acutely and with placebo for 6 weeks in the management of unstable coronary artery disease. Fragmin in unstable coronary artery disease study (FRISC). *Circulation* 1997;**96**: 61–8.

10. Cohen M, Demers C, Gurfinkel EP, Turpie AGG, Fromell GJ, Goodman S, et al for the Efficacy and Safety of Subcutaneous Enoxaparin in Non-Q-Wave Coronary Events Study Group. Low molecular weight heparin versus unfractionated heparin for unstable angina and non-Q wave myocardial infarction. *N Eng J Med* 1997;**337**:447–52.

11. TIMI 11B. Results presented at the European Congress of Cardiology, Vienna, Austria, August 1998.

12. The FRAXIS Investigators. Results presented at the European Congress of Cardiology, Vienna, Austria, August 1998.

13. The Global Use of Strategies to Open Occluded Coronary Arteries (GUSTO) IIb Investigators. A comparison of recombinant hirudin with heparin for the treatment of acute coronary syndromes. *N Eng J Med* 1996; **335**:775–82.

14. Effects of recombinant hirudin (lepirudin) compared with heparin on death, myocardial infarction, refractory angina, and revascularisation procedures in patients with acute myocardial ischemia without ST elevation: a randomised trial. Organisation to Assess Strategies for Ischemic Syndromes (OASIS-2) Investigators. *Lancet* 1999;**353**:429–38.

15. Meijer A, Verheugt F, Weter C, Lie K, van der Pol JM, von Femige MJ. Aspirin versus coumadin in the prevention of reocclusion and recurrent ischemia after successful thrombolysis: a prospective placebo-controlled angiographic study. Results of the APRICOT study. *Circulation* 1993;**87**: 1524–30.

16. Coumadin, Aspirin, Reinfarction Study (CARS) Investigators. Randomized, double-blind trial of fixed low dose warfarin with aspirin after myocardial infarction. *Lancet* 1997;**350**:389–96.

17. Organization to Assess Strategies for Ischemic Syndromes (OASIS) Investigators. Comparison of the effects of two doses of recombinant hirudin compared with heparin in patients with acute myocardial ischemia without ST elevation. A pilot study. *Circulation* 1997;**96**: 769–77.

18. Williams MJA, Morison IM, Parker JH, and Steward RAH. Progression of the culprit lesion in unstable coronary artery disease with warfarin and aspirin versus aspirin alone: preliminary study. *J Am Coll Cardiol* 1997;**30**: 364–9.

19. The Medical Research Council's General Practice Research Framework. Thrombosis Prevention Trial: randomized trial of low intensity oral anticoagulation with warfarin and low-dose aspirin in the primary prevention of ischemic heart disease in men at increased risk. *Lancet* 1998;**351**:233–41.

20. The ASPECT Research Group. Effect of long-term oral anticoagulant treatment on mortality and cardiovascular morbidity after myocardial infarction. Anticoagulants in the Secondary Prevention of Events in Coronary Thrombosis (ASPECT) Research Group. *Lancet* 1994; **343**:499–503.

21. The Medical Council's General Practice Research Framework. Thrombosis Prevention Trial: randomized trial of low-intensity oral anticoagulation with warfarin and low-dose aspirin in the primary prevention of ischaemic heart disease in men at increased risk. *Lancet* 1998;**351**:233–41.

22. The GUSTO Investigators. The effects of tissue plasminogen activators, streptokinase, or both on coronary artery patency, ventricular function, and survival after acute myocardial infarction. *N Engl J Med* 1993;**393**:1615–22.

23. The GUSTO Investigators. An international randomized trial comparing four thrombolytic strategies for acute myocardial infarction. *N Engl J Med* 1993;**393**:673–82.

24. Hsia J, Hamilton W, Kleiman N, Roberts R, Chaitman BR, Ross AM for the HART Investigators. A comparison between heparin and low-dose aspirin as adjunctive therapy with tissue plasminogen activator for acute myocardial infarction. *N Engl J Med* 1990; **323**:1433–7.

25. Bleich S, Nichols TC, Schumacher RR, Cooke DH, Tate DA, Teichman SL. Effects of heparin on coronary artery patency after thrombolysis with tissue plasminogen activator for acute myocardial infarction. *Am J Cardiol* 1990;**66**:1412–17.

26. The ISIS Pilot Study Investigators. Randomized factorial trial of high-dose intravenous streptokinase, of oral aspirin, and of intravenous heparin in acute myocardial infarction. *Eur Heart J* 1987;**8**:634–42.

27. The ISIS Pilot Study Investigators. Randomized factorial trial of high-dose intravenous streptokinase, of oral aspirin, and of intravenous heparin in acute myocardial infarction. *Eur Heart J* 1987;**8**:634–42.

28. The ISIS-2 (Second International Study of Infarct Survival). Randomised trial of intravenous streptokinase, oral aspirin, both, or neither among 17 187 cases of suspected acute myocardial infarction: ISIS-2. *Lancet* 1988;**2**: 349–360.

29. Eisenberg P, Sherman L, Jaffe A. Paradoxic elevation of fibrinopeptide A: Evidence for continued thrombosis despite intensive fibrinolysis. *J Am Coll Cardiol* 1987;**10**:527–9.

30. Owen J, Freidman K, Grossman B, et al. Thrombolytic therapy with tissue plasminogen activator or streptokinase induces transient thrombin activity. *Blood* 1988;**72**:616–20.

31. The ISIS-3 Collaborative Group. A randomized trial of streptokinase vs anistreptlase and of aspirin plus heparin vs aspirin alone among 41 299 cases of suspected acute myocardial infarction. *Lancet* 1992;**339**:753–70.

32. The GISSI-2 Collaborative Group. GISSI-2: A factorial randomized trial of alteplase versus streptokinase and heparin versus no heparin among 12 490 patients with acute myocardial infarction. *Lancet* 1990;**336**:65–71.

33. Collins R, Peto R, Baigent C, and Sleight P. Aspirin, heparin, and fibrinolytic therapy in suspected myocardial infarction. *N Eng J Med* 1997;**336**:847–60.

34. Canon C, McCabe C, Henry T, for the TIMI V investigators. A pilot trial of recombinant desulfatohirudin compared with heparin in conjunction with tissue-type plasminogen activator and aspirin for acute myocardial infarction: results of the Thrombolysis in Myocardial Infarction (TIMI) 5 trial. *Circulation* 1994;**86**: I-268.

35. Glick A, Kornowski R, Michowich Y, et al. Reduction of reinfarction and angina with use of low molecular weight heparin administered prior to streptokinase in patients with acute myocardial infarction. *Am J Cardiol* 1996;**77**: 1145–8.

36. Cannon C, McCabe C, Henry T, for the TIMI V investigators. A pilot trial of recombinant desulfatohirudin compared with heparin in conjunction with tissue-type plasminogen activator and aspirin for acute myocardial infarction: results of the Thrombolysis in Myocardial Infarction (TIMI) 5 trial. *Circulation* 1994;**86**: I-268.

37. Neuhaus K, Niederer W, Wagner J, Maurer W, for the ALKK-Study Group. HIT (Hirudin for the improvement of thrombolysis): results of a dose-escalation study. *Circulation* 1993; **88**: I-292.

38. Lee L, for the TIMI VI Investigators. Initial experience with hirudin and streptokinase in acute myocardial infarction (TIMI VI) trial. *Am J Cardiol* 1995;**75**:7–13.

39. Antman E, for the TIMI 9A Investigators. Hirudin in acute myocardial infarction. Safety report from the Thrombolysis and Thrombin Inhibition in Myocardial Infarction (TIMI) 9A Trial. *Circulation* 1994;**90**:1624–30.

40. The GUSTO IIa Investigators. Randomized trial of intravenous heparin versus recombinant hirudin for acute coronary syndromes. The Global Use of Strategies to Open Occluded Coronary Arteries (GUSTO) IIa Investigators. *Circulation* 1994;**90**:1631–7.

41. Neuhaus K, van Essen R, Tebbe U, for the ALKK investigators. Safety observations from the pilot phase of the randomized r-Hirudin for improvement of thrombolysis (HIT-III) Study. *Circulation* 1994;**92**:2374–80.

42. The GUSTO IIb Investigators. A comparison of recombinant hirudin with heparin for the treatment of acute coronary syndromes. *N Engl J Med* 1996;**335**:775–82.

43. Antman EM. Hirudin in acute myocardial infarction. Thrombolysis and Thrombin Inhibition in Myocardial Infarction (TIMI) 9B trial. *Circulation* 1996;**94**:911–21.

44. Lidon R-M, Theroux P, Lesperance J, Adelman B, Bonon R, Duval D, et al. A pilot, early angiographic patency study using a direct thrombin inhibitor as adjunctive therapy to streptokinase in acute myocardial infarction. *Circulation* 1994;**89**:1567–72.

45. Theroux P, Perez-Villa F, Waters D, Lesperance J, Shabain F, Bonan R. Randomized double-blind comparison of two doses of hirulog with heparin as adjunctive therapy to streptokinase to promote early patency of the infarct-related artery in acute myocardial infarction. *Circulation* 1995;**91**:2132–9.

46. White HD, Aylward PE, Frey MJ, Adgey AA, Nair R, Hillis WS, Shalev Y et al. Randomized, double-blind comparison of hirulog versus heparin in patients receiving streptokinase and aspirin for acute myocardial infarction (HERO). Hirulog Early Perfusion/Occlusion Trial Investigators. *Circulation* 1997;**96**:2155–61.

47. The TRIM Study Group. A low-molecular weight, selective thrombin inhibitor, inogatran, vs heparin, in unstable coronary artery disease in 1209 patients. *Eur Heart J* 1997;**18**: 1416–25.

48. Roux S, Christeller S, Ladin E. Effects of aspirin on coronary reocclusion and recurrent ischemia after thrombolysis: a meta analysis. *J Am Coll Cardiol* 1992;**19**:671–7.

49. Ohman E, Kleiman N, Talley J. Simultaneous platelet glycoprotein IIb/IIIa integrin blockade with accelerated tissue plasminogen activator in acute myocardial infarction. *Circulation* 1994;**90**:I-564.

50. Kleiman N, Ohman E, Califf R, George BS, Kereiakes D, Aguirre FU, et al. Profound inhibition of platelet aggregation with monoclonal antibody 7E3 Fab after thrombolytic therapy: results of the Thrombolysis in Myocardial Infarction (TAMI) 8 pilot study. *J Am Coll Cardiol* 1993;**22**:381–9.

51. Brener S, Barr L, Burchenal J, Katz S, George BS, Jones AA. A randomized, placebo-controlled trial of abciximab with primary angioplasty for acute MI. The RAPPORT Trial. *Circulation* 1997;**96**:I-473.

52. Ohman E, Kleiman N, Gacioch G, et al. Combined accelerated tissue plasminogen activator and platelet glycoprotein IIb/IIIa integrin receptor blockade with integrelin in acute myocardial infarction: results of a randomized, placebo-controlled, dose-ranging trial. *Circulation* 1997;**95**:846–54.

53. Moliterno D, Harrington R, Krucoff M, et al. More complete and stable reperfusion with platelet IIb/IIIa antagonism plus thrombolysis for AMI: the PARADIGM Trial [Abstract]. *Circulation* 1996;**94**:I-553.52.

54. The RAPT Investigators. Randomized trial of ridogrel a combined thromboxane synthase inhibitor and thromboxane A_2/prostaglandin endoperoxide receptor antagonist, versus aspirin as adjunct to thrombolysis in acute myocardial infarction: the ridogrel versus aspirin patency trial (RAPT). *Circulation* 1993;**89**:I-595.

55. Topol E, Ellis S, Califf R, et al. Combined tissue-type plasminogen activator and prostacyclin therapy in acute myocardial infarction: thrombolysis and angioplasty In Myocardial Infarction (TAMI) 4 study group. *J Am Coll Cardiol* 1989;**64**:S-877.

56. Sharma B, Wyeth B, Gimenez H, et al. Intracoronary prostaglandin E_1 plus streptokinase therapy in acute myocardial infarction. *J Am Coll Cardiol* 1986;**58**:1161–6.

57. Bar F, Meyer J, Michels R, et al. The effect of taprostene in patients with acute myocardial infarction treated with thrombolytic therapy: results of the START study. Saruplase Taprostene Acute Reocclusion Trial. *Eur Heart J* 1993;**14**:1118–26.

58. The EPILOG Investigators. Platelet glycoprotein IIb/IIIa receptor blockade and low-dose heparin during percutaneous coronary revascularization. *N Eng J Med* 1997;**336**:1689–96.

59. Theroux P, Kouz S, Roy L, Knudtson ML, Diodati JG, Marguis JF, et al. Platelet membrane receptor glycoprotein IIb/IIIa antagonism in unstable angina. The Canadian Lamifiban Study. *Circulation* 1996;**94**:899–905.

60. The PARAGON Investigators. A randomized trial of potent platelet IIb/IIIa antagonism, heparin, or both in patients with unstable angina: the PARAGON Study. *Circulation* 1996;**94(Suppl.)**:I-553.

61. The Platelet Receptor Inhibition in Ischemic Syndrome Management (PRISM) Study Investigators. A comparison of aspirin plus tirofiban with aspirin plus heparin for unstable angina. *N Eng J Med* 1998;**338**:1498–505.

62. The Platelet Receptor Inhibition in Ischemic Syndrome Management in Patients Limited by Unstable Signs and Symptoms (PRISM-PLUS) Study Investigators. Inhibition of the platelet glycoprotein IIb/IIIa receptor with tirofiban in unstable angina and non-Q-wave myocardial infarction. *N Eng J Med* 1998;**338**:1488–97.

63. The PURSUIT Investigators. A randomized comparison of the platelet glycoprotein IIb/IIIa peptide inhibitor eptifibatide with placebo in patients without persistent ST-segment elevation acute coronary syndromes. *N Eng J Med*, 1998;**7**:436–43.

64. Balsano F, Rizzon P, Violi F, Scrutinio D, Cimminiello C, Aguglia F, et al. Antiplatelet treatment with ticlopidine in unstable angina. *Circulation* 1990;**82**:17–26.

65. CAPRIE Steering Committee. A randomized, blinded, trial of clopidogrel versus aspirin in patients at risk of ischaemic events. *Lancet* 1996;**348**:1329–39.

19

Beyond platelet glycoprotein IIb/IIIa antagonists: targeting glycoprotein Ib, tissue factor and selectins

James T Willerson, Vincenzo Pasceri, Zhi-Qang Chen, and Pierre Zoldhelyi

Introduction

Platelet glycoprotein IIb/IIIa receptor antagonists are recognized as being useful in the treatment of patients with acute coronary heart disease syndromes.[1–8] Monoclonal antibodies, synthetic peptides, and small-molecular weight inhibitors of the GPIIb/IIIa receptors have been shown to be useful in reducing the risk of myocardial infarction (MI), death, and the need for second interventional procedure in patients undergoing interventional procedures, including angioplasty and stents. GPIIb/III antagonists have also been shown to reduce the risk of death, MI and the need for intervention in patients with unstable angina pectoris.[6–8] However, while these have been successful and have provided clear advances in the protection of patients with acute coronary syndromes, they have not been completely protective and there are patients who develop major and minor bleeding episodes and sometimes thrombocytopenia with their use.[1–8] Thus, it is worthwhile to identify other additive or alternative therapeutic approaches.

The GPIIb/IIIa receptor antagonists inhibit platelet aggregation in response to the agonists that accumulate at sites of vascular injury and promote platelet aggregation and dynamic vasoconstriction (Figure 19.1). However, they do not generally prevent platelet adhesion at sites of vascular injury, they do not diminish platelet activation or secretion, they may not inhibit the effect of tissue factor expressed in the media and toward the intima of injured arteries, and they do not reduce inflammation, which can be intimately related to the development of thrombosis.[9,10] Thus, opportunities exist for additional forms of therapy.

Platelet adhesion

With arterial injury, in the form of ulceration or rupture of atherosclerotic plaques, from interventional procedures such as angioplasty or atherectomy, and with other forms of arterial injury, platelets attach or adhere to the injured artery and this is followed subsequently by the build-up of a platelet-initiated thrombus through platelet aggregation. Platelet adhesion is not diminished by the GPIIb/IIIa receptor antagonist. Platelet adhesion occurs as a result of platelets binding to exposed collagen beneath the subendothelium and to the von Willebrand binding domain on the endothelium through platelet GPIb receptors.[11–14] This provides a pharmacological opportunity to inhibit the platelet adherence

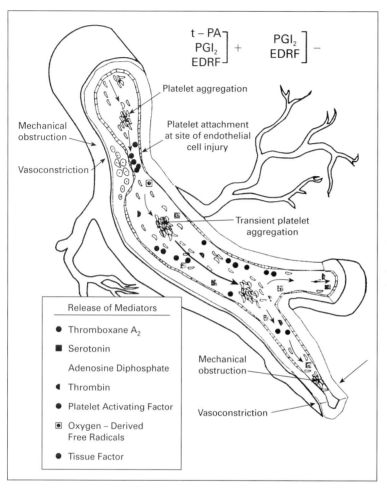

$$\left.\begin{array}{l} t-PA \\ PGI_2 \\ EDRF \end{array}\right] + \qquad \left.\begin{array}{l} PGI_2 \\ EDRF \end{array}\right] -$$

Platelet aggregation

Mechanical obstruction

Platelet attachment at site of endothelial cell injury

Vasoconstriction

Transient platelet aggregation

Release of Mediators

● Thromboxane A₂

■ Serotonin

Adenosine Diphosphate

◀ Thrombin

● Platelet Activating Factor

▣ Oxygen – Derived Free Radicals

● Tissue Factor

Mechanical obstruction

Vasoconstriction

Figure 19.1

With endothelial vascular injury in the form of atherosclerotic plaque fissuring or ulceration, platelets aggregate and release potent mediators of further platelet aggregation, thrombosis, vasoconstriction, and fibroproliferation, including thromboxane A_2, serotonin, ADP, and platelet-activating factor. Local increases in thrombin, oxygen-derived free radicals and tissue factor at the same sites contribute to a potent prothrombotic environment, as do local decreases in nitric oxide, prostacyclin, and tissue plasminogen activator, the levels of which are decreased at sites of vascular injury. Modified and reproduced with permission from Willerson et al.[44]

to injured vascular endothelium using inhibitors of the GPIb receptors. Fragments isolated from von Willebrand factor have been shown to bind to the platelet membrane glycoprotein Ib receptor and inhibit the interaction of von Willebrand factor with these receptors.[15,16] This inhibition has led to inhibiting platelet adhesion and thrombosis.[15,16] VCL (made by Bio-Technology General Inc., Israel) is a recombinant fragment of von Willebrand factor, Leu[504]-Lys[728], with a single intrachain disulfide bond that links residues Cys[509] and Cys[695].[15,16] Two different experimental animal models have been used to determine the effect of VCL on the development of arterial thrombosis.[15,16]

In the initial studies, a canine model was used to determine the effect of VCL on:

(1) The formation of intracoronary thrombosis; and

(2) Reocclusion of coronary arteries after thrombolysis with tissue plasminogen activator.[16]

In these studies, VCL delayed thrombus formation and reocclusion of coronary arteries when a thrombolytic agent had been given. Two main protocols were used—Protocol 1 and Protocol 2.

Protocol 1

In this Protocol the effect of VCL on intracoronary thrombus formation was evaluated. VCL was begun 30 min before electrical stimulation of the coronary arteries. Three different groups of animals were studied. In the control group (Group 1, $n = 12$), saline was given intravenously at 1 ml/min. In one experimental group (Group 2, $n = 7$), VCL was given intravenously at 4 mg/kg body weight as a bolus dose and at 2 mg/kg/h as a continuous infusion until the end of the study. This dose of VCL is enough to inhibit more than 50% of platelet aggregation induced by botrocetin and asialo-von Willebrand factor. In the other experimental group (Group 3, $n = 8$), aspirin was given intravenously at 5 mg/kg body weight as a bolus dose. The change in coronary blood flow before and after electrical stimulation was monitored carefully. The amount of time elapsed from the beginning of electrical stimulation to total occlusion of the coronary arteries was recorded. All animals were given tissue plasminogen activator (TPA) (Genentech, Inc) intravenously 3 h after total occlusion of coronary arteries at 80 µg/kg body weight as a bolus dose and at 8 µg/kg/min as a continuous infusion for 90 min. This treatment provided thrombolysis of the thrombi formed in the coronary arteries.

A thrombus was considered to be lysed (and the artery reperfused) when the flow velocity of the coronary artery returned to at least 70% of the value that existed before thrombus formation. The amount of time elapsed from TPA administration to reperfu-

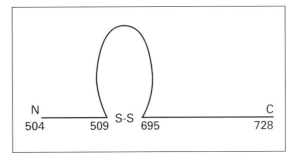

Figure 19.2
Schematic representation of the VCL peptide. Diagram of VCL illustrating the large internal bridge held in place by a disulfide bride (S–S). N, N-terminal; C, C-terminal. Reproduced by permission of the American Heart Association and McGhie et al 1994.[15]

sion was recorded as thrombolysis or reperfusion time. Dogs in whom reperfusion had not occurred after 90 min of TPA infusion were excluded from further study. Dogs in whom reperfusion occurred were monitored further until either the coronary arteries reoccluded or 180 min had elapsed without reocclusion. The time from reperfusion to reocclusion was recorded as the reocclusion time. Dogs in whom coronary arteries had not reoccluded after 180 min of reperfusion were considered not to have reoccluded. Dogs in whom reocclusion occurred were monitored for 30 min to verify persistent reocclusion.

Protocol 2

In Protocol 2, the effect of VCL on thrombolysis and reocclusion was evaluated in additional animals treated 3 h after the occlusion of coronary arteries. These animals were assigned to one of four additional groups: TPA and heparin (Group 4, $n = 7$); TPA, heparin, and VCL (Group 5, $n = 7$); TPA, heparin, and aspirin (Group 6, $n = 8$); and TPA, heparin, VCL, and aspirin (Group 7, $n = 8$). Heparin was given at 200 U/kg as an intravenous bolus. TPA, VCL, and aspirin were given at the same dose as for Protocol 1. The follow-up for thrombolysis and reocclusion was also the same as for protocol 1.

Insertion of the electrode needle into the coronary artery caused some stenosis in the arteries of all animals, as determined by reduction of blood flow velocity to approximately 65% of the baseline level. After electrical stimulation, all animals developed total occlusion of the affected coronary arteries. In Protocol 1, the elapsed time from electrical stimulation to total occlusion of the coronary arteries was significantly longer in dogs treated with VCL ($p < 0.001$) and aspirin ($p < 0.05$) than in dogs treated with saline (Figure 19.3). In all animals, aortic blood pressures and heart rates changed slightly after the occlusion of coronary arteries.

In Protocol 1, 3 h after the occlusion of coronary arteries, only TPA was given to the animals. The administration of TPA resulted in thrombolysis in 4/12 saline-treated dogs (33%), 5 out of 7 VCL-treated dogs (71%), and 4/8 aspirin-treated dogs (50%). The average elapsed time from TPA treatment to thrombolysis (thrombolysis time) was significantly shorter in VCL-treated than in saline-treated dogs (47 ± 12 min versus 81 ± 4 min, $p < 0.05$, Figure 19.4).

In protocol 2, dogs were not pretreated before their coronary arteries were occluded, and 3 h after the occlusion of coronary arteries, they received thrombolytic treatment as follows:

(1) TPA- and heparin-induced thrombolysis in 5/7 dogs (71%);
(2) TPA-, heparin-, and VCL-induced thrombolysis in 6/7 dogs (86%);

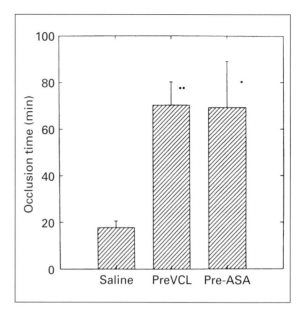

Figure 19.3
Elapsed times from electrical injury to the formation of occlusive thrombi in coronary arteries of animals pretreated with saline, VCL, and aspirin (ASA) intravenously (Protocol 1). Compared with saline, *p < 0.05; **p < 0.001. Reproduced by permission of the American Heart Association and Yao et al 1994.[16]

(3) TPA-, heparin-, and aspirin-induced thrombolysis in 7 out of 8 dogs (85%); and
(4) TPA-, heparin-, VCL-, and aspirin-induced thrombolysis in 8 out of 8 dogs (100%).

The average thrombolysis time in dogs treated with TPA, heparin, VCL, and aspirin was slightly more than half that in dogs treated only with TPA and heparin (23.5 ± 4 min versus 45 ± 12 min). The difference, however, was not statistically significant (Figure 19.5). Mean aortic pressure had decreased by approximately 20 mm Hg at 3 h after throm-

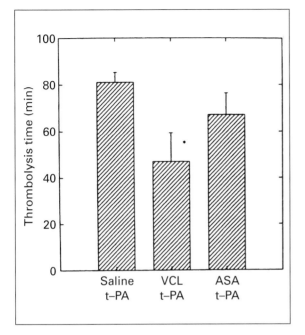

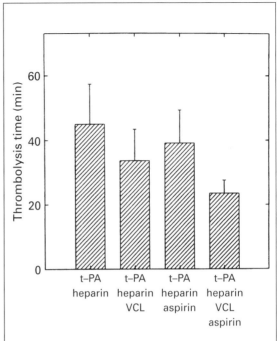

Figure 19.4
Elapse times from tissue plasminogen activator (t-PA) administration to thrombolysis in coronary arteries of animals pretreated with saline, VCL, and aspirin (ASA) intravenously (Protocol 1). Compared with saline, *p < 0.05. Reproduced by permission of the American Heart Association and Yao et al 1994.[16]

Figure 19.5
Elapsed times from intravenous administration of thrombolytic agents to thrombolysis in coronary arteries of animals that were not pretreated (Protocol 2). t-PA indicates tissue plasminogen activator. Reproduced by permission of the American Heart Association and Yao et al 1994.[16]

bolysis in dogs treated with TPA, heparin, and VCL or TPA, heparin, VCL, and aspirin.

After thrombolysis, many animals developed reocclusion of the coronary arteries during the 3-h monitoring period. In Protocol 1, the frequency of reocclusion was not significantly different among dogs pretreated with saline (4/4), aspirin (4/4), or VCL (4/5). However, the average time from thrombolysis to reocclusion (reocclusion time) was significantly longer in dogs pretreated with VCL (114 ± 18 min) than in dogs pretreated with saline (42 ± 4 min) or aspirin (55 ± 14 min) (p < 0.05, Figure 19.6).

In Protocol 2, coronary artery reocclusion developed in 5/5 dogs treated with TPA and heparin, and the addition of aspirin did not change the frequency of reocclusion (7/7). The addition of VCL to TPA and heparin significantly reduced the frequency of reocclusion in the reperfused coronary arteries of dogs (2/6; p < 0.05 compared with the TPA and heparin group). The addition of VCL and aspirin also significantly reduced the frequency of reocclusion (1/8; p < 0.01 compared with the TPA, heparin, VCL group). The average reocclusion time was also significantly longer in

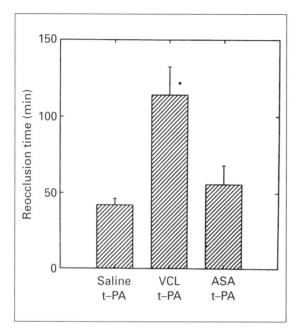

Figure 19.6
Elapsed times from thrombolysis to reocclusion
of coronary arteries in animals pretreated with
saline, VCL, and aspirin (ASA) (Protocol 1).
Compared with saline plus tissue plasminogen
activator (t-PA) and aspirin plus t-PA, *p < 0.05.
Reproduced by permission of the American Heart
Association and Yao et al 1994.[16]

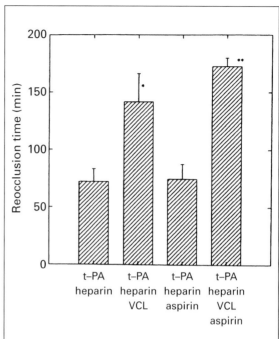

Figure 19.7
Elapsed times from thrombolysis to reocclusion
of coronary arteries of animals treated with tissue
plasminogen activator (t-PA), heparin, VCL, and
aspirin (Protocol 2). Compared with t-PA plus
heparin and t-PA plus heparin plus aspirin,
*p < 0.05; **p < 0.001. Reproduced by permission
of the American Heart Association and Yao et al
1994.[16]

VCL-treated dogs than in dogs who did not
receive VCL (Figure 19.7).

A plasma concentration of VCL of
20.6±0.6 µg/ml was detected at 10 min after
VCL was injected as an intravenous bolus at
4 mg/kg. Thereafter, the VCL level decreased
as shown in Figure 19.8. The half-life of VCL
was 24 min. After the injection and continuous infusion of VCL (4 mg/kg + 2 mg/kg/h),
the level of VCL reached a plateau in 60 min
at approximately 10 µg/ml (Figure 19.9).

In dogs treated with TPA alone, bleeding
around the surgical area was not significant.
The addition of VCL or aspirin caused mild
bleeding along the incisions. The combination
of TPA, heparin, VCL, and aspirin resulted in
moderate-to-severe bleeding around the surgical areas. Nevertheless, the hematocrit did not
change significantly in any group after TPA
treatment, nor did hemoglobin change significantly after treatment with TPA, heparin, and
VCL (12.9 ± 0.3% of control versus
14 ± 0.9% at 3 h after treatment). The platelet
count decreased slightly from 293 × 1000/mm³

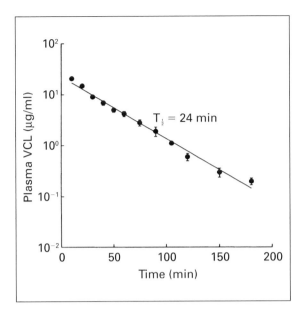

Figure 19.8
Plasma VCL concentration after administration at 4 mg/kg given as an intravenous bolus. Three animals were studied. Each sample was tested three times. Values are the average of three mean values of each sample. Reproduced by permission of the American Heart Association and Yao et al 1994.[16]

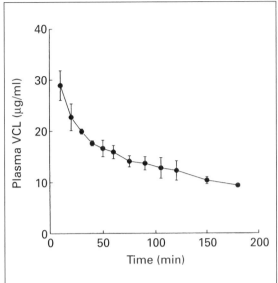

Figure 19.9
Plasma VCL concentration after 4 mg/kg given as an intravenous bolus plus 2 mg/kg/h as a continuous intravenous infusion. Reproduced by permission of the American Heart Association and Yao et al 1994.[16]

(baseline) to $262 \times 1000/mm^3$ at 30 min, $265 \times 1000/mm^3$ at 1 h, $270 \times 1000/mm^3$ at 2 h, and $269 \times 1000/mm^3$ at 3 h after treatment with TPA, heparin, and VCL ($p > 0.05$).

Activated clotting time was significantly prolonged immediately following TPA and heparin administration (to a peak of 6 times the baseline value in 10 min). It returned to 1.5 times the baseline value 1 h after treatment and to just above the baseline value 3 h after treatment. The addition of aspirin, VCL, or aspirin and VCL did not affect activated clotting time.

Ex vivo platelet aggregation induced by ADP was not affected by VCL infusion, but it was slightly reduced by aspirin injection (Figures 19.10 and 19.11). The botrocetin-induced platelet aggregation was completely inhibited by VCL treatment (Figure 19.10), and arachidonic acid-induced platelet aggregation was completely inhibited by aspirin injection (Figure 19.11).

Additional studies

Additional studies were also performed using VCL. The following hypotheses were tested:

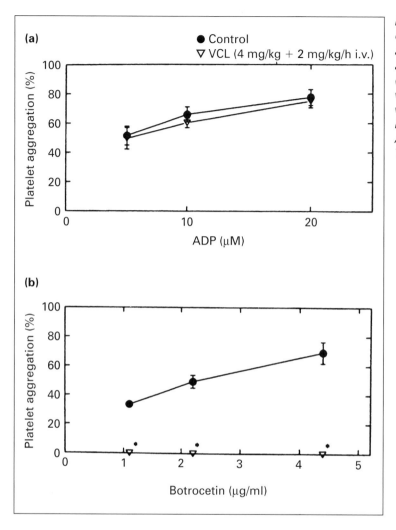

Figure 19.10

Changes in ex vivo platelet aggregation induced by (a) ADP and (b) botrocetin before (control) and after the treatment with intravenous VCL. Compared with control, *p < 0.001. Reproduced by permission of the American Heart Association and Yao et al 1994.[16]

(1) after in vivo administration, an antagonist of the von Willebrand-glycoprotein Ib binding domain attenuates or abolishes cyclic flow variations in stenosed, endothelium-injured coronary arteries in nonhuman primates; and

(2) in vivo administration of VCL reduces botrocetin-induced platelet aggregation in vitro.[15]

The aim of these studies was to evaluate the in vivo effects of the inhibitor of the platelet glycoprotein Ib receptor in a model of coronary artery stenosis with endothelial injury.

Anesthetized, open-chest male baboons (*n* = 18) were studied.[15] Catheters were inserted into a femoral artery and vein for measurement of aortic blood pressure and for drug and fluid administration, respectively. A

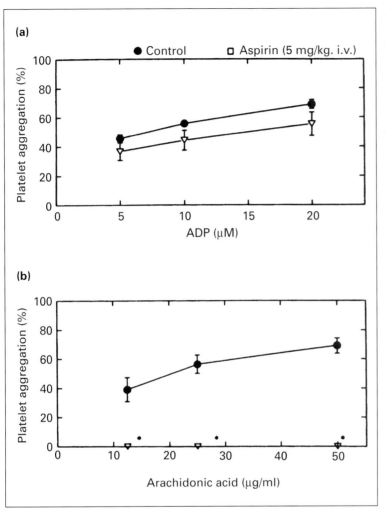

Figure 19.11
*Changes in ex vivo platelet aggregation induced by **(a)** ADP and **(b)** arachidonic acid before (control) and after treatment with intravenous aspirin. Compared with control, *p < 0.0001. Reproduced by permission of the American Heart Association and Yao et al 1994.[16]*

left-sided thoracotomy was performed, and the heart was suspended in a pericardial cradle. A 1- to 2-cm segment of the left anterior descending coronary artery was carefully isolated. An ultrasonic Doppler flow probe was placed around the proximal portion of the isolated segment of the left anterior descending coronary artery to measure coronary blood flow. Hemodynamics, including heart rate, systolic and diastolic arterial pressures, and mean and phasic coronary blood flow velocities, were recorded continuously on an eight-channel recorder. Cyclic flow variations were induced by gently squeezing the left anterior descending coronary artery with cushioned forceps to damage the endothelium and by placing a plastic constrictor around the injured portion of the artery. Once cyclic flow variations were induced, the animals were observed for a further 60 min to confirm the establishment of cyclic flow variations.

The baboons were divided into three groups. One group ($n = 4$) received placebo (90-min infusion of N saline), and two groups received VCL. One group ($n = 8$) received VCL as a bolus of 4 mg/kg followed by a 90-min infusion of 6 mg/kg/h (Schedule A), and the other received a bolus of 2 mg/kg followed by a 90-min infusion of 3 mg/kg/h (Schedule B). The baboons were observed for 3 h after the end of the infusion.

Four baboons received a placebo infusion of N saline. There was no significant change in the number of cyclic flow variations during the control period, 16 ± 4.2, compared with 24 ± 8.9 cycles/h at the end of the infusion period. In 7/8 baboons that received the VCL

infusion, cyclic flow variations were completely abolished after 33 ± 18 min and became markedly attenuated in one animal. The frequency of cyclic flow variations was reduced from 18 ± 9.4 cycles per hour during the control period to 1 ± 2.5 cycle/h after the 90-min infusion period, $p < 0.002$ (Figure 19.12). No statistically significant differences between the hematocrits, heart rates, or systolic or diastolic arterial pressures were observed. In 2 of the baboons, cyclic flow variations returned within 2.5 h after the infusion had ended. In 5/7 remaining baboons, cyclic flow variations remained abolished for over 3 h. An infusion of epinephrine (adrenaline) was administered to 4/5 of these baboons and resulted in the restoration of cyclic flow variations in 3 animals.

Pharmacokinetic studies were performed in

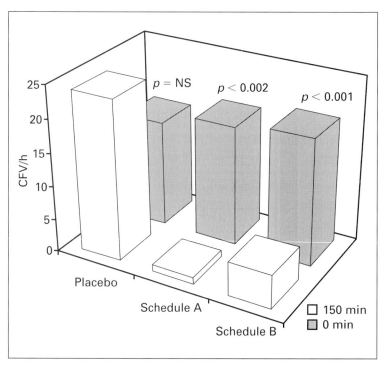

Figure 19.12
The effect of VCL on cyclic flow variations. Number of cyclic flow variations per hour (CFV/h) during control period (0 min) and after treatment (150 min). Reproduced by permission of the American Heart Association and McGhie et al 1994.[15]

3 baboons during dosing Schedule A. Blood samples (5 ml) were drawn 1, 5, 10, 15, 20, 30, 42, 50, 70, and 90 min after the onset of infusion and at 2, 5, 10, 15, 20, 30, 40, 60, 90, 120, 160, and 180 min after cessation of the infusion. Plasma concentrations of VCL were determined by ELISA. A mean concentration of VCL during the infusion was 44 ± 2.0 μg/ml VCL. After cessation of VCL infusion, the peptide was cleared rapidly, with a clearance half-time from the plasma of 29 min.

In 3/6 baboons receiving the different dosing schedule of VCL (i.e. 2 mg/kg bolus and 3 mg/kg/h with a 90-min infusion), cyclic flow variations were completely abolished after a mean of 20 ± 17 min and were markedly attenuated in the remaining animals. The number of cyclic flow variations fell from 17 ± 4.8 cycles during the control period to 5 ± 4.9 cycles per hour after the onset of VCL infusion (see Figure 19.12). No statistically significant differences between the hematocrits, heart rates, or systolic or diastolic arterial pressures were observed. In the 3 baboons in whom the cyclic flow variations were completely abolished, all returned spontaneously (mean, 38.0 ± 40 min).

Blood samples were drawn in all baboons for determination of VCL levels during dosing Schedule B. Samples were drawn at 5, 30, 60, and 90 min after the onset of infusion and at 10, 15, 20, 30, 40, 45, 60, 90, 120, 150, and 180 min after cessation of the infusion. The mean plasma concentration of 25 ± 3.5 μg/ml VCL was measured during the infusion. After cessation of the infusion, the clearance half-time of VCL from the plasma was 22 min.

The main findings from these studies were that, in dogs, VCL prolongs the time of development of intracoronary thrombus and enhances TPA-induced thrombolysis and also delays coronary artery reocclusion. In the non-human primates, VCL abolishes cyclic flow variations in stenosed and endothelium-injured coronary arteries and its in vivo administration decreased botrocetin-induced platelet aggregation.

In addition, von Willebrand factor plays an important role in hemostasis and its absence results in von Willebrand disease, an inherited bleeding disorder. Recent studies have shown that von Willebrand factor is essential for the formation of platelet thrombi, especially under flow conditions characterized by high shear stress, such as occurs in stenosed coronary arteries. von Willebrand factor interacts with GPIb receptors on the platelet membrane to initiate platelet adhesion and to activate platelet release of ADP, thromboxane A_2 and serotonin, which cause platelet aggregation and thrombus formation. In addition, there is increasing evidence that the interaction between von Willebrand factor and the GPIb receptor results in activation of the GPIIb/IIIa receptor, leading to binding of fibrinogen and ultimately to platelet aggregation. Therefore, inhibition of the initial contact between platelet GPIb receptor and von Willebrand factor may be effective in preventing platelet activation and subsequent thrombus formation.

Tissue factor

Tissue factor (TF) is a cellular initiator of thrombin generation and blood coagulation in hemostasis and thrombosis.[17–20] Tissue factor pathway inhibitor (TFPI) is an endogenous inhibitor of tissue factor and of factor X_a[20] that has been reported to prevent thrombin generation, thrombosis, and restenosis after experimental arterial injury when given systemically.[21–24] Whether systemic administration of TFPI provides lasting protection after vascular injury or percutaneous revascularization in patients with atherosclerotic disease is uncertain, unless its administration can be extended for some days after vascular injury. Continuous systemic administration of TFPI, however, may be associated with some increased hemorrhagic risk. The ideal way to administer TFPI when longer protection against tissue factor-mediated thrombosis and its consequences is needed may be locally.[17]

A recombinant, replication-deficient adenovirus encoding a full-length human TFPI cDNA has been used as a strategy to prevent thrombosis. Using this form of gene therapy it is possible to transfect normal and atherosclerotic experimental animal arteries, with protection against thrombosis in the subsequent several days thereafter.[17]

Future studies are needed in humans to determine the relative safety and efficacy of this form of gene therapy in attenuating or preventing tissue factor (TF)-mediated thrombosis and restenosis after vascular injury, including interventional therapies such as angioplasty and stenting. Such human studies are anticipated in the future.

Cox-1 and nitric oxide gene therapy

Several workers have used Cox-1 gene therapy to replenish prostacyclin concentration in injured porcine arteries.[25] In these studies, a cDNA for prostaglandin-H-synthase S-1 (Cox-1) and a cytomegalovirus promoter were used to demonstrate the ability to restore prostacyclin concentration after crush injury in porcine carotid arteries and following angioplasty injury to non-atherosclerotic porcine carotid arteries.[25] In these studies, the pig carotid artery was either crushed or injured by angioplasty using a human protocol. The gene therapy was allowed a 30-min dwell time

following the carotid injury, with reversible ligation of the proximal and distal ends of the carotid artery above and below the site of injury.[25] In the angioplasty studies, a coronary artery constrictor was left above the site of angioplasty injury and a Doppler flow probe was left proximal to the constrictor so that coronary blood flow could be monitored for the subsequent 10 days. A higher titer (6×10^{10} units/ml) not a lower titer (1×10^{10} units/ml) of plaque-forming units markedly inhibited thrombus development following angioplasty injury in this experimental model.[25]

Others have used the cDNA for nitric oxide synthase to replenish nitric oxide in arteries injured by angioplasty in experimental animal models and have shown an ability to restore nitric oxide at the site of injury and to protect subsequently against thrombosis.[26]

In the above studies, excessive hemorrhage was not identified and the duration of the protective gene therapy using the prototype adenoviral vector utilized in these studies was approximately 10–14 days.

Inflammation and thrombosis

The selectins are a family of calcium-dependent cell-adhesion molecules that bind carbohydrate ligands and share structural homology. Each selectin is composed of an amino terminal lectin domain, an epidermal growth factor-like region, and a variable number of complement receptor-like binding domains. L-selectin is expressed constitutively on the surface of circulating leukocytes, binds to inducible ligands on postcapillary venules and endothelial venules of lymph nodes, and is rapidly shed from the cell surface after leukocyte activation.[10,27–29] Neutrophil L-selectin is a ligand for E- and P-selectin[29,30] and mediates, co-operatively with P-selectin glycoprotein ligand-1, the initial attachment of neutrophils to P- and E-selectin under flow.[30,31] E-selectin is restricted to endothelial cells, where it is only expressed upon activation by cytokines, including interleukin-1, tumor necrosis factor-α and oxygen-derived free radicals.[32,33] The expression of E-selectin, which binds to ligands on myeloid cells and a subset of lymphocytes, requires de novo transcription and protein synthesis, and is detectable for 2–3 h after activation of endothelial cells. P-selectin is stored in the α-granules of platelets and the Weibel-Palade bodies of endothelial cells.[34] P-selectin binds to and is inhibited by heparin and sialylated Lewis-X, a carbohydrate antigen. In response to agonists, including thrombin, histamine, and oxygen radicals, P-selectin rapidly translocates to the cell surface where it mediates cell interactions.[35–37]

The role of the selectins in blood coagulation and blood cell-vessel wall interactions has been recognized,[38–40] as has their involvement in the pathogenesis of myocardial reperfusion injury.[41,42] The role of selectins in coronary thrombus formation has been investigated in a canine model of severe arterial injury and stenosis, to test the hypothesis that the inhibition of these selectins by systemic or local application of a small-molecular-weight inhibitor, methoxybenzoylpropionic acid (MBPA), might prevent coronary artery thrombosis.[9] In these studies of dogs, the hypothesis that combined blockade of L-, E- and P-selectin by MBPA exerts antithrombotic activity was tested. A canine coronary Folts' model[43] was used and it was found that recurrent coronary vasoconstriction and thrombus deposition were severely attenuated or abolished by both systemic or local administration of the MBPA.[9] A P-selectin specific antibody partially reproduced the antithrombotic effect found in these studies, thereby indicating an important role for P-selectin and the combined selectins in mediating coronary thrombosis and inflammation after vascular injury.[9]

Summary

In summary, this chapter discusses how platelet GPIb receptors, tissue factor, and E-, P-, and L-selectins may be future targets for new antithrombotic therapy. In addition, the possibility of restoring prostacyclin and nitric oxide to injured vessels also represents a potential form of antithrombotic therapy, with, potentially, a minimal risk of systemic bleeding. Furthermore, combinations of these therapies with inhibitors of platelet GPIIb/IIIa receptors might provide an even greater degree of protection against thrombosis and its consequences after vascular injury in the future.

References

1. The EPIC Investigators. Use of a monoclonal antibody directed against the platelet glycoprotein IIb/IIIa receptor in high-risk coronary angioplasty. *N Engl J Med* 1994;**330**:956–61.

2. Topol EJ, Califf RM, Weisman HF, Ellis SG, Tcheng JE, Worley S, et al on behalf of the EPIC Investigators. Randomised trial of coronary intervention with antibody against platelet IIb/IIIa integrin for reduction of clinical restenosis: results at six months. *Lancet* 1994;**343**:881–6.

3. The EPILOG Investigators. Platelet glycoprotein IIb/IIIa receptor blockade and low-dose heparin during percutaneous coronary revascularization. *N Engl J Med* 1997;**336**:1689–96.

4. Topol EJ, Ferguson JJ, Weisman HF, Tcheng JE, Ellis SG, Kleiman NS, et al for the EPIC Investigator Group. Long-term protection from myocardial ischemic events in a randomized trial of brief integrin β_3 blockade with percutaneous coronary intervention. *J Am Med Assoc* 1997;**278**:479–84.

5. The IMPACT-II Investigators. Randomised placebo-controlled trial of effect of eptifibatide on complications of percutaneous coronary intervention: IMPACT-II. *Lancet* 1997;**349**:1422–8.

6. The CAPTURE Investigators. Randomised placebo-controlled trial of abciximab before and during coronary intervention in refractory unstable angina: the CAPTURE study. *Lancet* 1997;**349**:1429–35.

7. The RESTORE Investigators. Effects of platelet glycoprotein IIb/IIIa blockade with tirofiban on adverse cardiac events in patients with unstable angina or acute myocardial infarction undergoing coronary angioplasty. *Circulation* 1997; **96**:1445–53.

8. The Platelet Receptor Inhibition in Ischemic Syndrome Management in Patients Limited by Unstable Signs and Symptoms (PRISM-PLUS) Study Investigators. Inhibition of the platelet glycoprotein IIb/IIIa receptor with tirofiban in unstable angina and non-Q-wave myocardial infarction. *N Engl J Med* 1998;**338**:1488–97.

9. Zoldhelyi P, Ober JC, McNatt JM, Akhtar S, Bjercke R, Ahmed M, et al. Prevention of coronary thrombosis after arterial injury by selectin inhibition. (Submitted for publication.)

10. Bevilacqua MP, Nelson RM. Selectins. *J Clin Invest* 1993;**91**:379–87.

11. Ruggeri ZM. Inhibition of platelet-vessel wall interaction: platelet receptors, monoclonal antibodies, and synthetic peptides. *Circulation* 1990;**81**(Suppl. I):I-35–I-39.

12. Weiss HJ, Turitto VT, Baumgartner HR. Effect of shear rate on platelet interaction with subendothelium in citrated and native blood, I: shear rate-dependent decrease of adhesion in von Willebrand's disease and the Bernard-Soulier syndrome. *J Lab Clin Med* 1978;**92**:750–64.

13. Gralnick HR, Williams SB, Coller BS. Asialo von Willebrand factor interactions with platelets: interdependence of glycoproteins Ib and IIb/IIIa for binding and aggregation. *J Clin Invest* 1985;**75**:19–25.

14. De Marco L, Girolami A, Russel S, Ruggeri ZM. Interaction of asialo von Willebrand factor with glycoprotein Ib induces fibrinogen binding to the glycoprotein IIb/IIIa complex and mediates platelet aggregation. *J Clin Invest* 1985;**75**:1198–203.

15. McGhie AI, McNatt J, Ezov N, Cui K, Mower LK, Hagay Y, et al. Abolition of cyclic flow variations in stenosed, endothelium-injured coronary arteries in nonhuman primates with a peptide fragment (VCL) derived from human plasma von Willebrand factor–glycoprotein Ib binding domain. *Circulation* 1994;**90**:2976–81.

16. Yao S-K, Ober JC, Garfinkel LI, Hagay Y, Ezov N, Ferguson JJ, et al. Blockade of platelet membrane glycoprotein Ib receptors delays intracoronary thrombogenesis, enhances thrombolysis, and delays coronary artery reocclusion in dogs. *Circulation* 1994; **89**:2822–8.

17. Zoldhelyi P, McNatt J, Ober JC, Shelat HS,

Dillard PM, Willerson JT. Gene transfer of human tissue factor pathway inhibitor in vitro and to severely atherosclerotic arteries in vivo. (Submitted for publication.)

18. Edgington TS, Mackman N, Brank K, Ruf W. The structural biology of expression and function of tissue factor. *Thromb Haemost* 1991;**66**:67–79.

19. Gailani D, Broze GJ Jr. Factor XI activation in a revised model of blood coagulation. *Science* 1991;**253**:909–12.

20. Broze GJ Jr. TFPI and the revised theory of coagulation. *Ann Rev Med* 1995;**46**:103–12.

21. Haskel EJ, Torr SR, Day KC, Palmier MO, Wun TC, Sobel BE. Prevention of arterial reocclusion after thrombolysis with recombinant lipoprotein-associated coagulation inhibitor. *Circulation* 1991;**84**:821–7.

22. Abendschein DR, Meng YY, Torr-Brown S, Sobel BE. Maintenance of coronary patency after fibrinolysis with tissue factor pathway inhibitor. *Circulation* 1995;**92**:944–9.

23. Jang Y, Guzman LA, Lincoff M, Topol EJ. Influence of blockade at specific levels of the coagulation cascade on restenosis in a rabbit atherosclerotic femoral artery injury model. *Circulation* 1995;**92**:3041–50.

24. Abendschein DR. Inhibition of tissue factor-mediated coagulation markedly attenuates stenosis after balloon-induced arterial injury in minipigs. *Circulation* 1997;**96**:646–52.

25. Zoldhelyi P, McNatt J, Xu XM, Loose-Mitchell D, Meidell R, Cluff FJ, et al. Prevention of arterial thrombosis by adenovirus-mediated transfer of cyclooxygenase gene. *Circulation* 1996;**93**:10–17.

26. von der Leyen HE, Gibbons GH, Morishita R, Lewis NP, Zhang L, Nakajima M, et al. Gene therapy inhibiting neointimal vascular lesion: in vivo transfer of endothelial cell nitric oxide synthase gene. *Proc Natl Acad Sci USA* 1995;**92**:1137–41.

27. Kishimoto TK. The selectins. *Structure, Function, and Regulation of Molecules Involved in Leukocyte Adhesion.* (New York, Springer-Verlag, 1993) 107–34.

28. Springer TA. Traffic signals for lymphocyte recirculation and leukocyte emigration. The multistep paradigm. *Cell* 1994;**76**:301–14.

29. Picker LJ, Warnock RA, Burns AR, Doerschuk CM, Berg EL, Butcher EC. The neutrophil selectin LECAM-1 presents carbohydrate ligands to the vascular selectins ELAM-1 and GMP-140. *Cell* 1991;**66**:921–33.

30. Patel KD, Moore KL, Nollert MU, McEver RP. Neutrophils use both shared and distinct mechanisms to adhere to selectins under static and flow conditions. *J Clin Invest* 1995;**94**:1887–96.

31. Lawrence MB, Bainton DF, Springer TA. Neutrophil tethering to and rolling on E-selectin are separable by requirement for L-selectins. *Immunity* 1994;**1**:137–45.

32. Bevilacqua MP, Stengelin S, Gimbrone MA, Seed B. Endothelial-leukocyte adhesion molecule-1: an inducible receptor for neutrophils related to complement regulatory proteins and lectins. *Science* 1989;**243**:1160–65.

33. Pober JS, Cotran RS. The role of endothelial cells in inflammation. *Transplantation* 1990;**50**:537–44.

34. McEver RP, Beckstead JH, Moore KL, Marshall-Carison L, Bainton DF. GMP-140, a platelet alpha-granule membrane protein, is also synthesized by vascular endothelial cells and is localized in Weibel-Palade bodies. *J Clin Invest* 1989;**84**:92–9.

35. Bonfani R, Furie BC, Furie B, Wagner DD. PAGDEM (GMP-140) is a component of Weibel-Palade bodies of human endothelial cells. *Blood* 1989;**73**:1109–12.

36. Patel KD, Zimmerman GA, Prescott SM, McEver RP, McIntyre TM. Oxygen radicals induce human endothelial cells to express GMP-140 and bind neutrophils. *J Biol Chem* 1991;**112**:749–59.

37. Sugama Y, Tiruppathi C, Janakidevi K, Andersen TT, Fenton JW II, Malik AB. Thrombin-induced expression of endothelial P-selectin and intercellular adhesion molecule-1: a mechanism for stabilizing neutrophil adhesion. *J Cell Biol* 1992;**119**(4):935–44.

38. Palabrica T, Lobb R, Furie BC, Aronovitz M, Benjamin C, Hsu YM, et al. Leukocyte accumulation promoting fibrin deposition is mediated in vivo by P-selectin on adherent platelets. *Nature* 1992;**359**:848–51.

39. Jang Y, Lincoff AM, Plow EF, Topol EJ. Cell adhesion molecules in coronary artery disease. *J Am Coll Cardiol* 1994;**24**:1591–601.

40. Frenette PS, Wagner DD. Adhesion molecules-part II: blood vessels and blood cells. *N Engl J Med* 1996;335:43–5.

41. Lefer AM. Role of the selectins in reperfusion injury. *Ann Thor Surg* 1995; **60**:73–777.

42. Mihelcic D, Schleiffenbaum B, Tedder TF, Sharar SR, Harlan JM, Winn RK. Inhibition of leukocyte L-selectin function with a monoclonal antibody attenuates reperfusion injury to the rabbit ears. *Blood* 1994;84:2322–8.

43. Folts JD, Gallagher K, Rowe GG. Blood flow reductions in stenosed canine coronary arteries: vasospasm or platelet aggregation. *Circulation* 1982;**65**:248–55.

44. Willerson JT, Colimo P, Erdt J, Campbell WB, Buja LM. Specific platelet mediators and unstable coronary artery lesions. Experimental evidence and potential clinical implications. *Circulation* 1989;80:198–205.

Index

Note: Page reference in *italic* text denote figures or tables